Aggregatibacter actinomycetemcomitans — Gram-Negative Bacterial Pathogen

Aggregatibacter actinomycetemcomitans—Gram-Negative Bacterial Pathogen

Editors

Anders Johansson
Joseph M. DiRienzo

MDPI • Basel • Beijing • Wuhan • Barcelona • Belgrade • Manchester • Tokyo • Cluj • Tianjin

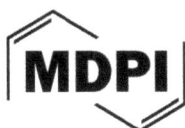

Editors
Anders Johansson
Umeå University
Sweden

Joseph M. DiRienzo
University of Pennsylvania
USA

Editorial Office
MDPI
St. Alban-Anlage 66
4052 Basel, Switzerland

This is a reprint of articles from the Special Issue published online in the open access journal *Pathogens* (ISSN 2076-0817) (available at: https://www.mdpi.com/journal/pathogens/special_issues/Aggregatibacter_actinomycetemcomitans).

For citation purposes, cite each article independently as indicated on the article page online and as indicated below:

LastName, A.A.; LastName, B.B.; LastName, C.C. Article Title. *Journal Name* **Year**, *Article Number*, Page Range.

ISBN 978-3-03943-376-6 (Pbk)
ISBN 978-3-03943-377-3 (PDF)

© 2020 by the authors. Articles in this book are Open Access and distributed under the Creative Commons Attribution (CC BY) license, which allows users to download, copy and build upon published articles, as long as the author and publisher are properly credited, which ensures maximum dissemination and a wider impact of our publications.

The book as a whole is distributed by MDPI under the terms and conditions of the Creative Commons license CC BY-NC-ND.

Contents

About the Editors vii

Preface to "*Aggregatibacter actinomycetemcomitans***—Gram-Negative Bacterial Pathogen"** . . ix

Jan Oscarsson, Joseph M. DiRienzo and Anders Johansson
Editorial Comments to the Special Issue: "*Aggregatibacter actinomycetemcomitans*—Gram-Negative Bacterial Pathogen"
Reprinted from: *Pathogens* **2020**, *9*, 441, doi:10.3390/pathogens9060441 1

Daniel H. Fine, Helen Schreiner and Senthil Kumar Velusamy
Aggregatibacter, a Low Abundance Pathobiont That Influences Biogeography, Microbial Dysbiosis, and Host Defense Capabilities in Periodontitis: The History of a Bug, and Localization of Disease
Reprinted from: *Pathogens* **2020**, *9*, 179, doi:10.3390/pathogens9030179 7

Niels Nørskov-Lauritsen, Rolf Claesson, Anne Birkeholm Jensen, Carola Höglund Åberg and Dorte Haubek
Aggregatibacter Actinomycetemcomitans: Clinical Significance of a Pathobiont Subjected to Ample Changes in Classification and Nomenclature
Reprinted from: *Pathogens* **2019**, *8*, 243, doi:10.3390/pathogens8040243 33

Georgios N. Belibasakis, Terhi Maula, Kai Bao, Mark Lindholm, Nagihan Bostanci, Jan Oscarsson, Riikka Ihalin and Anders Johansson
Virulence and Pathogenicity Properties of *Aggregatibacter actinomycetemcomitans*
Reprinted from: *Pathogens* **2019**, *8*, 222, doi:10.3390/pathogens8040222 51

Alexandra Stähli, Anton Sculean and Sigrun Eick
JP2 Genotype of *Aggregatibacter actinomycetemcomitans* in Caucasian Patients: A Presentation of Two Cases
Reprinted from: *Pathogens* **2020**, *9*, 178, doi:10.3390/pathogens9030178 75

Ellen S. Ando-Suguimoto, Manjunatha R. Benakanakere, Marcia P.A. Mayer and Denis F. Kinane
Distinct Signaling Pathways Between Human Macrophages and Primary Gingival Epithelial Cells by *Aggregatibacter actinomycetemcomitans*
Reprinted from: *Pathogens* **2020**, *9*, 248, doi:10.3390/pathogens9040248 85

Sanae Akkaoui, Anders Johansson, Maâmar Yagoubi, Dorte Haubek, Adnane El hamidi, Sana Rida, Rolf Claesson and OumKeltoum Ennibi
Chemical Composition, Antimicrobial activity, In Vitro Cytotoxicity and Leukotoxin Neutralization of Essential Oil from *Origanum vulgare* against *Aggregatibacter actinomycetemcomitans*
Reprinted from: *Pathogens* **2020**, *9*, 192, doi:10.3390/pathogens9030192 99

Edward T Lally, Kathleen Boesze-Battaglia, Anuradha Dhingra, Nestor M Gomez, Jinery Lora, Claire H Mitchell, Alexander Giannakakis, Syed A Fahim, Roland Benz and Nataliya Balashova
Aggregatibacter actinomycetemcomitans LtxA Hijacks Endocytic Trafficking Pathways in Human Lymphocytes
Reprinted from: *Pathogens* **2020**, *9*, 74, doi:10.3390/pathogens9020074 113

Bruce J. Shenker, Lisa M. Walker, Ali Zekavat, Robert H. Weiss and
Kathleen Boesze-Battaglia
The Cell-Cycle Regulatory Protein p21$^{CIP1/WAF1}$ Is Required for Cytolethal Distending Toxin (Cdt)-Induced Apoptosis
Reprinted from: *Pathogens* 2020, 9, 38, doi:10.3390/pathogens9010038 137

Natalia O. Tjokro, Weerayuth Kittichotirat, Annamari Torittu, Riikka Ihalin,
Roger E. Bumgarner and Casey Chen
Transcriptomic Analysis of *Aggregatibacter actinomycetemcomitans* Core and Accessory Genes in Different Growth Conditions
Reprinted from: *Pathogens* 2019, 8, 282, doi:10.3390/pathogens8040282 157

Arzu Beklen, Annamari Torittu, Riikka Ihalin and Marja Pöllänen
Aggregatibacter actinomycetemcomitans Biofilm Reduces Gingival Epithelial Cell Keratin Expression in an Organotypic Gingival Tissue Culture Model
Reprinted from: *Pathogens* 2019, 8, 278, doi:10.3390/pathogens8040278 171

Signe Nedergaard, Carl M. Kobel, Marie B. Nielsen, Rikke T. Møller, Anne B. Jensen and
Niels Nørskov-Lauritsen
Whole Genome Sequencing of *Aggregatibacter actinomycetemcomitans* Cultured from Blood Stream Infections Reveals Three Major Phylogenetic Groups Including a Novel Lineage Expressing Serotype a Membrane O Polysaccharide
Reprinted from: *Pathogens* 2019, 8, 256, doi:10.3390/pathogens8040256 181

Anne Birkeholm Jensen, Marianne Lund, Niels Nørskov-Lauritsen, Anders Johansson,
Rolf Claesson, Jesper Reinholdt and Dorte Haubek
Differential Cell Lysis Among Periodontal Strains of JP2 and Non-JP2 Genotype of *Aggregatibacter actinomycetemcomitans* Serotype B Is Not Reflected in Dissimilar Expression and Production of Leukotoxin
Reprinted from: *Pathogens* 2019, 8, 211, doi:10.3390/pathogens8040211 191

Anders Johansson, Rolf Claesson, Carola Höglund Åberg, Dorte Haubek, Mark Lindholm,
Sarah Jasim and Jan Oscarsson
Genetic Profiling of *Aggregatibacter actinomycetemcomitans* Serotype B Isolated from Periodontitis Patients Living in Sweden
Reprinted from: *Pathogens* 2019, 8, 153, doi:10.3390/pathogens8030153 205

Nataliya Balashova
In Memoriam: Edward "Ned" Lally
Reprinted from: *Pathogens* 2020, 9, 177, doi:10.3390/pathogens9030177 219

About the Editors

Anders Johansson (Ph.D., Associate Professor) is a docent in experimental periodontology and has been active for several decades at Umeå university. His major research topics have been interactions between *A. actinomycetemcomitans* and leukocytes. Dr. Johansson and his co-workers have discovered active processes in the leukocytes that have been induced by the leukotoxin, like neutrophil degranulation and inflammasome activation in macrophages. His research has also involved clinical studies that contributed to clarifying the role of enhanced leukotoxin production for disease progression.

Joseph M. DiRienzo (Ph.D., Emeritus Professor) received a Ph.D. in Microbiology from McGill University and postdoctoral training in the Department of Biochemistry at the State University of New York at Stony Brook. He recently retired, after 40 years of teaching and research, from the School of Dental Medicine at the University of Pennsylvania. Dr. DiRienzo studied the role of bacteria in the pathogenesis of periodontal diseases using molecular biology and biochemical approaches to identify and characterize virulence genes and their gene products from *Aggregatibacter (Actinobacillus) actinomycetemcomitans*. Studies were focused on the characterization of the cytolethal distending toxin and its effects on oral epithelial cells. Dr. DiRienzo also studied the role of horizontal gene transfer in the dissemination of virulence genes in *A. actinomycetemcomitans*.

Preface to "*Aggregatibacter actinomycetemcomitans*—Gram-Negative Bacterial Pathogen"

Aggregatibacter actinomycetemcomitans, a member of the Gram-negative taxonomic family Pasteurellaceae, has attracted considerable attention as a potentially important pathogen in specific forms of periodontal disease and has earned a reputation as a member of the HACEK group of bacteria associated with some cases of infective endocarditis. The bacterium has acquired an impressive virulence-related armamentarium, including two well-characterized cytotoxins, exoenzymes, adhesins, and signaling molecules that promote its colonization and the perturbation of the tissues, structural cells, and inflammatory cells of the human oral cavity. This Special Issue focuses on the properties and activities of *A. actinomycetemcomitans* that promote its function as an infectious agent, that is, its ability to target specific host populations and define its interactions with specific mucosal tissues and cells. The objective is to present a complete picture of the participation of this bacterium in disease by presenting both in vitro and in vivo experimental and clinical studies. A comprehensive view of the contribution of this bacterium to the mechanisms of infection and disease should also provide a basis for the development of new control strategies that move beyond the classical antibiotics.

Anders Johansson, Joseph M. DiRienzo
Editors

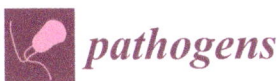

Editorial

Editorial Comments to the Special Issue: "*Aggregatibacter actinomycetemcomitans*—Gram-Negative Bacterial Pathogen"

Jan Oscarsson [1], Joseph M. DiRienzo [2] and Anders Johansson [1,*]

1. Department of Odontology, Umeå University, S-901 87 Umeå, Sweden; jan.oscarsson@umu.se
2. Department of Basic and Translational Sciences, School of Dental Medicine, University of Pennsylvania, Philadelphia, PA 19104-6030, USA; dirienzo@upenn.edu
* Correspondence: anders.p.johansson@umu.se; Tel.: +46-90-7856291

Received: 29 May 2020; Accepted: 2 June 2020; Published: 4 June 2020

Abstract: *Aggregatibacter actinomycetemcomitans* is a periodontal pathogen colonizing the oral cavity in many individuals of the human population. It is equipped with several potent virulence factors that can cause cell death and induce or evade the host inflammatory response. Both harmless and highly virulent genotypes of the bacterium have emerged because of the large genetic diversity within the species. The oral condition and age, as well as the geographic origin of the individual, influence the risk to be colonized by a virulent genotype of the bacterium. In the present editorial, the different genetic and virulence properties of *A. actinomycetemcomitans* will be addressed in relation to the publications in this Special Issue.

Keywords: *Aggregatibacter actinomycetemcomitans*; leukotoxin; cytolethal distending toxin; lipopolysaccharides; cytokine binding factors; horizontal gene transfer; outer membrane vesicles; biofilm; proteomics

---

1. Overview

In the light of three different reviews, various aspects of the pathobiont *Aggregatibacter actinomycetemcomitans* have been addressed. The role of this gram-negative facultatively anaerobic bacterium is described by Fine and co-workers [1]. They proposed that the host response can confine local damage by restricting bacteremic translocation of members of the oral microbiota to distant organs, thus constraining the morbidity and mortality of the host. The battery of virulence factors released from *A. actinomycetemcomitans*, as well as the many virulence mechanisms, support that the local and systemic host defense is a life insurance for the colonized individuals. The many weapons that the bacterium can use to evade host response and induce disease are reviewed by Belibasakis and collaborators [2]. Unique for *A. actinomycetemcomitans* among the oral bacteria is the production of two exotoxins, a leukotoxin (LtxA) and a cytolethal distending toxin (CDT). LtxA is considered to be a major virulence factor in aggressive forms of periodontitis, where it protects the bacterium from phagocytosis by killing the defense cells and induces a pro-inflammatory response in exposed macrophages. CDT can enter the nucleus and cleave double stranded DNA in the host cells, which leads to a prompt growth arrest. In an alternative mode of action, the toxin functions as a phosphatase that can contribute to the progression of an apoptotic pathway.

Both toxins can be secreted from the bacteria to the surrounding tissues and can also be spread through the release of toxin loaded outer membrane vesicles. *A. actinomycetemcomitans* is one of the human pathogens that can bind host cytokines, such as IL-1β, IL-8, and IL-6, and internalize them, which leads to changes in the biofilm properties, decreasing the metabolic activity and changing the composition of the extracellular matrix. In polymicrobial biofilm models, it has been shown that the presence of *A. actinomycetemcomitans* changes the profile of the secreted proteins. Due to the large genetic diversity of *A. actinomycetemcomitans*, there is a substantial intraspecies variation in the ability to produce virulence factors, an aspect reviewed by Nørskov-Lauritsen [3]. It is no doubt that this bacterium exists as both harmless commensals, as well as opportunistic pathogens with strong pathogenic potential. The well-studied JP2 genotype of this bacterium has enhanced production of LtxA and is shown to significantly increase the risk for onset of periodontitis in the colonized individuals. *A. actinomycetemcomitans* can be detected by both culture and PCR techniques and the characteristic 530-bp deletion in the leukotoxin promoter of the JP2 genotype function as a suitable marker for detection of highly leukotoxic genotypes. The prevalence of this bacterium is estimated to be 20% for periodontally healthy juveniles, 36% for healthy adults, 50% for adult periodontitis patients, and 90% for young periodontitis patients. The highly leukotoxic JP2 genotype, together with other virulent genotypes, are mainly detected among the young periodontitis patients.

2. Clinical Findings

The JP2 genotype of *A. actinomycetemcomitans* with enhanced leukotoxic activity is mostly present in individuals of North and West African origin, however, with the increasing number of reports of detection also in individuals of non-African origin [3]. In one paper of this Special Issue, two cases of Caucasians diagnosed with the JP2 genotype are presented. Both are middle-aged females with severe periodontitis [4]. Microbiological diagnostics revealed the presence of *A. actinomycetemcomitans* JP2 genotype, but not *Porphyromonas gingivalis* in the subgingival samples from the patients. Both patients were successfully treated with adjunctive antibiotics and the JP2 genotype was eliminated. The authors claim that the microbiological diagnosis was the key for the successful treatment with adjunctive antibiotics.

3. Phenotypic and Genotypic Characterization

The JP2 genotype of *A. actinomycetemcomitans* is the classical pathogen with enhanced leukotoxin production and enhanced prevalence in subgingival sites of adolescents with periodontitis [2]. By further genotypic and phenotypic characterization of isolates from periodontitis patients living in Sweden, another virulent type of this bacterium, *cagE*, was discovered by Johansson and collaborators [5]. This genotype is, like JP2, exclusively found in serotype b and has an enhanced leukotoxicity, but frequently lacks the JP2-like 530 bp leukotoxin promoter deletion. Interestingly, however, all hitherto identified JP2 genotype strains share the *cagE* genotype. The authors suggested therefore, and due to other common genetic features, that this genotype may be the ancestor of JP2.

The *A. actinomycetemcomitans* genome can be divided into an accessory gene pool that is found in some strains, and a core gene pool, found in all strains. Tjokro and co-workers [6] hypothesize that the accessory genes confer critical functions for the bacterium in vivo. The authors showed that these genes exhibited distinct patterns of expression from the core genes and may play a role in the survival of *A. actinomycetemcomitans* in nutrient-limited environments. These genes coded for some important virulence factors and were located both in genomic islands and in the chromosome.

Whole genome sequencing (WGS) has been introduced for characterization of the *A. actinomycetemcomitans* and has separated the species into five different clades [3]. In the largest study, 30 oral human *A. actinomycetemcomitans* strains were sequenced and characterized. In their paper within this Special Issue, Nedergard et al. [7] reported on the serotyping and genome sequencing of 29 strains of *A. actinomycetemcomitans* cultured from blood stream infections of patients in Denmark. The authors concluded that WGS data add valuable information for further classification. They suggested that the population structure of this bacterium is more accurately described by a division of the species into three phylogenetic lineages, I–III.

4. Host–Parasite Interactions

The host response induced by *A. actinomycetemcomitans* is a challenge for the host and mimic several mechanisms that are associated with processes of degenerative diseases, such as periodontitis [1,2]. In aggressive forms of periodontitis, the dysbiotic microbiota in the subgingival crevice is abundant in *A. actinomycetemcomitans*. Ando-Sugimoto et al. [8] report in this Special Issue that the interactions of the bacterium, with extra-and intracellular receptors of host cells, leads to exacerbated inflammation and subsequent tissue destruction. In interactions with macrophages and human gingival epithelial cells, *A. actinomycetemcomitans* induces a signaling cascade that is involved in inflammasome and inflammatory responses. Differences in host cell responses between gingival epithelial cells and macrophages led the authors to suggest that survival of *A. actinomycetemcomitans* in periodontal tissues may be favored by its ability to differentially activate host cells. The most well-studied virulence factor expressed by this bacterium is LtxA, which specifically interacts with human leukocytes [1,2]. Several important discoveries on this toxin have been made by Edward ("Ned") Lally, who sadly passed away last year, and is a topic of an In Memoriam in this issue [9]. Lally and his co-workers discovered the receptor for LtxA (LFA-1), as well as mapped the domains of the toxin that were responsible for the interaction with its receptor. These findings explained the specificity of LtxA for leukocytes and have created a foundation for the subsequent delineation of the mechanisms in which the toxin affect various target cells. In one paper of this Special Issue, Lally et al. [10] show that LtxA enters the cytosol of lymphocytes without evidence of plasma membrane damage, utilizing receptor-mediated endocytic mechanisms. The authors suggest that LtxA can accompany LFA-1 in its recycling pathway and apparently dissociate from the receptor in endocytic vesicles and independently follow the degradative pathway. LtxA-delivery to the terminal point of this route results in the lysosomal membrane rupture. The ability of *A. actinomycetemcomitans* to express LtxA is closely linked to the capacity to kill leukocytes [2]. There is no golden standard available for quantification of LtxA production in different strains from this bacterium. Jensen and co-workers [11] applied three different methods for analyses of LtxA production in a collection of serotype b isolates. The results showed that that the JP2 genotype of *A. actinomycetemcomitans* had an enhanced LtxA production, even though there was a substantial variation between the examined isolates. The production of LtxA in the non-JP2 serotype b isolates was, in general, lower and that of JP2. However, a few non-JP2 isolates exhibited a higher LtxA production than some of the JP2 isolates. They also found a significant correlation between the levels of transcription of the leukotoxin genes and of the produced LtxA protein.

As described above, the CDT is the other exotoxin produced by *A. actinomycetemcomitans* [2]. In their paper in the present Special Issue, Shenker and co-workers [12] report on the mechanism for CDT-induced apoptosis in T-lymphocytes. Their data demonstrate that toxin-induced apoptosis is dependent upon increased levels of specific intracellular signaling, and conclude that that the ability of CDT to impair lymphocyte proliferation and promote cell death therefore compromises the host response to CDT-producing organisms. The effect of *A. actinomycetemcomitans* on epithelial cells has also been examined in a paper of this Special Issue [13]. Beklen and collaborators show that *A. actinomycetemcomitans* biofilms release outer membrane vesicles, which can be found in close contact with the epithelium. After exposure to the bacterial products, gingival epithelial cells might lose their membrane integrity and become more vulnerable to bacterial infection. In the case of an *A. actinomycetemcomitans* infection with a highly virulent variant of the bacterium, the treatment strategy often involves antibiotics [4]. Akkaoui and co-workers [14] demonstrated the efficiency of an essential oil from the plant *Origanum vulgare* in preventing *A. actinomycetemcomitans* growth in vitro. The authors found that this effect of the oil was substantially stronger than that of the tested antibiotics. The oil did not inhibit the leukotoxicity of *A. actinomycetemcomitans*, but the authors demonstrated the possibility of including leukotoxin neutralization agents in mixtures with the oil.

5. Conclusions

A. actinomycetemcomitans is a pathobiont that expresses several virulence factors with the capacity to cause imbalance in the host response and subsequently disease. The large genetic diversity of the bacterium related to its pathogenicity varies from harmless to highly virulent. *A. actinomycetemcomitans* could be isolated from the oral cavity of in many individuals of the human population, but can also sometimes be found in the bloodstream. In the oral cavity, this species is an important cause of periodontitis that affects young individuals and it is also associated with an increased risk for several systemic diseases. The present Special Issue provides insights into the various characteristics and activities *A. actinomycetemcomitans*. This information will enhance the development of valuable tools for limiting the negative health effects associated with this bacterium.

Author Contributions: Conceptualization, A.J., J.O. and J.D.; Writing—Original draft preparation, A.J. and J.O.; Writing—Review and Editing, A.J., J.O. and J.D. All authors have read and agreed to the published version of the manuscript.

Funding: This work was supported by TUA grants from the County Council of Västerbotten, Sweden (A.J.; 7003193, and J.O.; 7002667).

Acknowledgments: We acknowledge all the authors of the fourteen papers for their contribution, which made this Special Issue a valuable and comprehensive work. We thank the European Network for *A. actinomycetemcomitans* Research (https://projects.au.dk/aggregatibacter/) for encouraging us to initiate this Special Issue.

Conflicts of Interest: The authors declare no conflict of interest.

References

1. Fine, D.H.; Schreiner, H.; Velusamy, S.K. Aggregatibacter, a Low Abundance Pathobiont That Influences Biogeography, Microbial Dysbiosis, and Host Defense Capabilities in Periodontitis: The History of A Bug, And Localization of Disease. *Pathogens* **2020**, *9*, 179. [CrossRef] [PubMed]
2. Belibasakis, G.N.; Maula, T.; Bao, K.; Lindholm, M.; Bostanci, N.; Oscarsson, J.; Ihalin, R.; Johansson, A. Virulence and Pathogenicity Properties of *Aggregatibacter actinomycetemcomitans*. *Pathogens* **2019**, *8*, 222. [CrossRef] [PubMed]
3. Nørskov-Lauritsen, N.; Claesson, R.; Birkeholm Jensen, A.; Åberg, C.H.; Haubek, D. *Aggregatibacter actinomycetemcomitans*: Clinical Significance of a Pathobiont Subjected to Ample Changes in Classification and Nomenclature. *Pathogens* **2019**, *8*, 243. [CrossRef] [PubMed]
4. Stähli, A.; Sculean, A.; Eick, S. JP2 Genotype of *Aggregatibacter actinomycetemcomitans* in Caucasian Patients: A Presentation of Two Cases. *Pathogens* **2020**, *9*, 178. [CrossRef] [PubMed]
5. Johansson, A.; Claesson, R.; Höglund Åberg, C.; Haubek, D.; Lindholm, M.; Jasim, S.; Oscarsson, J. Genetic Profiling of *Aggregatibacter actinomycetemcomitans* Serotype B Isolated from Periodontitis Patients Living in Sweden. *Pathogens* **2019**, *8*, 153. [CrossRef] [PubMed]
6. Tjokro, N.O.; Kittichotirat, W.; Torittu, A.; Ihalin, R.; Bumgarner, R.E.; Chen, C. Transcriptomic Analysis of *Aggregatibacter actinomycetemcomitans* Core and Accessory Genes in Different Growth Conditions. *Pathogens* **2019**, *8*, 282. [CrossRef] [PubMed]
7. Nedergaard, S.; Kobel, C.M.; Nielsen, M.B.; Møller, R.T.; Jensen, A.B.; Nørskov-Lauritsen, N. Whole Genome Sequencing of *Aggregatibacter actinomycetemcomitans* Cultured from Blood Stream Infections Reveals Three Major Phylogenetic Groups Including a Novel Lineage Expressing Serotype a Membrane O Polysaccharide. *Pathogens* **2019**, *8*, 256. [CrossRef] [PubMed]
8. Ando-Suguimoto, E.S.; Benakanakere, M.R.; Mayer, M.P.A.; Kinane, D.F. Distinct Signaling Pathways Between Human Macrophages and Primary Gingival Epithelial Cells by *Aggregatibacter actinomycetemcomitans*. *Pathogens* **2020**, *9*, 248. [CrossRef] [PubMed]
9. Balashova, N. In Memoriam: Edward "Ned" Lally. *Pathogens* **2020**, *9*, 177. [CrossRef] [PubMed]
10. Lally, E.T.; Boesze-Battaglia, K.; Dhingra, A.; Gomez, N.M.; Lora, J.; Mitchell, C.H.; Giannakakis, A.; Fahim, S.A.; Benz, R.; Balashova, N. *Aggregatibacter actinomycetemcomitans* LtxA Hijacks Endocytic Trafficking Pathways in Human Lymphocytes. *Pathogens* **2020**, *9*, 74. [CrossRef] [PubMed]

11. Jensen, A.B.; Lund, M.; Nørskov-Lauritsen, N.; Johansson, A.; Claesson, R.; Reinholdt, J.; Haubek, D. Differential Cell Lysis Among Periodontal Strains of JP2 and Non-JP2 Genotype of *Aggregatibacter actinomycetemcomitans* Serotype B Is Not Reflected in Dissimilar Expression and Production of Leukotoxin. *Pathogens* **2019**, *8*, 211. [CrossRef] [PubMed]
12. Shenker, B.J.; Walker, L.M.; Zekavat, A.; Weiss, R.H.; Boesze-Battaglia, K. The Cell-Cycle Regulatory Protein p21(CIP1/WAF1) Is Required for Cytolethal Distending Toxin (Cdt)-Induced Apoptosis. *Pathogens* **2020**, *9*, 38. [CrossRef] [PubMed]
13. Beklen, A.; Torittu, A.; Ihalin, R.; Pöllänen, M. *Aggregatibacter actinomycetemcomitans* Biofilm Reduces Gingival Epithelial Cell Keratin Expression in an Organotypic Gingival Tissue Culture Model. *Pathogens* **2019**, *8*, 278. [CrossRef] [PubMed]
14. Akkaoui, S.; Johansson, A.; Yagoubi, M.; Haubek, D.; El Hamidi, A.; Rida, S.; Claesson, R.; Ennibi, O. Chemical Composition, Antimicrobial activity, in Vitro Cytotoxicity and Leukotoxin Neutralization of Essential Oil from *Origanum vulgare* against *Aggregatibacter actinomycetemcomitans*. *Pathogens* **2020**, *9*, 192. [CrossRef] [PubMed]

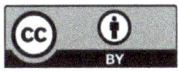

© 2020 by the authors. Licensee MDPI, Basel, Switzerland. This article is an open access article distributed under the terms and conditions of the Creative Commons Attribution (CC BY) license (http://creativecommons.org/licenses/by/4.0/).

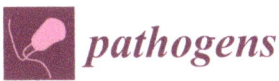

Review

Aggregatibacter, a Low Abundance Pathobiont That Influences Biogeography, Microbial Dysbiosis, and Host Defense Capabilities in Periodontitis: The History of a Bug, and Localization of Disease

Daniel H. Fine *, Helen Schreiner and Senthil Kumar Velusamy

Department of Oral Biology, Rutgers School of Dental Medicine, Room C-830110 Bergen Street, Newark, NJ 07103, USA; hschrein@sdm.rutgers.edu (H.S.); velusase@sdm.rutgers.edu (S.K.V.)
* Correspondence: finedh@sdm.rutgers.edu; Tel.: +1-973-972-3728

Received: 16 January 2020; Accepted: 26 February 2020; Published: 2 March 2020

Abstract: *Aggregatibacter actinomycetemcomitans*, the focus of this review, was initially proposed as a microbe directly related to a phenotypically distinct form of periodontitis called localized juvenile periodontitis. At the time, it seemed as if specific microbes were implicated as the cause of distinct forms of disease. Over the years, much has changed. The sense that specific microbes relate to distinct forms of disease has been challenged, as has the sense that distinct forms of periodontitis exist. This review consists of two components. The first part is presented as a detective story where we attempt to determine what role, if any, *Aggregatibacter* plays as a participant in disease. The second part describes landscape ecology in the context of how the host environment shapes the framework of local microbial dysbiosis. We then conjecture as to how the local host response may limit the damage caused by pathobionts. We propose that the host may overcome the constant barrage of a dysbiotic microbiota by confining it to a local tooth site. We conclude speculating that the host response can confine local damage by restricting bacteremic translocation of members of the oral microbiota to distant organs thus constraining morbidity and mortality of the host.

Keywords: *Aggregatibacter actinomycetemcomitans*; leukotoxin; localized aggressive periodontitis: animal studies: human studies; landscape ecology; damage/response framework; bacteremia; horseshoe crab

1. Introduction

This review is written as an overall appraisal of a field of research that has been part of a personal journey related to a specific microorganism (*Aggregatibacter actinomycetemcomitans*) and its relationship to a specific form of periodontal disease (Localized Aggressive Periodontitis, LAgP). The review is not presented as a systematic review of the literature (several reviews on this topic already exist [1–6]) but rather as a critical but broad interpretation of the field of research based on studies done by members of our laboratory and others in the field. The review offers novel ways of assessing infectious diseases from the point of view of the microbe, its host, and particularly interactions between the microbe and its host. It is the authors' hope that the review challenges current concepts and stimulates scientific discourse.

The review has been written in two parts. The first part is written as if it were a detective story with a suspect (a specific bacteria) and a victim (a specific host). The second part endeavors to interpret the story from the perspective of the victim (its host). The characters in the story consist of a protagonist or suspect (*Actinobacillus*), a crime (periodontal disease), and a crime scene (the oral cavity). At the conclusion or denouement, the suspect (*Actinobacillus*) is loosely associated with the crime (first named

Periodontosis), but this connection is still unresolved, the suspect remains unconvicted, and the crime itself contested.

The story begins in 1912 with the discovery of the protagonist *Actinobacillus actinomycetemcomitans*, a Gram-negative coccobacillus heretofore unknown to humankind. Even at the time of its discovery, the protagonist of this drama (*Actinobacillus*) was not accused of criminality but was considered an associate or an accessory to a rare, invasive/disruptive offense (a disease called Actinomycosis; i.e., lumpy jaw disease). *Actinobacillus* was thought of as an accomplice, one of two suspects, alongside its partner *Actinomyces israelii*, itself typically considered as an innocuous bystander [7]. The newly discovered co-conspirator, *Actinobacillus*, is therefore provided with the given name of actinomycetemcomitans—working in common with *Actinomyces*. However, this is not the crime of interest and the crime and the protagonist (*Actinobacillus*) remain unconnected for several years.

The crime in this story (Periodontosis) was disclosed 11 years later in 1923 by Dr. Bernhard Gottlieb, a Viennese physician, who described a distinctive condition related to youthful Viennese soldiers who were afflicted by a rare form of periodontal disease that showed minimal inflammation and advanced bone loss around first molars [8]. However, the crime (Periodontosis; reputedly a degenerative disease) and the suspected protagonist (*Actinobacillus*) were not linked until 1976 when two independent investigators, one in Europe and one in the United States, made the association between the microbe and its disease [9,10].

Over the last 50 years, confusion reigns and both the crime and the suspect undergo multiple identity shifts making the association more complicated. As for the disease, several name changes have occurred, including but not limited to: Periodontosis (also referred to as advance alveolar atrophy), Localized Juvenile Periodontitis, Generalized Juvenile Periodontitis, Early Onset Periodontitis, Localized Aggressive Periodontitis (LAgP), and Generalized Aggressive Periodontitis [11]. Even presently, the suspected perpetrator's defense attorneys have cleverly changed the laws (disease classification) and have stated that there never was a crime (disease) and if not how can there be a suspect [12]?

As for the perpetrator, first called *Actinobacillus* and then *Haemophilus*, it is now named *Aggegatibacter actinomycetemcomitans* with several closely related cousins that show remarkable physiological and genetic similarities, making the association even more difficult to demonstrate [13]. Never before has there been such clever manipulation of the legal system (disease classification) that has thrown such disciplined jurors (scientists) into this level of confusion [12].

The first part of the story begins with a trial seeking evidence to link the suspect (*Actinobacillus*, the microbe) with the crime (disease, LAgP) and the crime scene (the oral cavity). However, prior to the start of the drama, both the crime (disease) and the suspect (*Actinobacillus*) are described in detail. The investigation begins and the detectives examine: (1) evidence of the crime (examination of the crime scene, described as observational studies); (2) re-enactment of the crime (described as experimental or interventional (animal) studies); and (3) DNA evidence (described as molecular studies associated with the suspect).

The second part of the story (the epilogue) looks at the crime (local periodontitis) in a completely different manner or framework and offers the possibility that the victim (host) is a holobiont (the host composed of mammalian cells, bacteria, protozoa, yeast, and viruses). Survival (lack of systemic disease resulting from infection derived from members of the oral microbiota), it is proposed, is conditioned by a consistent retreat of local orally derived host cells that distance themselves from pathobionts that form an advancing front acquiring more of root territory in the process. The host response translates into tissue damage at the local site (periodontal disease); however, it could also be interpreted as a host (holobiont) defense strategy protecting host survival by surrendering local territory. The story concludes conjecturing that the purported disease (periodontitis) is part of a host protective mechanism where the tissue responds by attempting to prevent members of the oral microbiome from transmigrating from the local site (the tooth-surface) via the bloodstream where oral microorganisms previously thought to be innocuous can participate in morbidity and mortality of the host by spreading to distant organs.

2. The Disease

LAgP is a phenotypically distinct clinical entity that has several unique features that show: (1) rapid-excessive bone loss relative to patient age; (2) bone loss with a molar/incisor distribution; (3) minimal overall plaque levels relative to clinical levels of disease, (4) onset of disease at a young age (anywhere from preadolescence to adolescence); (5) minimal proximal decay; and (6) greater prevalence in adolescents of African descent [14] (Figure 1).

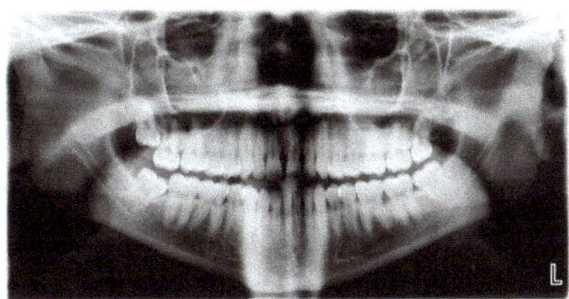

Figure 1. Radiograph of subject with Localized Aggressive Periodontitis: Panoramic radiograph showing extreme bone loss in first molar on left side in a 19-year-old patient.

2.1. The Dispute

While these clinical characteristics are universally agreed upon, in a recent consensus conference of world experts, it was argued that this condition should not be classified as a distinctive disease entity because genetic, pathobiologic, and microbiological evidence is not sufficient to categorize this as a unique disease, and therefore LAgP should be considered as a subset of traditional chronic periodontitis [14].

2.2. The Counter Argument

The counter argument to this dispute is formidable. In terms of genetics, the evidence is incontrovertible that there is familial aggregation, powerfully suggesting that there is a genetic pre-disposition for this disease. While several genes have been implicated as unique to those with LAgP (using the restrictive definition outlined above), data are limited because of: (1) the rarity of the disease; and (2) the use of broad inaccurate definitions of the disease. If the disease is limited to adolescents of African descent showing the distinctive clinical pattern of disease described above, then there are several genes of interest but these have not been substantiated due to the issues described above [15–18] (Table 1; only GWAS with over 1000 cases are included).

Table 1. Genes Associated with Aggressive Periodontitis: GWAS studies.

Gene Symbol	Gene Name	SNP Region	Reference
PTGR1	Prostaglandin reductase	rs758534	[15]
DGKD	Diacylglycerol kinase delta 130 kDa	rs10980953	[15–17]
INPP5F	Inositol polyphosphate phosphatase 1F	rs17680667	[15–17]
HTR1D	5-hydoxytryptamine (serotonin) receptor 1D, G protein coupled	rs16828047	[15–17]
LUZP1	Lucine zipper protein1	rs94266589	[15,17]
PLG	Plasminogen *	rs4252120	[18]

found in both chronic and aggressive periodontitis.

3. The Microbe: *Aggregatibacter actinomycetemcomitans*

Work related to *A. actinomycetemcomitans* (also referred to as *Actinobacillus*) began about 40 years ago when it was projected that this microbe was directly associated with a phenotypically distinct form of periodontitis then called Localized Juvenile Periodontitis (LJP). *Aggregatibacter* (formerly *Acitnobacillus*) was first isolated from patients with LJP in 1976 [9]. It was characterized as a Gram-negative, non-motile, coccobacillus that was either a facultative anaerobe or was capnophilic [10]. *A. actinomycetemcomitans* has been shown to possess several virulence factors, the most relevant of which are adherence factors, leukotoxin, cytolethal distending toxin, complement resistance factors, and moonlighting proteins, among other factors that account for its successful adaptation to a variety of environments [1,2]. Since there have been excellent review papers that describe these factors in detail, they do not form the basis of this review. Instead, this review highlights a few specific virulence and survival factors that *A. actinomycetemcomitans* possesses in the context of its host.

3.1. The Dispute

From the time of its discovery, it was shown that *A. actinomycetemcomitans* was found in two distinctly different colonial morphologies: a sessile adherent colonial form and a planktonic minimally adherent form [19]. The sessile form when isolated from subjects with LAgP showed a colony with a star on its top and with an irregular border. When this colony was removed from agar, it left a pit in the agar. The planktonic form emerged after serial passage of clinical isolates in the laboratory. This distinctive form proved to be minimally adherent with no star and with regular borders that left no pit when removed from the agar [19]. This contrast created significant confusion relative to molecular studies and was particularly relevant to our group since we selected adherence as the *A. actinomycetemcomitans* trait we wished to study [20]. Only after we and others learned how to maintain the rough sessile form by careful transfer from plate to plate could we study the adherent phenotype. In the process of conversion to the smooth phenotype, the minimally adherent form lost its fimbriation [20]. The number of passages in broth for this conversion was not predictable but this transformation created a great deal of confusion because the smooth/star negative strain failed to adhere to salivary coated hydroxyapatite and failed to show coaggregation, but still produced leukotoxin [21]. However, the well maintained clinically isolated parental strain was largely ignored early on and thus *A. actinomycetemcomitans* was characterized as a tertiary colonizer [22]. After a period of neglect, effort was made to compare the rough and smooth phenotypes derived from the same parental strain [19]. These comparisons showed that the lipo-oligosaccharide differed as did the lipopolysaccharide activity as well as its effect on fibroblasts. Adherence was reversed by periodate treatment as opposed to protease treatment suggesting that *A. actinomycetemcomitans* adherence was due to carbohydrates, which qualified it as a biofilm former [23]. A conundrum developed when efforts made to identify gene mutations were misinterpreted because conversion to the non-fimbriated phenotype occurred spontaneously. As such, the planktonic form outgrew their rough fimbriated parental strains, which was falsely interpreted as a successful gene knock-out. Eventually, it was learned that passage from plate to broth encouraged the overgrowth of the planktonic (afimbriated) form since its generation time was much faster than that of the sessile form (Figure 2).

Ultimately, several studies including work by Inoue et al. [24], Haase et al. [25], and Planet et al. [26] established that adherence was dependent on a 14 gene operon, the *tad* operon, that was widespread in nature [27]. Pieces of this important operon were found in most microbes that had pathogenic potential as well as all archae sequenced to date, suggesting the biological significance of this operon in nature [26].

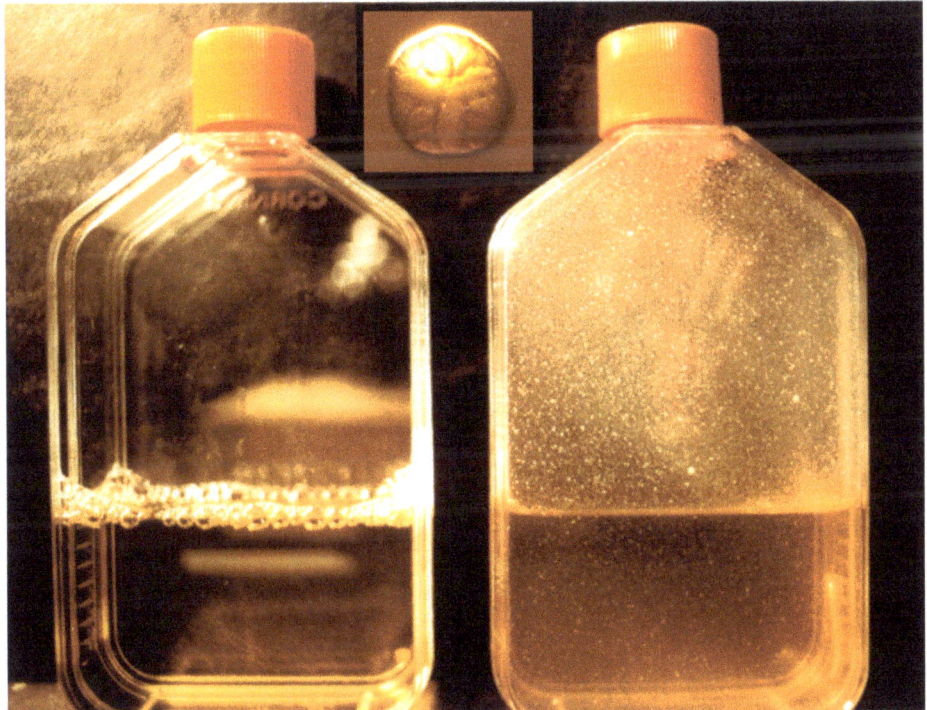

Figure 2. *A. actinomycetemcomitans* abiotic surfaces. *A. actinomycetemcomitans* was inoculated into a flask and allowed to grow on the side of the flask for three days. The flask on the left is an un-inoculated control. The flask on the right shows binding of *A. actinomycetemcomitans* to the side of the flask and no microbes can be found in the media. The insert in the center is the colonial morphology of *A. actinomycetemcomitans* showing star on top and rough colonial outer surface.

3.2. The Counter Argument

It was argued that the switch from the rough to smooth phenotype was due to phase variation and some even proposed that the smooth non-piliated variant was more pathogenic than the rough form, as was the case for *Neisseria gonorrhea* [28]. It had been proposed that *N. gonorrhea* pili removal permitted the microbe to invade cells, which was theorized to result in consequential gonococcal infections [28]. The switch from the piliated adherent to the non-piliated invasive phenotype was thought to be due to phase variation, as facilitated by slipped strand mis-pairing of repeat sequences in the promoter region or in gene repeat numbers altering translation or transcription [29]. Expression of opacity surface proteins and Lipo-oligosaccharides of *Neisseria* species were also considered as part of the invasive process [30]. This was thought to be true for *N. meningitidis* as well; however, much is still to be determined and the invasive phenotype is still unclear [31].

In the case of *A. actinomycetemcomitans*, only in one instance was there a modest and partial reversion from the smooth to the rough strain in vitro. In all other work in hundreds of passages in the laboratory in numerous paired strains (rough and smooth), this reversion has never been observed. Work by Chen and his group has clearly shown that smooth variants of *A. actinomycetemcomitans*, such as ATCC strain Y-4, and other smooth strains lack a region within the promoter sequence of the *tad* operon that affects expression of the *flp*1 gene. Lack of expression of Flp appears to result in a smooth variant [32]. Further, this work showed that knocking in the promoter region in the Y-4 strain restores its adherent and fimbriated characteristics, implying that the slipped strand mis-pairing was improbable in *A. actinomycetemcomitans* [33]. Further colonization and persistence of rough and smooth variants derived from the same parental strain of *A. actinomycetemcomitans* inoculated into a rat model supported this conclusion. Thus, while four of eight rats inoculated with the smooth strain colonized for one week, and two of eight colonized for four weeks, none were seen after eight weeks, and none of the smooth strains ever reverted to their rough textured fimbriated phenotype. In contrast, all of the inoculated rough strains colonized over the eight-week period maintained their rough phenotype, and none reverted to the smooth strain in the animal model [34]. Thus, as seen in the laboratory, the process of phase variation did not occur in vivo. The importance of the *flp* and *tad* genes relative to colonization have also been confirmed in an animal model of colonization and bone loss where it was shown that deletion of either *tad*A or *flp*1 in *A. actinomycetemcomitans* prevented colonization and bone loss in a rat model, whereas the parental wild-type strain caused bone loss over a 12-week period [35].

4. The Evidence Linking the Microbe to the Disease

4.1. A. actinomycetemcomitans as an Amphibiont or Pathobiont

As has been done in many instances prior to the decision to study the relationship of a specific microbe to a specific disease, the following question was posited: "Is there sufficient evidence to warrant an in depth exploration of this microbe and the disease it was purported to cause?" Attributes or "virulence factors" possessed by the microbe in question were expected to provide it with a unique phenotype that could link the microbe to the disease. Molecular studies were designed to determine *A. actinomycetemcomitans*'s ability to attach, since attachment was considered to be the necessary first step in the infectious process. An animal model was developed, whereby specific virulence genes of interest could be studied in a host environment. A human observational model was developed to provide evidence that carriage of *A. actinomycetemcomitans* at a specific tooth site preceded disease. Each approach is defined below in the context of *A. actinomycetemcomitans* and the disease LAgP [36]. What follows are lessons learned over the years.

4.2. Molecular Approach

These studies were designed to assess the effect of relevant genes in the suspected pathogen to determine the putative effect of "virulence related" genes in a controlled simplified environment. Studies of attachment genes and leukotoxin are presented as examples of selected genetic studies since these are important virulence attributes that appear to be linked and could provide clues for relevant interventions.

4.2.1. Adherence Genes: Abiotic Adherence

After discovery of the sequence of the *flp*1 gene and then the assembly of the 14-gene operon termed the *tad* (tight adherence) operon, it was discovered that this operon was widespread in nature [27]. Phylogenetic analysis revealed that many Gram-negative and -positive pathogens and/or pathobionts had significant portions of this operon as did all archae sequenced to date [27]. These findings indicate that this operon should have biological significance in long-term survival since the operon is ever-present (hence, its name the widespread colonization island) and functionally it appears to be responsible for non-specific adherence to abiotic surfaces [37]. The *tad* genes encode a macromolecular system responsible for biogenesis of Flp, pili that bundle to form fibrils that are related to biofilm formation, that also show an association with surface related polysaccharides [2]. Further, elegant work by Wang et al. pointed to specific genes in the *tad* operon and their effect on extracellular matrix material such as vesicles, exopolysaccharides, and fimbriae [33]. The *tad* genes appear to have evolved via a specific horizontal transfer event and appear to provide a region relevant to disease in species as divergent as *Haemophilus ducreyi* (Hd), *Pasteurella multocida* (Pm), *Pseudonmonas aeruginosa* (Pa), *Yersinia pestis* (Yp) *Burkohoderia pasudomallei* (Bp), and *Caulobacter cresentus* (Cc) (Figure 3) [27].

In vitro studies indicate that *A. actinomycetemcomitans* binds in a linear fashion to salivary coated hydroxyapatite, shows minimal specificity, and thus never reaches a saturation point relative to surface binding [23,38]. Further, it has been shown that these fibrils provided a surface for glycoprotein and/or polysaccharide accumulation that also participates in the attachment process (Figure 3) [27,39].

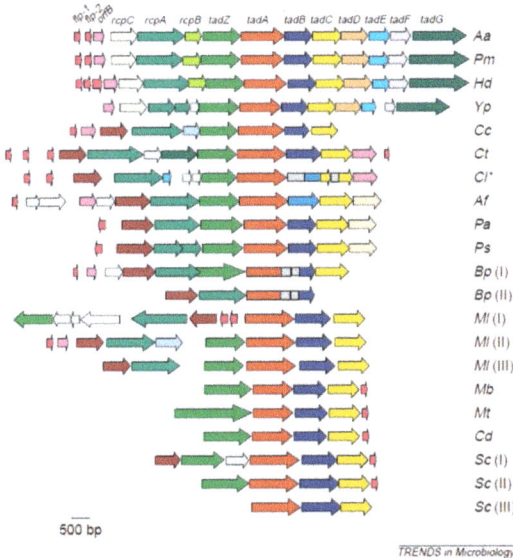

Figure 3. Phylogenetic analysis of the *tad* operon in a various microbial species. Illustration of the widespread colonization island (wci). WCI is a 14-gene operon. The top three microorganisms have the complete *tad* operon. The others have portions of it. WCI is present in many pathobionts and all archae sequenced to date.

4.2.2. Adherence Genes: Receptor/Adhesin related Adherence

Efforts to examine host bacterial interactions in an animal model initially showed that, despite possessing powerful attachment genes (i.e., *tad* genes), *A. actinomycetemcomitans* failed to colonize in a mouse model [40]. This led to the assessment of the specificity of attachment of *A. actinomycetemcomitans* to cells derived from a variety of mammals. Buccal epithelial cells (BECs) were obtained from the cheek of various mammals and *A. actinomycetemcomitans* was shown to bind to BECs obtained from Old World primates, humans, cows, and rats; minimally to mice; and not to dogs, cats, pigs, sheep, or New World primates (Figure 4) [38].

Binding was linked to an outer membrane protein called Aae that was dependent on the specificity of the interaction of the receptor (on the BEC)/adhesin (on the surface of *A. actinomycetemcomitans*) that was saturable and thus reached a plateau. Aae bound to BECs from Old World primates but had no effect on BECs from rats and cows, suggesting another adhesin or outer membrane protein existed apart from Aae (Figure 4). It turned out that this second adhesin, another autotransporter protein, was OMP 100 or ApiA, which also bound to BECs with a high level of specificity but at a significantly higher multiplicity of infection (MOI), requiring at least a ratio of 100,000 *A. actinomycetemcomitans* to 1 BEC [41].

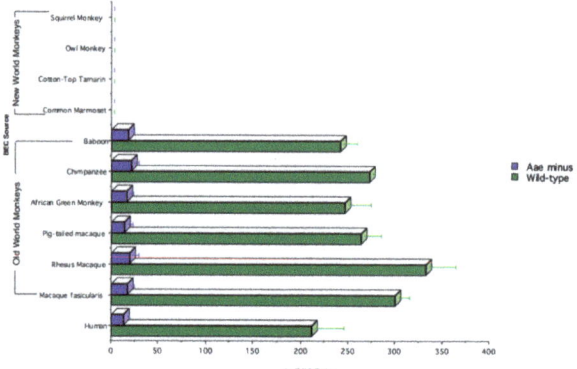

Figure 4. Binding of human *A. actinomycetemcomitans* to buccal epithelial cells (BECs). *A. actinomycetemcomitans* binds to BECs from Old World primates but not from New World primates. Mutation of the *aae* gene significantly reduces binding in these primates.

Figure 5 shows the kinetics of binding: (1) of wild type *A. actinomycetemcomitans* (black); (2) of *A. actinomycetemcomitans* with a deletion in the *flp* gene (red); and (3) with a deletion in the *aae* gene blue (blue). Note that the *flp* knock-out reaches a plateau while the wild type shows linear binding due to Flp. In the bottom curve, the *aae* knock-out does not show binding until almost 1,000,000 microbes are added, suggesting that another adhesin is present and that this adhesin clumps due to the linearity of curve.

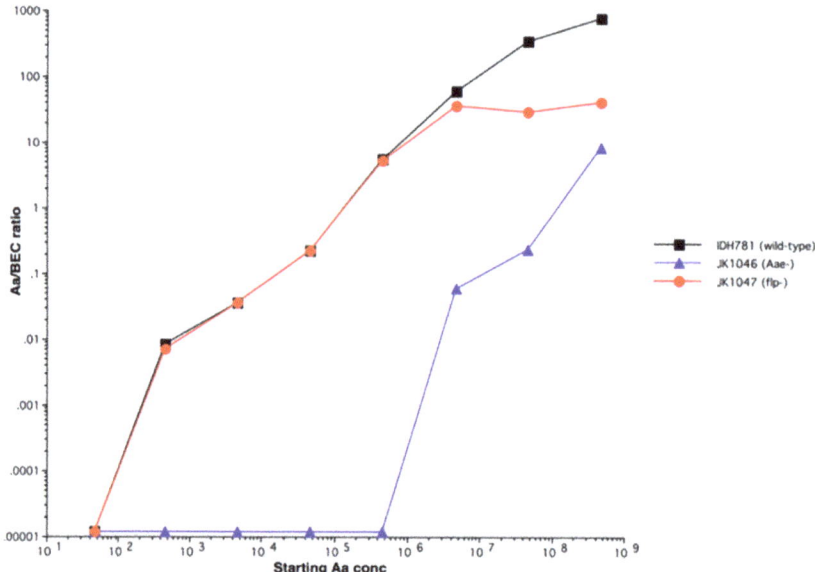

Figure 5. Kinetics of binding of *A. actinomycetemcomitans* to buccal epithelial cells (BECs).

ApiA had additional functions that included complement resistance. It was our assumption based on the MOI differential that Aae was important in initial stages of binding, while ApiA is expressed later. Since *A. actinomycetemcomitans* is found in pre-dentate children, it is our assumption that *A. actinomycetemcomitans* moves via Aae from BECs to teeth. We also have evidence from both in vivo and in vitro experiments that *A. actinomycetemcomitans* does not move from hard to soft tissue and thus once tooth bound it remains until it disperses [42].

Conclusions: Bacterial attachment in the oral cavity is of primary importance. *A. actinomycetemcomitans* has to resist the forces of mastication and the swift flows of saliva so that both abiotic and adhesin/receptor binding mechanisms are important. However, colonization models in animals (rodents and primates) suggest that the *tad* genes and abiotic binding to teeth are critical for persistence.

4.2.3. Leukotoxin

Leukotoxin (Ltx) was first described 40 years ago by Baehni et al. [43], members of the Taichman lab; and then characterized and purified by Tsai et al. [44]. The toxin was shown to be a 113 kDa protein derived from *A. actinomycetemcomitans* that killed leukocytes. The DNA sequence of the structural gene (*ltxA*) was defined by both Lally et al. [45] and Kolodrubetz et al. [46] as a member of the RTX toxin family. The discovery of an altered promoter region missing 530 base pairs upstream from the structural (*ltxA*) gene (termed the JP2 promoter region), which led to increased leukotoxin production, has sparked a great deal of interest [47]. In fact, substantial evidence has emerged showing that individuals who have *A. actinomycetemcomitans* with the JP2 promoter region have an increased relative risk for disease [48]. This association seen mostly in individuals from either West or North Africa provides convincing evidence that this form of *A. actinomycetemcomitans* is related to increased disease susceptibility [48]. The leukotoxin operon consists of a four-gene sequence such that *ltxC* is followed by the structural gene (*ltxA*), in turn followed by *ltxB* and *ltxD*. As such, the C gene helps activate the structural gene, which is transcribed and transported by the B and D genes. The toxin is both secreted and vesicle bound [49]. The secreted version appears to effect a LFA receptor on the surface of leukocytes and causes pore formation, leakage, and cell death [49]. Alternatively, the blebs containing Ltx appear to be internalized and cause inner disruption of cell function. Secretion of the toxin appears to be dependent on a TdeA protein (toxin and drug export; similar to TolC in *E. coli*) that works in concert with *ltxB* and *ltxD* [49].

Many reviews describe the Ltx operon in detail. Three recent discoveries may have an impact on future understanding of *A. actinomycetemcomitans* virulence. First, recent disclosure indicates that specific serotype b strains of *A. actinomycetemcomitans* that contain a *CagE* presence and a complete *cdtABC* gene operon are more pathogenic than strains that lack this genotype [50]. It is proposed that these strains could serve as a risk marker for aggressive disease and produce levels of leukotoxin that are comparable to JP2 promoter region strains through some mechanism as yet to be described [50]. This finding takes the emphasis off the JP2 strain type and places the focus on leukotoxin levels as a key virulence determinant [50]. Second, a recent discovery shows that the JP2 promoter region contains a 100 base pair segment closest to the *ltxC* gene that has a weak terminator [51]. Thus, detection of this 100 base pair region, as opposed to the entire 530 base pair promoter region, could be a main reason for lower levels of leukotoxin. Targeting this region with a more powerful terminator could significantly reduce leukotoxin production. Third, leukotoxin expression has recently been linked, in some unknown manner, to the *flp* and *tad* genes and thus deletion or reduction in Ltx reduces *A. actinomycetemcomitans* attachment, another potential focus for intervention.

Conclusion: First, leukotoxin stands as a critical determinant of increased risk for disease. The more we understand about how to modulate leukotoxin production, the better chances we have in controlling its action. Secondarily, some as of yet understood linkage between leukotoxin and *flp* genes appear to exist and thus strains devoid of leukotoxin (through gene deletion) barely express *flp*, do not attach in vivo, and barely attach in vitro. Further, strains showing elevated levels of Ltx attach to a greater extent than non-JP2 promoter strains both in vivo and in vitro. Understanding this linkage could prove to be an important way to modulate *A. actinomycetemcomitans'* participation in disease.

4.3. Interventional Studies

These animal studies were designed to examine the most likely genetic variants of the suspected pathogen in an effort to study the effect of a specific gene in a complex environment that resembles that seen in humans [52].

Inoculation of Rifampin-labeled *A. actinomycetemcomitans* strains containing *tadA* and *flp1* knock-outs in a rat colonization model showed no *A. actinomycetemcomitans* colonization, significantly less antibody to *A. actinomycetemcomitans*, and significantly less bone loss than the Rifampin-labeled wild type parental colonizing strain [35]. Studies of genetically distinct rat strains indicated that inoculation of the same strain of *A. actinomycetemcomitans* showed different levels of disease in the genetically different rat strains [53]. Further, inoculation of different strains of *A. actinomycetemcomitans* into genetically similar rat strains showed different levels of disease [40]. Taken together, these two sets of experiments emphasized the importance of considering both the host as well as the microbe in determination of pathogenicity (the Damage/Response Framework discussed below). In all cases, inoculated *A. actinomycetemcomitans* was seen at a low abundance since *A. actinomycetemcomitans* formed a minor component of the total microbial flora [35].

Due to the similarity between human and primate microbiota and anatomy, we began investigating a primate model of disease. In these studies, we learned that inoculation of a labeled *A. actinomycetemcomitans* strain of human origin could not colonize and sustain itself in a Rhesus (Rh) monkey model [54]. In contrast, a strain derived from Rh monkeys could colonize and survive over a 4-5-week period [54]. Using that same parental Rh *A. actinomycetemcomitans* strain, we also found to our surprise that deletion of *ltxA* resulted in a failure of the *ltx* knock-out strain to colonize. This *ltx* gene deletion resulted in a complete lack of attachment in vivo and reduced binding to hydroxyapatite in vitro, resulting from reduced expression of genes in the *tad* operon [55]. This linkage between *ltx* genes and *flp* genes was confirmed in another model, which showed that, when *A. actinomycetemcomitans* was stressed, four genes were linked: *flp*, *ltx*, *pgA*, and *tfox* [56].

Conclusion: Different strains of *A. actinomycetemcomitans* cause different levels of disease in the same rat strain and the same strain of *A. actinomycetemcomitans* causes different levels of bone loss in different rat strains, supporting the concept that both the host and the microbe need to be considered in pathogenesis of disease. Once again, *flp* and *tad* appear important in *A. actinomycetemcomitans* persistence, and *flp* is linked in some undisclosed manner to leukotoxin.

4.4. Observational Studies

These studies were designed to examine the relationship of the specific unaltered microbe (now named *Aggregatibacter*) in a susceptible well-defined patient population (healthy adolescents susceptible to LAgP), in a time related manner that moves from relative health to early disease so as to provide meaningful data related to disease causation. Further, these studies were designed to determine if *A. actinomycetemcomitans* was seen at the specific site of disease prior to the start of the disease, following the rules of disease temporality (contamination, infection, clinical manifestation of disease, and recuperation).

A two-phase study was initiated. Due to the projected level of prevalence of LAgP in African American adolescent communities (2%), we sought to determine whether combining carriage of *Aggregatibacter* in African American adolescents in Newark, New Jersey would provide us with a higher level of susceptibility to LAgP in this "vulnerable" population. As such, we launched a cross-sectional study of 1075 subjects and found that 42 subjects had one molar proximal site with one pocket greater than 6 mm with greater than 2 mm of clinical attachment loss (CAL). We considered this to be the early stage of LAgP. Of those 42 subjects, 66.7% had *A. actinomycetemcomitans*. If we then refined the definition to the Loe Brown definition of disease (two molars and added teeth with disease [57]), then 2% of African American adolescents had LAgP and 67.9% of these subjects had *A. actinomycetemcomitans* [58].

In an attempt to examine disease progression over a one-year period, we followed 96 subjects from borderline healthy (one 5-mm pocket) to disease progression over the year in two groups, one *A. actinomycetemcomitans* positive and one negative [58]. Subjects were considered borderline healthy if they had one pocket or fewer with a probing depth of 5 mm or less. Subjects who remained at one 5-mm pocket or less were considered as survivors over the one-year period. Subjects who progressed to clinical conditions with more than one 5-mm pocket to two or more pockets were considered as non-survivors. Subjects who did not survive over the year were divided into four categories as follows. In Category 1, subjects failed to survive if they had two 5-mm pockets and 90% of these were in the *A. actinomycetemcomitans* positive group. In Category 2, subjects failed to survive if they had three 5-mm pockets and 80% of these were in the *A. actinomycetemcomitans*-positive group. In Category 3 were subjects with one 6-mm pocket and CAL of 2 mm or greater and 85% were *A. actinomycetemcomitans*-positive. In Category 4 were subjects with detectable bone loss and all eight of these adolescents were *A. actinomycetemcomitans*-positive. No *A. actinomycetemcomitans*-negative subjects developed bone loss and a maximum of 20% of *A. actinomycetemcomitans*-negative adolescents were found in any group [58]. In virtually all cases, *A. actinomycetemcomitans* was found as a low abundance microbe relative to total recovery. If one considers that disease develops from pocket depth to CAL to bone loss, then this model suggested that carriage of *A. actinomycetemcomitans* at a particular site was indicative of progression of disease from relative health to pocket depth to bone loss [58]. Thus, while *A. actinomycetemcomitans* could be considered as an initiator of disease, we felt more comfortable suggesting that *A. actinomycetemcomitans* was a marker of risk for LAgP [58]. Our results indicate that subject susceptibility to LAgP, as we defined it, increased from 2% to 25% if the subjects had *A. actinomycetemcomitans* prior to the start of the one-year observation period, even at a low abundance, in this vulnerable population [58].

The second longitudinal study reflected learning from the first study and started with a balanced group of *A. actinomycetemcomitans* positive and *A. actinomycetemcomitans* negative subjects from 11 to 17 years of age from the Newark community who were considered healthy if they had one pocket of 4 mm or less [59]. Further clinical examinations were coupled with molar bite-wing X-rays and included the collection of saliva, subgingival microbial samples, and crevice fluid. Subgingival samples obtained from all first molar sites were stored frozen for future analysis. When radiographic evidence of bone loss was seen, saliva and samples taken from the first molars (healthy and diseased) 6–9 months prior to bone loss were thawed for testing. In addition, samples were taken from bone loss sites at the time bone loss was detected and from sites in the same subject that remained healthy for comparison in the microbiome analysis. In addition to microbiome analysis, crevice fluid samples and salivary samples were assessed for cytokine analysis.

Of the 2058 subjects entered into the study, 71 *A. actinomycetemcomitans*-negative and 63 *A. actinomycetemcomitans*-positive subjects were followed every six months for 2–3 years or until bone loss was detected at any site. In the initial cross-sectional analysis of the 2058 subjects, there were 64 subjects who had one 6-mm pocket with >2 mm of clinical attachment loss (CAL) and 67.2% had *A. actinomycetemcomitans*; 27 had two pockets of 6 mm or greater with >2 mm of CAL and 81.2% had *A. actinomycetemcomitans*; and 12 subjects had bone loss, 11 of whom had *A. actinomycetemcomitans*. The average age of the subjects was approximately 15 years of age. These subjects did not participate in the longitudinal study. The principal findings of the 2–3-year longitudinal study showed 23 subjects with one 6-mm pocket or greater with >2 mm of CAL, 86.9% of whom had *A. actinomycetemcomitans*, and 8 subjects with two pockets of 6 mm or more with >2 mm of CAL, 100% of whom had *A. actinomycetemcomitans*. These subjects were approximately 13 years of age. As for bone loss, there were 16 subjects and 18 sites that developed radiographic evidence of bone loss, all had *A. actinomycetemcomitans*, and they were approximately 14 years of age. Further, all sites with bone loss had *A. actinomycetemcomitans* prior to bone loss; however, healthy sites also had *A. actinomycetemcomitans* so that the sensitivity of the test was 100% and the specificity was 62%.

There were several other microorganisms that were elevated at the diseased sites prior to disease and these were *Filifactor alocis, Streptococcus parasanguinis*, a *Veillonella* cluster, a Fusobacterial cluster, and *Porphyromonas gingivalis* HOT-619 probe AA93. We then calculated the three most likely consortia for their presence at sites prior to bone loss and for their absence at sites without bone loss. We found that *A. actinomycetemcomitans*, *S. parasanguinis*, and *F. alocis* were found with a sensitivity of 89%, a specificity of 99%, a confidence interval of 95%, a positive predictive value of 94%, and a negative predictive value of 98%.

Further cytokine data from both saliva and crevice fluid indicated that MIP-1α and IL-1β were significantly elevated prior to bone loss at both the subject and site levels. Since both MIP-1α and IL-1β can play a biologically prominent role in activation of osteoclasts, we felt that this could potentially provide a diagnostic tool to examine bone loss at both the patient and site level prior to X-ray evidence in the future [60]. The association of MIP-1α with disease has been confirmed in salivary studies of patients with chronic periodontitis [61].

Conclusions:

(1) In cross-sectional studies, isolation and characterization of *Aggregatibacter* in a vulnerable adolescent population who were of African or Hispanic descent increased the susceptibility of that population for disease from 2% to 25%.

(2) In preliminary one-year longitudinal studies, a powerful correlation existed in adolescents who started with one 5-mm pocket and carriage of *A. actinomycetemcomitans* and disease progression in subjects who also developed bone loss as compared to matched subjects who did not carry *Aggregatibacter*.

(3) In longitudinal studies over a 2–3-year period, *A. actinomycetemcomitans* was deemed as necessary but not sufficient to be seen as causative. Association of *A. actinomycetemcomitans* with *F. alocis* and *S. parasanguinis* significantly increased predictability that disease would occur at a specific site. As with all the interventional studies, in the observational studies as well, *A. actinomycetemcomitans* was seen at low levels relative to the overall flora.

Taken together, these studies suggest that *A. actinomycetemcomitans* was necessary but not sufficient to cause disease but is a likely determinant of dysbiosis. We speculate that *A. actinomycetemcomitans* can suppress the local host defense system by virtue of leukotoxin and complement resistance, thus allowing other community members to overgrow.

5. The Defense: Novel Ways of Assessing Periodontitis as an Infectious Disease; Update: "War No More"

In the remainder of the review, evidence related to host and environmental disturbances that effect microbial/host interactions is examined. We speculate as to whether damage to the local site (i.e., by *A. actinomycetemcomitans*) is detrimental to the overall survival of the host. Further, we hypothesize that local host defenses can limit the extent of overall host damage and/or survival caused by the bacterial assault.

In the last century, infectious diseases have been portrayed as a war between the invading hordes of bacteria and the host's ability to protect its epithelial barrier by mounting a defensive strategy. Bacteria were envisioned as the hostile aggressors and the hosts job was to wall off the challenge by promoting a successful homeostatic defense. Bacteria were armed with adhesins, invasins, toxins, enzymes, and siderophores, while the host was armed with resistance factors such as IgA proteases, leukotoxins, and complement. Host defenses supplemented the natural epithelial barrier with innate non-specific factors such as phagocytes, cytokines, and complement, and adaptive immune response elements such as antibodies and lymphocytes. Perhaps the earliest example of the change in our view of the "war analogy" was put forth in a book by Rosebury "Life on Man" which exposed us to the idea that bacteria were not our enemies but were partners in our co-evolution. Scientist as renown as Joshua Lederberg indicated that we should say "war no more" relative to our bacterial partners and we should be encouraged to read Rosebury's " little book" that is "best source to learn more about this obscure category ... contained within a now out of print 'cult favorite'" Life on Man [62]. Stanley Falkow stated that "Rosebury reminded us ... years ago that we are a single community and that it would be a good idea to stop thinking of ... our unicellular companions as repulsive ... " [63].

This battleground analogy was further complicated by the AIDS pandemic where it became obvious that patients were dying of typically harmless microorganisms that were endemic such as *Cryptosporidia* and *Pneumococcus*. The AIDS crisis challenged many infectious disease specialists to change their approach to studying contagious diseases. One distinctive approach was developed at Einstein Medical School in New York City by Casadevall and Pirofski [64]. In an effort to teach medical students to think differently about infectious diseases they developed what they called the Damage/Response Framework. Their rationale was that previous concepts of infectious diseases failed to take the host into consideration in discussions of pathogenicity. It became obvious to these researchers that HIV infected patients were dying of typically harmless microorganisms that were part of the endemic microbiota. These pathobionts were successful in causing disease because the host was so totally overwhelmed by HIV compromised immune non-responsiveness. In efforts to put this into the context of pathogenesis, Casadevall and Pirofski felt it was mandatory to include the host as a critical component in the framework of microbial pathogenicity. As opposed to other systems (Henle/Koch postulates and Bradford Hill Criteria), pathogenicity in the Damage/Response Framework demanded that microbial pathogenic potential could not be defined if the host was minimized or excluded. The Framework was especially informative in helping understand how typically innocuous agents, such as *Candida*, *Crytococcus*, etc., could lead to morbidity and mortality in an HIV infected patient. It illustrated how the host response framework played a critical role in pathogenicity. In further support of the "war no more" philosophy, the importance of the commensal microbiota has been highlighted. It was put forward that early on we are inoculated by indigenous members of our microbiota that train our immune responsiveness. This novel way of looking at our microbiota initially called the hygiene hypothesis has been re-stated as the "Old Friends" hypothesis [65]. Recently, Dahlen et al. mentioned the Damage/Response Framework in reference to dental disease, during which time they highlighted the prominence of *A. actinomycetemcomitans* as a potential pathogen, which prompted this review [3].

5.1. The Microbial Point of View: Biogeography, Landscape Ecology in the Oral Cavity

Some microbiologists are of the belief that bacteria are everywhere and form communities in environments that best support their growth. However, other microbial ecologists believe that communities form in a random manner [66]. The term biogeography is a broad term that has been used to describe how the physical environment affects plant and animal species in their worldly distribution. Recent elegant studies by Mark Welsh et al. have illustrated in great detail the biogeography of dental plaque [67]. As seen in this work, the aggregate biogeography is composed of multiple communities (metacommunities) of species (animals, plants, or in our case microbes). Overall, the general consensus is that community form is based on selection centered around how species distribute themselves (dispersal), how they interact (fitness), and how they compete for substrates to gain territory (abundance) [68]. A metacommunity is formed by a series of interacting communities within the overall biogeography and further subdivisions of these metacommunities are termed patches. A patch is a dimensionally distinct region that supports growth and persistence of lifeforms contained within the patch, bordered by a matrix that influences survival of lifeforms outside the patch. In microbial ecology, each patch contains a community of microbes that change as a result of dispersal of microbes from one patch to another patch [68].

There are essentially four models that attempt to describe patch development and diversity: patch dynamics, species sorting, source sink dynamics, and the neutral model. The patch dynamic model suggests that less competitive species within one patch disperse to a lower density patch (anaerobic fastidious species find their way to environments that exclude oxygen; e.g., movement from the supra- to the subgingival domain). The species sorting model suggests that the environment in one patch is better for a specific species than another patch (e.g., one patch has a low pH and favors acid producing and acid loving species). The source sink model states that a high-quality habitat shows elevated populations, whereas a low-quality habitat (sink) shows a decrease in population diversity and level (e.g., a high carbohydrate environment favors microbes that metabolize carbohydrates and minimizes those that are assarcharolytic). The neutral model states that biodiversity arises randomly and thus sympatric species compete for the same resources and in this case some species are more successful than others [69].

The oral environment consists of several habitats, domains, or landscapes that present microorganisms with specific colonizing surfaces, nutritional options, and mechanical interferences that are unique to each landscape. The overall environment of the oral cavity is composed of complex geographies made up of a variety of hard non-shedding tooth surfaces and soft tissue surfaces, some keratinized, others pseudo-keratinized and others non-keratinized [70]. This is exemplified by differences in the filiform and fungiform surfaces of the ventral surface of the tongue as opposed to the dorsal surface, the cheek mucosa, the palatine tonsils, the gingival epithelium, and sulcular and junctional epithelium. These differing habitats are suitable for colonization of yeast, bacteria, and viruses [69]. Moreover, hard tissue non-shedding tooth surfaces permit bacteria to adhere and resist removal from the swift flows of saliva and the forces of mastication. Even among the tooth surfaces there are significant differences. There is the bell-shaped tooth surface of molars that differs from relatively flat incisor surfaces. Further, the more coronal surface of molars and premolars differ from the surfaces below the protruding bell-shaped mid-surface, which forms protection for the supra-gingival region. Hidden occlusal pit and fissure surfaces are tortuous, deep, and unreachable by mechanical cleansing methods and are completely different from buccal, lingual, and proximal smooth surfaces of enamel that are exposed and cleansable. Exposed enamel is bathed by saliva while enamel below the gum line is bathed by gingival crevice fluid, a serum transudate. Overall, this complex biogeography precludes simple ecological analysis and thus each biogeography has to be analyzed individually [71].

5.1.1. Landscapes and Proximal Caries

To illustrate this point, we compare two major dental diseases caries and periodontal diseases that occur in neighboring landscapes. Landscape ecology examines the spatial configuration of natural environments and is used by ecologists to study spatial patterns of plants, bacteria, and forms of life in complex environments. This system of analysis illustrates "patches" of unique homogenous areas that for specific biological reasons permit or encourage the growth of defined populations of lifeforms. The lifeforms examined and the confining biogeography depend on spatial patterns considering time as well as space as defining conditions [72]. This systematic way of examining microbiology has been introduced into the infectious disease literature by Proctor and Relman as applied to the nose, mouth, and throat [73]. The two experiments below highlight the role of amphibionts (now called pathobionts, i.e., members of the indigenous microbiota that can influence disease) in the two most prominent dental diseases. Questions arise as to what makes these habitats distinct environments and how do these distinctive environments support the growth of similar or different microbial communities and cause a different Damage/Response pathway. What is particularly attractive about landscape ecology as it applies to dental disease is that it can be relevant to a specific location in the oral cavity that harbors a distinctive microbiota and disease phenotype that is uniquely different from its neighboring landscape. For a comprehensive review of this topic with respect to periodontal disease, see Proctor et al. (2019) [69].

In the mid-1960s in Denmark, Harald Loe and colleagues conducted a seminal experiment that highlighted the relevance of the accumulation of dental plaque and its effect on gingival health [74]. This simple but elegant experiment caught the attention of the clinical and research community and changed the way in which developing dental plaque (a true biofilm) was henceforth studied. In these experiments, dental students with healthy gingiva were asked to abstain from all oral hygiene for a period of three weeks, during which time plaque developed on their teeth and healthy gingiva became clinically inflamed, often exhibiting punctate areas of bleeding. Resumption of oral hygiene immediately thereafter removed the accumulated supragingival plaque and the inflamed and bleeding gingiva returned to its previously healthy condition. These studies of experimentally induced gingivitis led to an exploration of the structured sequence of events in microbial plaque development but also established a sense that the massive accumulation of plaque led to disease (in this case gingivitis). It was clear that inflammation arose from the vasculature directly below the sulcular or junctional epithelium and that the serum transudate derived from this inflammatory response was directly related to the accumulating supragingival plaque that extended to the subgingival domain. Collection of fluid from the crevice between the teeth and the gum line showed that the transudate contained complement and polymorphonuclear leukocytes. Furthermore, after removal of the tooth accumulated plaque, both the volume and the components of the transudate were reduced as the microbial challenge was reduced. Studies followed that used this model to determine the exact sequence of events relative to colonization, highlighting pioneer colonizers that attached to salivary coated enamel surfaces, followed by a succession of secondary and tertiary colonizers, always documenting how these sequential events could be replicated, characterized, and extended to the subgingival habitat [75,76].

Not long thereafter, Von der Fehr et al. (1970) augmented the original experimental gingivitis study by adding nine daily rinses of 10 mL of 50% sucrose to the routine of abstaining from brushing maxillary anterior teeth now for a 23-day period [77]. In this case, instead of just gingivitis, the dental students who abstained also developed early caries or white spot lesions on their anterior incisors. Thus, the result was a shift in the plaque microbiota from one that was primarily responsible for gingivitis to one that was responsible for early caries. This exaggerated sucrose challenge clearly demonstrated the effect of the imposition of one environmental hazard (abstinence and development of a climax community of members of the commensal microbiota) on another environmental hazard (frequent sucrose rinsing which shifted the commensal flora to one that favored a acidophilic/aciduric flora) on the outcome of dental disease. Thus, the power of the environment clearly won out and the entire shift in disease activity was committed by amphibionts that overgrew or overpowered homeostasis to create an ecological catastrophe (or simply put members of the commensal microbiota under exaggerated circumstances, bloom or overgrew, and became involved in dysbiosis and disease) [77].

Caries is caused by the direct microbiological damage to its adjacent host tissue landscape. In proximal caries, microorganisms that are acid producing and live in a viscous biofilm matrix emit acids which are in direct contact with the enamel surface. The acid in the viscous matrix is derived from the commensal microbiota [78]. Within this landscape of acid producing bacteria, there can be microbes that consume acids (lactic acid). Species sorting occurs within the matrix, and, as more and more sticky carbohydrates are consumed, the acidophilic and aciduric organisms become predominant. Moreover, the metabolic byproduct of microbes living within this landscape are microbes such as *Streptococcus mutans* that consume sucrose and can provide lactic acid, a mandated carbon source for the growth and survival of Veillonella, a Gram-negative microbe that can live in association with *S. mutans* [79,80]. Recent evidence suggests that *A. actinomycetemcomitans* can also thrive on lactate as its main carbon source, thus eliminating competition for glucose as an energy source with pioneer colonizers such as Streptococci [36,81].

A well-controlled dual-species biofilm animal experiment as described below illustrates this symbiosis best. Here, a group of animals fed a high sucrose containing diet in conjunction with *S. mutans* were co-inoculated with *Veillonella* spp., which consumed lactic acid. The addition of Veillonella caused an increase in the biofilm pH and thus reduced caries levels when compared to the animal inoculated with *S. mutans* alone [80]. Several other experiments have shown that caries is a multifactorial disease that depends on an acid producing microbiota, a high carbohydrate diet, and teeth. The microbial landscape or patch within the landscape can be modified by environmental factors such as saliva and diet over time, while the damage can be influenced by lactic acid consuming bacteria as well as arginine and ammonia producing bacteria within the biofilm matrix [71].

Further in keeping with the damage response framework, the host, which is in this case the enamel, begins to shed mineral from its sub-surface after repeated attacks by acid producing bacteria when the pH dips below 5.5. The host is also capable of interfering with (responding to) this attack by buffering the acid produced by bacteria, by providing calcium that can heal the wounded enamel, or by protecting the host tissue from damage by the production of salivary antibodies or antibacterial factors [82]. Moreover, bacteria within the plaque biofilm matrix such as *Veillonella* spp., limit the potential damage. Here, we see a good example of how disease (dental caries) has to be assessed by examining both the damage and the response framework in order to determine the end-point, i.e., disease, in this case caries [83].

Conclusion: There are at least two points to consider when describing caries. First, there is a direct attack by bacterial byproducts (damage) on the host tissue (enamel). Second, the pathobionts (acidophiles) in this case survive in an ecology where diversity has been reduced by the hazardous environmental threat of a severely reduced pH. These two points may differ when we explore periodontal disease.

5.1.2. Landscapes and Proximal Periodontitis

Periodontitis occurs just below the gingival margin in the inter-proximal region. The disease takes place as a result of microbial accumulation that begins at or slightly above the gingival margin with the initial colonization of Gram-positive Streptococci that form parallel rows of palisading layers of microbes that attach to enamel and project from the tooth surface. Interspersed between the parallel rows are anaerobic Gram-negative cocci that form a complex community that overtime forms a mixed population of *Corynibacteria, Streptococci, Actinomyces, Neisseria, Fusobacteria, Vibrios, Tanerella*, and ultimately *Spirochetes* and *Porphyromonads* [84]. In essence, a complex climax community is developed that projects from above the gumline to below the gumline. The bacteria above the gumline derive their nutrition from saliva where the major carbon source is supplied by glucose, whereas the nutrition below the gumline is derived from bacterial byproducts from supragingival bacteria and serum proteins and small chain fatty acids below the gingival margin [82].

In another series of ground-breaking studies, Moore studied the supra- and subgingival plaque microbiota in well-characterized volunteers using a non-biased system of anaerobic microbiology to capture the micro-organisms that thrived above and below the gum-line [85,86]. Using a sensitive Roll-Tube method, an enriched non-selective agar, picking every fifth colony and then carefully characterizing each colony, they found that there were some bacteria that thrived in the supragingival plaque of healthy subjects as opposed to some that thrived in the subgingival domain. Of interest was the fact that there were some bacteria that were capable of thriving in both environments. This dynamic illustrates the potential for microbes to disperse and show fitness for domains or landscapes that are environmentally unique. Further, they found that some microbes were dominant in health and some were dominant in disease but others were capable of thriving in either condition, once again demonstrating the keen adaptability of microbes for landscapes of extremely different nutritional and competitive conditions [87]. These experiments demonstrate that, even in environments (landscapes or patches) that are demonstrably different, subpopulations of bacteria have capabilities of adaptation permitting them to overcome these extremes. Newer DNA-based methods have supported these observations, but it should not be overlooked that microbial induced infectious diseases typically require some determination of live bacteria for initiation of disease.

As the plaque biofilm moves from the supragingival landscape to the subgingival landscape, the biofilm impinges on the epithelium lining the gingiva, which elicits an inflammatory response from the blood vessels directly subjacent to the basal layer of the junctional epithelium. The $^{(a)}U^{(b)}$ shaped sulcus or crevice, is composed of an inner junctional epithelium on one surface (a), which is attached to and derived from the enamel and the outer sulcular surface (b) that covers the connective tissue (Figure 6). The base or the bottom of the U is typically formed by junctional epithelial cells that are basal in nature [88,89]. Microbes can migrate from above the gum into the sulcus where they reach the base of the U-shaped sulcus. Here microbial products form an antigenic overload that elicits an osmotic gradient, encouraging cells to migrate from subjacent vessels. The white cells contained within these vascular networks undergo stagnation, margination, diapedesis, and chemotaxis of polymorphonuclear leukocytes (PMNs) into the sulcus. Ultimately, after the sulcus is packed with biofilm containing microbes, the PMNs line the base of the sulcus to form a poly band, protecting the underlying connective tissue from microbial or microbial product invasion [90].

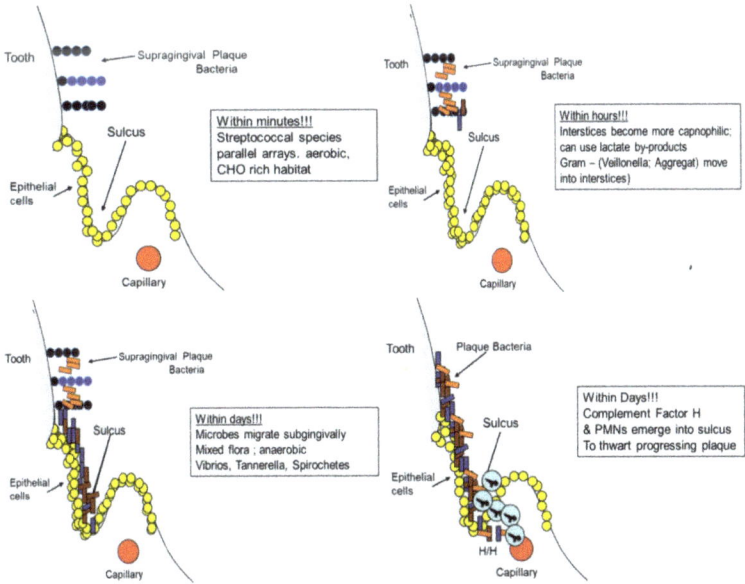

Figure 6. Microbial plaque development over time. Plaque starts above the gingival margin and progresses to the subgingival environment where it eventually encounters polymorphonuclear leukocytes (PMNs) along with complement in an attempt by the host to limit the accumulating biofilm from invading the underlying tissue.

During this challenging period, complement is found as a prominent protein in the crevice fluid. In this manner, complement and PMNs form the first line of defense in the Damage/Response scenario. At this stage, the innate immune response, probably in conjunction with fibrinogen-like proteins, plays a significant role in protecting the host from microbial invasion [91] (Figure 6). Once this inflammatory response is in full force, eating hard foods can cause a pumping action on the tooth in its socket, creating a bacteremic challenge for the vulnerable junctional epithelial barrier that, unchecked, can force the packed subgingival microbiota through the damaged basement membrane into the underlying vasculature, leading to a transient bacteremia. This transient bacteremia can translocate otherwise innocuous members of the commensal microbiota to organs distant from the oral cavity that might now contribute to damage of host tissue in a less protected framework at that distant site [92].

Conclusion: Damage/Response Framework in Periodontitis: In the case of LAgP, the damage occurs at the interface between the soft tissue surface and bone. Unlike the damage seen in caries, the damage in periodontal disease is not directly derived from bacteria but appears to be related to bacterial effects on the modulation of the host response. In the case of LAgP, *A. actinomycetemcomitans*, a low abundance pathobiont, represses the local innate immune response and allows microbes to overgrow that would ordinarily be killed by PMNs, macrophages, complement, or antibody. *A. actinomycetemcomitans* has a profound effect on the initial host response framework at the local site, providing the ability of a consortium of potentially damaging microorganism to survive and thrive in the absence of host interference. Thus, it has been proposed that periodontitis is a disease caused by an increased diversity of microorganisms due to an inadequate local host responsiveness, which may prove to be an unusual response compared to most infectious diseases [93]. This hypothesis, if further substantiated, distinguishes this disease from many other infections including caries.

5.2. The Host Point of View: Damage/Response Framework

5.2.1. Localization of Gingivitis and Periodontitis

In the 1980s, New York City was one of the epicenters of the AIDS crisis, and at Columbia, at the time, it was important to convince the dental faculty to wear protective masks and gloves. In the Preventive Dentistry Division, our group decided to design experiments to demonstrate the spread of microbes from patients to dentists by the aerosol back-spray generated by ultrasonic removal of supragingival plaque from patient's mouths [94]. In another set of demonstrations, we assessed the spread of plaque bacteria from the patient's tooth site to distant organs by means of bacteremia created by the aggressive effort (scaling) to remove subgingival plaque [92]. It was our hope that these demonstrations would be convincing enough to advance our public health policies. In the process, we learned things that were unexpected.

We fully expected that a procedure as aggressive as ultrasonic scaling in the subgingival area in a patient with periodontal pockets would generate bacteremias in all patients subjected to this procedure. Experiments were carefully controlled, and subjects were chosen who had incipient to minimal periodontitis in three quadrants. After abstaining from tooth-cleaning for 24 h, we assessed subjects for bacteremia in one quadrant after ultrasonic scaling. Of 25 subjects, 72% (18) showed bacteremia in one quadrant while 28% did not [92]. Bacteremia-positive subjects returned and had a second and third scaling with remaining pocketed quadrants in the following weeks. Pre-procedural subgingival irrigation was performed in the remaining diseased and pocketed quadrants followed by rinsing with an antiseptic mouthrinse. Those who were irrigated with the antiseptic showed significantly reduced bacteremia in all 18 test subjects, while all 18 in the placebo irrigated cross-over control group continued to have bacteremia [92]. A similar demonstration was conducted in subjects with gingivitis and no pockets and here only 30% of subjects screened showed bacteremia. In these experiments, we standardized the bacteremia test to include chewing a hard apple for 2 min, after which we took our peripheral blood sample. This time, test subjects who were positive for bacteremia after the apple test, rinsed for two weeks with an antiseptic rinse prior to the apple test and this once again reduced the bacteremia. However, once again, the controls who rinsed with a placebo rinse had bacteremia consistently in the apple test group [92]. A third study was designed to determine if subjects who had gingivitis and were resistant to bacteremia remained resistant to bacteremia after a second or third apple challenge. Once again, 30% of gingivitis subjects had bacteremias initially at the screening visit and continued to have bacteremias repeatedly while those who were initially resistant continued to be bacteremia-negative after the repeated apple tests. Experiments showing resistance to bacteremia have been reproduced in other labs where aggressive procedures such as scaling and tooth extraction did not produce bacteremias in specific groups of subjects [95].

Conclusion:

(1) A segment of the population is more resistant to transient bacteremia resulting from physical challenge while others are susceptible.

(2) The more aggressive is the challenge and the more advanced is the disease, the greater is the chances that bacteremia will occur.

(3) The overall consensus is that intact epithelium provides the protective barrier that resists the local bacterial challenge.

This logic does not appear to be consistent with the biology in the case of ultrasonic scaling and tooth extraction where the procedures performed are very disruptive and typically compromise the epithelial barrier. It appears as if something else is at play here. What can account for this resistance? What is the protective mechanism operating at the epithelial border? What prevents constant exposure of the underlying vasculature to bacteria adjacent to a physically disrupted epithelium from permitting bacteria from circulating to distant organs? Will these transiently circulating oral bacteria, which possess the ability to adhere as one of their main attributes, land on a distant organ (the heart, colon, appendix, etc. [96–98]), and then contribute to exacerbation of disease at that distant organ [99]? Some thought experiments described below might suggest different ways that periodontal disease can challenge host survival.

5.2.2. Toxin localization: The Horseshoe Crab and Periodontitis

The American horseshoe crab (*Limulus Polyphemus*) is estimated to be over 250 million years old. It has gained attention in the medical community in the last 40 years because of its utility in determining miniscule levels of endotoxin, lipoteichoic acids, and now B–D-glucan presence by coagulation mediated pathways [100]. In that capacity, the limulus lysate test has replaced Schwartzman reaction testing in rabbits as a means of detecting endotoxin to ensure that hospital instruments and supplies are free from low levels of endotoxin [101]. In the Schwartzman phenomenon, thrombosis is due to diffuse intravascular coagulation resulting in tissue necrosis [102]. As a replacement for Schwartzman testing, the horseshoe crab limulus lysate system was found to be significantly more sensitive and thus could serve as a replacement for animal testing. The process required that scientists bleed the horseshow crab, collect their hemolymph, separate the hemocytes, lyse them, and use the lysate for the assessment of nanogram to picogram levels of endotoxin. On an evolutionary level, it is conjectured that the horseshow crab has survived all this time for two basic reasons: (1) because of its hard outer shell that is virtually impenetrable; and (2) because of its primitive but highly successful innate immune system consisting of a one cell army of hemocytes. This primitive defense system operates as follows. If by chance the soft underbelly of the crab is penetrated and infected, then hemocytes chemotax to the origin of the infection. The migration of hemocytes would then come in contact with endotoxin, lyse, and then release granules from their cell bodies. These granules contain coagulogen, a large inactive precursor protein. The coagulogen is enzymatically attacked in a sequential manner, eventually by a proclotting enzyme, and then a clotting enzyme in order to degrade coagulogin to coagulin, which causes gelation of coagulation proteins that form an impenetrable barrier [103]. This gel-like substance produced at the site of the infection holds endotoxin at bay and prevents its migration from the infection site to any distant organ (heart, etc.) so as to protect the horseshoe crab from death. It has recently been shown that the clotting cascade can also produce antimicrobial agents similar to B defensins, suggesting that both clotting and killing can occur together. The fibrinogen/fibrin system in mammals is similar [104]. With these examples in mind, there are lessons to be learned from the horseshoe crab localization analogy that may play a role in the Damage/Response Framework we observe in the localization of dental infections in humans (Figure 7).

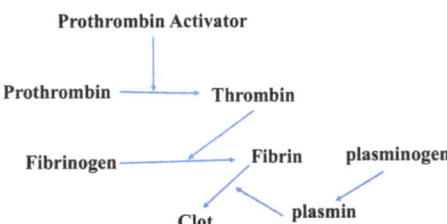

Figure 7. The fibrin cascade simplified. Prothrombin activator enzymatically cleaves prothrombin, which then activates thrombin that is now available to cleave fibrinogen to fibrin. Fibrin is acted on by plasmin to form a clot in a manner similar to that seen in the horseshoe crab.

6. Concluding Remarks: The Final Verdict, Lesion Localization/Host Survival via Disease Localization

A good example of the localization of dental infections occurs in periapical inflammatory responses to endodontic infections [105]. Pulpal infection can lead to periapical lesions (PAL) that can result in periapical cysts or granulomas that form a constrained measurable circular lesion extending below the apex of the tooth root. Localization of the PAL is thought to be due to IL-1β and TNF-α and their receptors expressed at the local site as well as the presence of Hageman factor, which can induce coagulation due to fibrin clot formation at the local site [106]. In IL-1β receptor knock-out mice challenged by root containing endotoxin, mice die due to the lack of confinement or localization of endotoxin [106]. Undoubtedly, PMNs, antibody, macrophages, and lymphocytes and their products play an important role in localization, but in this review our intent is to focus on the parallels between the primitive and successful horseshoe crab response and the human fibrin response. As such, host defense mechanisms that include coagulation factors (fibrin, Hageman factor, etc.) can act as a determinant in deterring systemic damage by localizing disease to the immediate area of challenge [107].

With respect to periodontitis, bacteria that form the subgingival microbial landscape are members of the commensal microbiota that are sampled by dendritic cells, macrophages, and lymphocytes throughout life [108]. As such, immune recognition of these antigens protects the body by localizing the infection to the specific site of attack. Even in the case of chronic periodontitis, the damage in the Damage/Response Framework is localized, minimal, indirect, and due to immune hyper-reactivity [109]. However, as time continues, the constant barrage of this antigenic challenge can undermine the supporting structures of the teeth unless attended to by preventive procedures [110].

Progressive damage of the connection between the tooth root and its fibrous union to the adjacent bone that holds the tooth in its socket deteriorates overtime to a degree such that the tooth becomes loosened, weakened, and lost. This typically occurs by virtue of years of neglect and failure to intervene [111,112]. In contrast to current beliefs, it may be useful to look at tissue destruction at the local site as localization of disease in an effort to limit the assault to teeth and prevent infection from occurring at a distant site (heart, gut, and kidney; see Table S1 for details). After years of a constant barrage of microbes that include bacteria, yeast, and viruses, periodontal disease continues to occur at a local site, in an incremental manner, and in the face of an ulcerated epithelium, rarely resulting in mortality or morbidity [113]. As we continue to study the oral cavity, especially the oral microbiome in light of infectious diseases, we can potentially learn more about where we came from and where we are heading in the future. We may even learn that periodontal disease in immunologically competent individuals provides a response framework that limits the overall damage to a vulnerable tissue complex that is continually under attack but responds by confining the damage to the local landscape. In our thought experiment, we postulate that a fibrinogen/fibrin-like network combined with defensins provide a Damage/Response Framework not too dissimilar to what is seen in the primitive horseshoe crab [16]. We hypothesize that this clot confining system should not be ignored and combined with cytokines and immunologic surveillance strategies can participate in restricting the microbial challenge to the local site so as to protect the host from its demise.

Supplementary Materials: The following are available online at http://www.mdpi.com/2076-0817/9/3/179/s1, Table S1: Selected Oral Bacteria found at distant sites related to extra-oral diseases.

Author Contributions: Conceptualization and writing, D.H.F.; review, comments, and animal studies, H.S., S.K.V., and D.H.F.; molecular studies, S.K.V., H.S., and D.H.F.; and initial draft, D.H.F. All authors have read and agreed to the published version of the manuscript.

Funding: This work was supported to the greatest extent by funds from the National Institute of Dental and Craniofacial Research (DHF; DE017968, DE021172, and DE016306).

Acknowledgments: We thank all our collaborators over the years who include but are not limited to David Furgang, Narayanan Ramasubbu, Scott Kachlany, Paul Planet, Jeffrey Kaplan, Maribasappa Karched, Robert DeSalle and especially David Figurski. We would also like to thank Dean Cecile Feldman for helping supplement funding for some of the primate studies. As a result of the focused nature of this review, there were manuscripts references not included. This was not intentional, and we apologize to those who have devoted time and effort to this area of research who we have failed to acknowledge.

Conflicts of Interest: The authors declare no conflict of interest.

References

1. Haubek, D.; Johansson, A. Pathogenicity of the highly leukotoxiic JP2 clone of Aggregatibacter actinomycetemcomitans and its geographic dissemination and role in aggressive periodontitis. *J. Oral Microbiol.* **2014**, 1–22. [CrossRef]
2. Belibasakis, G.N.; Maula, T.; Bao, K.; Lindholm, M.; Bostanci, N.; Oscarsson, J.; Ihalin, R.; Johansson, A. Virulence and Pathogenicity of Aggregatibacter actinomycetemcomitans. *Pathogens* **2019**, 222. [CrossRef] [PubMed]
3. Dahlen, D.; Basic, A.; Bylund, J. Importance of Virulence Factors for the Persisitence of Oral Bacterria in the Inflamed Gingival Crevice and in the Pathogenesis of Periodontal Disease. *J. Clin. Microbiol.* **2019**, *8*, 1339.
4. Fine, D.; Patil, A.; Velusamy, S. Aggregatibacter actinomycetemcomitans (Aa) Under the Radar: Myths and Misunderstandings of Aa and its Role in Aggressive Periodontitis. *Front Immunol.* **2019**, *25*. [CrossRef]
5. Nedergaard, S.; Kobel, C.M.; Nielsen, M.B.; Meller, R.T.; Jensen, A.B.; Norskov-Lauritsen, N. Whole Genome Sequencing of Aggregatibacter actinomycetemcomitans Cultured from Blood Stream Infections Reveals Three Major Phylogenetic Groups Including Novel Lineage Expressing Seerotype a Membrane Polysaccharide. *Pathogens* **2019**, *8*, 256. [CrossRef]
6. Tjokro, N.O.; Kittichotirat, W.; Torittu, A.; Ihalin, R.; Bumgarner, R.E.; Chen, C. Transcriptomic Analysis of Aggregatibacter actinomycetemcomitans Core and Accessory Genes in Different Growth Conditions. *Pathogens* **2019**, *8*, 282. [CrossRef]
7. Klinger, R. Untersuchungen uber enschliche aktinomykose. *Cent. Bacteriol.* **1912**, *62*, 191–200.
8. Fine, D.H.; Cohen, D.W.; Bimstein, E.; Bruckmann, C. A ninety-year history of periodontosis: The legacy of Professor Bernhard Gottlieb. *J. Periodontol.* **2015**, *86*, 1–6. [CrossRef]
9. Slots, J. The predominant cultivable organisms in juvenile periodontitis. *Scand. J. Dent. Res.* **1976**, *84*, 1–10. [CrossRef]
10. Newman, M.G.; Socransky, S.S.; Savitt, E.D.; Propas, D.A.; Crawford, A. Studies of the microbiology of periodontosis. *J. Periodontol.* **1976**, *47*, 373–379. [CrossRef]
11. Fine, D.H.; Patil, A.G.; Loos, B.G. Classification and diagnosis of aggressive periodontitis. *J. Periodontol.* **2018**, *89*, S103–S119. [CrossRef] [PubMed]
12. Papapanou, P.N.; Sanz, M.; Budunell, N.; Dietrich, T.; Feres, M.; Fine, D.H.; Flemmig, T.F.; Garcia, R.; Giannobile, W.V.; Graziani, F.; et al. Peridontitis: Consensus report of workgroup 2 of the 2017 World Workshop on the Classification of Periodontal Disease and Peri-Implant Disease and Conditions. *J. Periodontol.* **2018**, *89*, S173–S182. [CrossRef] [PubMed]
13. Norskov-Lauritsen, N. Classification, Identification, and Clinical Significance of Haemophilu and Aggregatibacter Species with Host Specificity for Humans. *Clin. Microbiol. Rev.* **2014**, *27*, 214–240. [CrossRef] [PubMed]
14. Baer, P.N. The case for periodontosis as a clinical entity. *J. Periodontol.* **1971**, *42*, 516–520. [CrossRef]
15. Offenbacher, S.; Divaris, K.; Barros, S.P.; Moss, K.L.; Marchesan, J.T.; Morelli, T.; Zhang, S.; Kim, S.; Sun, L.; Beck, J.D.; et al. Genome-Wide association study of biologically informed periodontal complex traits offers novel insights into the genetic basis for periodontal disease. *Hum. Mol. Genet.* **2016**, *25*, 2113–2129. [CrossRef]
16. Munz, M.; Richter, G.M.; Loos, B.G.; Jensen, S.; Divaris, K.; Offenbacher, S.; Teumer, A.; Holtfreter, B.; Kocher, T.; Bruckmann, C.; et al. Meta-analysis of genome-wide association studies of aggressive and chronic periodontitis identifies two novel risk loci. *Eur. J. Hum. Genet.* **2019**, *27*, 102–113. [CrossRef]
17. Nibali, L.; Almofareh, S.A.; Bayliss-Chapman, J.; Zhou, Y.; Vieira, A.R.; Divaris, K. Heritability of periodontitis: A systematic review of evidence from animal studies. *Arch. Oral Biol.* **2020**, *109*, 1–6. [CrossRef]
18. Munz, M.; Chen, H.; Jockel-Schneider, Y.; Adam, K.; Hoffman, P.; Berger, K.; Kocher, T.; Meyle, J.; Eickholz, P.; Doerfer, C.; et al. A haplotype block downstream of plasminogen is associated with chronic and aggressive periodontitis. *J. Clin. Periodontal.* **2017**, *44*, 962–970. [CrossRef]
19. Fine, D.H.; Furgang, D.; Schreiner, H.C.; Goncharoff, P.; Charlesworth, J.; Ghazwan, G.; Fitzgerald-Bocarsly, P.; Figurski, D.H. Phenotypic variation in Actinobacillus actinomycetemcomitans during laboratory growth: Implications for virulence. *Microbiology* **1999**, *145*, 1335–1347. [CrossRef]
20. Fine, D.H.; Kaplan, J.B.; Kachlany, S.C.; Schreiner, H.C. How we got attached to Actinobacillus actinomycetemcomitans: A model for infectious diseases. *Periodontol. 2000* **2006**, *42*, 114–157. [CrossRef]

21. Kachlany, S.C.; Fine, D.H.; Figurski, D.H. Secretion of RTX leukotoxin by Actinobacillus actinomycetemcomitans. *Infect. Immun.* **2000**, *68*, 6094–6100. [CrossRef] [PubMed]
22. Kolenbrander, P.E.; Palmer, R.J., Jr.; Periasamy, S.; Jakubovics, N.S. Oral multispecies biofilm development and the key role of cell-cell distance. *Nat. Rev. Microbiol.* **2010**, *8*, 471–480. [CrossRef]
23. Fine, D.H.; Furgang, D.; Kaplan, J.; Charlesworth, J.; Figurski, D.H. Tenacious adhesion of Actinobacillus actinomycetemcomitans strain CU1000 to salivary coated hydroxyapatite. *Arch. Oral Biol.* **1999**, *44*, 1063–1076. [CrossRef]
24. Inouye, T.; Ohta, H.; Kokeguchi, S.; Fukui, K.; Kato, K. Colonial variation and fimbriation of Actinobacillus actinomycetemcomitans. *FEMS Microbiol. Lett.* **1990**, *57*, 13–17. [CrossRef]
25. Haase, E.M.; Zmuda, J.L.; Scannapieco, F.A. Identification of rough-colony-specific outer membrane proteins in Actinobacillus actinomycetemcomitans. *Infect. Immun.* **1999**, *67*, 2901–2908. [CrossRef] [PubMed]
26. Planet, P.J.; Kachlany, S.C.; DeSalle, R.; Figurski, D.H. Phylogeny of genes for secretion of NTPases: Identification of the widespread tadA subfamily and development of a diagnostic key for gene classification. *Proc. Natl. Acad. Sci. USA* **2001**, *98*, 2503–2508. [CrossRef]
27. Planet, P.J.; Kachlany, S.C.; Fine, D.H.; DeSalle, R.; Figurski, D.H. The widespread colonization island of Actnobacillus actinomycetemcomitans. *Nat. Genet.* **2003**, *34*, 193–198. [CrossRef]
28. Makino, S.-I.; van Putten, J.P.M.; Meyer, T.F. Phase variation of the opacity outer membrane protein contrals invasion by Neisseria gonorrhea into human epithelial cells. *EMBO* **1991**, *10*, 1307–1315. [CrossRef]
29. Koomey, M.; Gotschlich, E.C.; Robbins, K.; Bergstrom, S.; Swanson, J. Effects of *recA* on Pilus Anrigenic Variation and Phase Transitions in *Neisseria Gonorrhoeae*. *Genetics* **1987**, *117*, 391–398.
30. Lenz, J.D.; Dillard, J.P. Pathogenesis of Neisseria gonorrhea and the Host Defense in Ascending Infections of Human Fallopian Tube. *Front. Immunol.* **2018**, *9*, 2710. [CrossRef]
31. Coureuil, M.; Join-Lambert, O.; Lecuyer, H.; Bourdoulous, S.; Marullo, S.; Nassif, X. Mechanism of meningeal invasion by Neisseria meningitides. *Virulence* **2012**, *3*, 164–172. [CrossRef] [PubMed]
32. Wang, Y.; Chen, C. Mutation analysis of the *flp* operon in *Actinobacillus actinomycetemcomitans*. *Gene* **2005**, *351*, 61–71. [CrossRef] [PubMed]
33. Wang, Y.; Lui, A.; Chen, C. Genetic basis for conversion of Rough-to-Smooth Colony Morphology in *Actinobacillus actinomycetemcomitans*. *Infect. Immun.* **2005**, *73*, 3749–3753. [CrossRef] [PubMed]
34. Fine, D.H.; Goncharoff, P.; Schreiner, H.C.; Chang, K.M.; Furgang, D.; Figurski, D. Colonization and persistence of rough and smooth colony variants of *Actinobacillus actinomycetemcitans* in the mouth of rats. *Arch. Oral Biol.* **2001**, *46*, 1065–1078. [CrossRef]
35. Schreiner, H.C.; Sinatra, K.; Kaplan, J.B.; Furgang, D.; Kachlany, S.C.; Planet, P.J.; Perez, B.A.; Figurski, D.H.; Fine, D.H. Tight-adherence genes of Actinobacillus actinomycetemcomitans are required for virulence in a rat model. *Proc. Natl. Acad. Sci. U S A* **2003**, *100*, 7295–7300. [CrossRef]
36. Fine, D.H.; Armitage, G.C.; Genco, R.J.; Griffen, A.L.; Diehl, S.R. Unique etiologic. demographic, and pathologic characteristics of localized aggressive periodontitis support classification as a distinct subcategory of periodontitis. *J. Am. Dent. Assoc.* **2019**, *150*, 922–931. [CrossRef]
37. Kachlany, S.C.; Planet, P.J.; Bhattacharjee, M.K.; Kollia, E.; DeSalle, R.; Fine, D.H.; Figurski, D.H. Nonspecific adherence by Actinobacillus actinomycetemcomitans requires genes widespread in bacteria and archaea. *J. Bacteriol.* **2000**, *182*, 6169–6176. [CrossRef]
38. Fine, D.H.; Velliyagonder, K.; Furgang, D.; Kaplan, J.B. The Actinobacillus actinomycetemcomitans autotransporter adhesin Aae exhibits specificity for buccal epithelial cells from humans and old world primates. *Infect. Immun.* **2005**, *73*, 1947–1953. [CrossRef]
39. Danforth, D.R.; Tang-Siegel, G.; Ruiz, T.; Mintz, K.P. A Nonfimbiral Adhesin of *Aggregatibacter actinomycetemcomitans* Mediates Biofilm Biogenesis. *Infect. Immun.* **2019**, *87*, 00704–00718.
40. Schreiner, H.; Li, Y.; Cline, J.; Tsiagbe, V.K.; Fine, D.H. A comparison of *Aggregatibacter actinomycetemcomitans* (Aa) virulence traits in a rat model for periodontal disease. *PLoS ONE*. **2013**, *8*, e69382. [CrossRef]
41. Yue, G.; Kaplan, J.B.; Furgang, D.; Mansfield, K.G.; Fine, D.H. A second *Aggregatbacter actinomycetemcomitans* autotransporter adhesin that exhibits specificity for buccal epithelial cells of humans and Old World Primates. *Infect. Immun.* **2007**, *75*, 4440–4448. [CrossRef]
42. Fine, D.H.; Markowitz, K.; Furgang, D.; Velliyagounder, K. *Aggregatibacter actinomycetemcomitans* as an early colonizer of oral tissues: Epithelium as a reservoir? *J. Clin. Microbiol.* **2010**, *48*, 4464–4473. [CrossRef]

43. Baehni, P.; Tsai, C.C.; Taichman, N.S.; McArthur, W.P. Interaction of inflammatory cells and oral microorganisms. V. Electron microscopic and biochemical study on the mechanisms of release of lysosomal constituents from human polymorphonuclear leukocytes exposed to dental plaque. *J. Periodontal. Res.* **1978**, *13*, 333–348. [CrossRef] [PubMed]
44. Tsai, C.C.; McArthur, W.P.; Baehni, P.C.; Hammond, B.F.; Taichman, N.S. Extraction and partial characterization of a leukotoxin from a plaque-derived Gram-negative microorganism. *Infect. Immun.* **1979**, *25*, 427–439. [CrossRef] [PubMed]
45. Lally, E.T.; Golub, E.E.; Kieba, I.R.; Taichman, N.S.; Rosenblum, J.; Rosenblum, J.C.; Gibson, C.W.; Demuth, D.R. Analysis of the *Actinobacillus actinomycetemcomitans* leukotoxin gene. *J. Biol. Chem.* **1989**, *264*, 15451–15456. [PubMed]
46. Koldrubetz, D.; Dailey, T.; Ebersole, J. Cloning and expression of the leukotoxin gene from Actinobacillus actinomycetemcomitans. *Infect. Immun.* **1989**, *57*, 1465–1469. [CrossRef]
47. Haubek, D.; Ennibi, O.K.; Poulsen, K.; Benzarti, N.; Baelum, V. The highly leukotoxic JP2 clone of Actinobacillus actinomycetemcomitans and progression of periodontal attachment loss. *J. Dent. Res.* **2004**, *83*, 767–770. [CrossRef] [PubMed]
48. Haubek, D.; Ennibi, O.K.; Poulsen, K.; Vaeth, M.; Poulsen, S.; Kilian, M. Risk of aggressive periodontitis in adolescent carriers of the JP2 clone of *Aggregatibacter (Actinobacillus) actinomycetemcomitans* in Morocco: A prospective longitudinal cohort study. *Lancet* **2008**, *371*, 237–242. [CrossRef]
49. Kachlany, S.C. *Aggregatibacter actinomycetemcomitans* leukotoxin from threat to therapy. *J. Dent. Res.* **2010**, *89*, 561–570. [CrossRef]
50. Johansson, A.; Claesson, R.; Aberg, C.H.; Haubek, D.; Lindholm, M.; Jasim, S.; Oscarsson, J. Genetic Profiling of *Aggragatibacter actinomycetemcomitans* Serotype B Isolated from Periodontitis Patients Living in Sweden. *Pathogens* **2019**, *8*, 153. [CrossRef]
51. Sampathkumar, V.; Velusamy, S.K.; Godboley, D.; Fine, D.H. Increased leukotoxin production: Characterization of 100 base pairs within the 530 base pair leukotoxin promoter region of *Aggregatibacter actinomycetemcomitans*. *Sci. Rep.* **2017**, *7*, 1887. [CrossRef] [PubMed]
52. Graves, D.T.; Fine, D.; Teng, Y.T.; Van Dyke, T.E.; Hajishengallis, G. The use of rodent models to investigate host-bacterial interactions related to periodontal diseases. *J. Clin. Periodontol.* **2008**, *35*, 89–105. [CrossRef] [PubMed]
53. Schreiner, H.C.; Markowitz, K.; Miryalkar, M.; Moore, D.; Diehl, S.; Fine, D.H. *Aggregatibacter actinomycetemcomitans*-Induced Bone Loss and Antibody Response in Three Rat Strains. *J. Periodontol.* **2011**, *82*, 142–150. [CrossRef] [PubMed]
54. Fine, D.H.; Karched, M.; Furgang, D.; Sampathkumar, V.; Velusamy, S.; Godboley, D. Colonization and Persistence of Labeled and Foreign Strains of Inoculated into the Mouths of Rhesus Monkeys. *J. Oral Biol. (Northborough)* **2015**, *2*. [CrossRef]
55. Velusamy, S.K.; Sampathkumar, V.; Godboley, D.; Fine, D.H. Profound Effects of *Aggregatibacter actinomycetemcomitans* Leukotoxin Mutation on Adherence Properties Are Clarified in in vitro Experiments. *PLoS ONE* **2016**, *11*, e0151361. [CrossRef]
56. Narayanan, A.M.; Ramsey, M.M.; Stacy, A.; Whiteley, M. Defining Genetic Fitness Determinants and Creating Genomic Resources for an Oral Pathogen. *Appl. Environ. Microbiol.* **2017**, *83*, e00797-17. [CrossRef]
57. Loe, H.; Brown, L.J. Early onset periodontitis in the United States of America. *J. Periodontol.* **1991**, *62*, 608–616. [CrossRef]
58. Fine, D.H.; Markowitz, K.; Furgang, D.; Fairlie, K.; Ferrandiz, J.; Nasri, C.; McKiernan, M.; Gunsolley, J. *Aggregatibacter actinomycetemcomitans* and its relationship to initiation of localized aggressive periodontitis: Longitudinal cohort study of initially healthy adolescents. *J. Clin. Microbiol.* **2007**, *45*, 3859–3869. [CrossRef]
59. Fine, D.H.; Markowitz, K.; Fairlie, K.; Tischio-Bereski, D.; Ferrendiz, J.; Furgang, D.; Paster, B.J.; Dewhirst, F.E. A consortium of *Aggregatibacter actinomycetemcomitans*, Streptococcus parasanguinis, and Filifactor alocis is present in sites prior to bone loss in a longitudinal study of localized aggressive periodontitis. *J. Clin. Microbiol.* **2013**, *51*, 2850–2861. [CrossRef]
60. Fine, D.H.; Markowitz, K.; Fairlie, K.; Tischio-Bereski, D.; Ferrandiz, J.; Godboley, D.; Furgang, D.; Gunsolley, J.; Best, A. Macrophage inflammatory protein-1alpha shows predictive value as a risk marker for subjects and sites vulnerable to bone loss in a longitudinal model of aggressive periodontitis. *PLoS ONE* **2014**, *9*, e98541. [CrossRef]

61. Al-Sabbagh, M.; Alladah, A.; Lin, Y.; Keyscio, R.J.; Thomas, M.V.; Ebersole, J.L.; Miller, C.S. Bone remodelling-associated biomarker MIP-1alpha distinguishes periodontal disease from health. *J. Periodontol. Res.* **2012**, *47*, 389–395. [CrossRef] [PubMed]
62. Fine, D.H. Dr. Theodor Rosebury: Grandfather of Modern Oral Microbiology. *J. Dent. Res.* **2006**, *85*, 990–995. [CrossRef] [PubMed]
63. Falkow, S. Is persistent bactarial infection good for your health? *Cell* **2006**, *124*, 699–702. [CrossRef] [PubMed]
64. Pirofski, L.; Casadevall, A. The Damage-Response Framework as a Tool for the Physician-Scientist to Understand the Pathogenesis of Infectious Diseases. *J. Infect. Dis.* **2018**, *218*, S7–S11. [CrossRef] [PubMed]
65. Rook, G.A.W.; Lowry, C.A.; Raison, C.L. Microbial Old Friends immunoregulation and stress resilience. *Evol. Med. Public Health* **2013**, *2013*, 46–64. [CrossRef] [PubMed]
66. Levin, S.A.; Paine, R.T. Disturbance, patch formation, and community struture. *PNAS* **1974**, *71*, 2744–2747. [CrossRef]
67. Mark Welch, J.L.; Dewhirst, F.E.; Borisy, G.G. Biogeographty of the Oral Microbiome: The Site-Specific Hyothesis. *Ann. Rev. Microbiol.* **2019**, *73*, 335–358. [CrossRef]
68. Picket, S.T.; Cadenasso, M.L. Landscape ecolotgy: Spatial heterogeneity in ecological systems. *Science* **1995**, *269*, 331–334. [CrossRef]
69. Proctor, D.M.; Shelef, K.M.; Gonzalez, A.; Davis, C.L.; Dethlefsen, L.; Burns, A.R.; Loomer, P.M.; Armitage, G.C.; Ryder, M.I.; Millman, M.E.; et al. Microbial biogeography and ecology of the mouth and implications for periodontal diseases. *Periodontol. 2000* **2019**, *82*, 26–41. [CrossRef]
70. Schroeder, H.E.; Listgarten, M.A. The gingival tissues: The architecture of periodontal protection. *Periodontol. 2000* **1997**, *13*, 91–120. [CrossRef]
71. Scannapieco, F. Saliva-bacterial interactions in oral microbial ecology. *Crit. Rev. Oral Biol. Med.* **1994**, *5*, 203–248. [CrossRef] [PubMed]
72. Wiens, J.A. *Landscape Mosaics and Ecological Theory*; Springer Netherland: London, UK, 1995.
73. Proctor, D.M.; Relman, D.A. The Landscape Ecology and Microbiota of the Ear, Nose and Throught. *Cell Host Microbe* **2017**, *21*, 421–432. [CrossRef] [PubMed]
74. Loe, H.; Theilade, E.; Jensen, S.B. Experimental Gingivitis in Man. *J. Periodontol.* **1965**, *36*, 177–187. [CrossRef] [PubMed]
75. Ritz, H.L. Microbial population shifts in developing human plaque. *Arch. Oral Biol.* **1967**, *12*, 1561–1568. [CrossRef]
76. Kolenbrander, P.E.; Palmer, R.J., Jr.; Rickard, A.H.; Jakubovics, N.S.; Chalmers, N.I.; Diaz, P.I. Bacterial interactions and successions during plaque development. *Periodontol. 2000* **2006**, *42*, 47–79. [CrossRef]
77. Von der Fehr, F.R.; Loe, H.; Theilade, E. Experimental caries in man. *Caries Res.* **1970**, *4*, 131–148. [CrossRef]
78. Marsh, P.D. Microbial ecology of dental plaque and its significance in health and disease. *Adv. Dent. Res.* **1994**, *8*, 263–271. [CrossRef]
79. Marsh, P.D.; Zaura, E. Dental biofilm: Ecological interactions in health and disease. *J. Clin. Periodontol.* **2017**, *44*, S12–S22. [CrossRef]
80. Van der Hoeven, J.S.; Toorop, A.I.; Mikx, F.H.M. Symbiotic Relationship of Veillonella alcalescens and Streptococcus mutans in Dental Plaque in Gnotobiotic Rats. *Caries Res.* **1978**, *12*, 142–147. [CrossRef]
81. Ramsey, M.M.; Rumbaugh, K.P.; Whiteley, M. Metabolite cross-feeding enhances virulence in a model polymicrobial infection. *PLoS Pathog.* **2011**, *7*, e1002012. [CrossRef]
82. Mandel, I.D. The functions of saliva. *J. Dent. Res.* **1987**, *66*, 623–627. [CrossRef] [PubMed]
83. Casadevall, A.; Pirofski, L.-A. Host-Pathogen Interactions: Redefining the Basic Concepts of Virulence and Pathogenicity. *Infect. Immun.* **1999**, *67*, 3703–3713. [CrossRef] [PubMed]
84. Jakubovics, N.S.; Kolenbrander, P.E. The road to ruin: The formation of disease-associated oral biofilms. *Oral Dis.* **2010**, *16*, 729–739. [CrossRef]
85. Moore, L.V.; Moore, W.E.; Cato, E.P.; Smibert, R.M.; Burmeister, J.A.; Best, A.M.; Ranney, R.R. Bacteriology of human gingivitis. *J. Dent. Res.* **1987**, *66*, 989–995. [CrossRef] [PubMed]
86. Moore, W.E.; Moore, L.H.; Ranney, R.R.; Smibert, R.M.; Burmeister, J.A.; Schenkein, H.A. The microflora of periodontal sites showing active destructive progression. *J. Clin. Periodontol.* **1991**, *18*, 729–739. [CrossRef] [PubMed]
87. Moore, W.E.C.; Moore, L.V.H. The bacteria of periodontal disease. *Periodontol. 2000* **1994**, *5*, 66–77. [CrossRef] [PubMed]

88. Listgarten, M.A. Ultrastructure of the dento-gingival junction after gingivectomy. *J. Periodontal Res.* **1972**, *7*, 151–160. [CrossRef] [PubMed]
89. Schroeder, H.E.; Listgarten, M.A. Fine structure of the developing epithelial attachment to teeth. *Monogr. Dev. Biol.* **1971**, *2*, 33–46.
90. Listgarten, M.A. The structure of dental plaque. *Periodontol. 2000* **1994**, *5*, 52–65. [CrossRef]
91. Page, R.C.; Schroeder, H.E. Pathogenesis of inflammatory periodontal disease. A summary of current work. *Lab. Invest.* **1976**, *34*, 235–249.
92. Fine, D.H.; Furgang, D.; McKiernan, M.; Tereski-Bischio, D.; Ricci-Nittel, D.; Zhang, P.; Araugo, M.W.B. An investigation of the effect of an essential oil mouthrinse on induced bacteremia: A pilot study. *J. Clin. Periodontol.* **2010**, *37*, 840–847. [CrossRef] [PubMed]
93. Griffen, A.L.; Beall, C.J.; Campbell, J.H.; Firestone, N.D.; Kumar, P.S.; Yang, Z.K.; Podar, M.; Leys, E.J. Distinct and complex bacterial profiles in human periodontitis and health revealed by 16S pyrosequencing. *ISME* **2012**, *6*, 1176–1185. [CrossRef]
94. Fine, D.H.; Korik, I.; Furgang, D.; Myers, R.; Olshan, A.; Barnett, M.L.; VIncent, J. Assessing Pre-Procedural Subgingival Irrigation and Rinsing with an Antiseptic Mouthrinse to Reduce Bacteremia. *JADA* **1996**, *127*, 641–646. [CrossRef] [PubMed]
95. Sreenivasan, P.K.; Tischio-Bereski, D.; Fine, D.H. Reduction in bacteremia after brushing with a triclosan/copolymer dentifrice-A randomized clinical study. *J. Clin. Periodontol.* **2017**, *44*, 1020–1028. [CrossRef] [PubMed]
96. Figuero, E.; Sanchez-Beltran, M.; Cuesta-Frechoso, S.; Tejerina, J.M.; del Castro, J.A.; Gutierrez, J.M.; Herrera, D.; Sanz, M. Detection of Periodontal Bacteria in Atheromatous Plaque by Nested Polymerase Chain Reaction. *J. Periodontol.* **2011**, *82*, 1469–1477. [CrossRef]
97. Lee, S.A.; Liu, F.; Riordan, S.; Lee, C.S.; Zhang, L.G. Global Investigations of Fusobacterium nucleatum in Human Colorectal Cancer. *Front. Oncol.* **2019**, *9*, 566. [CrossRef]
98. Roblin, X.; Neut, C.; Darfeuille-Michaud, A.; Colombel, J.F. Local appendiceal dysbiosis: The missing link between the appendix and ulcerative colitis? *Gut* **2012**, *61*, 635–636. [CrossRef]
99. Offenbacher, S.; Beck, J.D. Changing Paradigms in the Oral Disease-Systemic Disease Relationship. *J. Periodontol.* **2014**, *85*, 761–763. [CrossRef]
100. IIwanaga, S. Biochemical principle of *Limulus* test for detecting bacterial endotoxins. *Proc. Jpn. Acad. Ser* **2007**, *83*, 110–119. [CrossRef]
101. Levin, J.; Bang, F.B. Clottable protein in Limulus: Its localization and kinetics of its coagulation by endotoxin. *Thromb. Diath. Haemorrh.* **1968**, *19*, 186–194. [CrossRef]
102. Chalin, A.B.; Opal, J.M.; Opal, S.M. Whatever happened to the Schwartzman phenomenon? *Innate Immun.* **2018**, *24*, 466–479.
103. Young, N.S.; Levin, J.; Prendergast, R.A. An Invertebrate Coagulation System Activated by Endotoxin: Evidence for Enzymatic Mediation. *J. Clin. Investig.* **1972**, *51*, 1790–1797. [CrossRef]
104. Kweider, M.; Lowe, G.D.O.; Murray, G.D.; Kinane, D.F.; McGowan, D.A. Dental Disease, Fibringogen and White Cell Count; Links with Myocardial Infaction? *Scot. Med. J.* **1993**, *38*, 73–74. [CrossRef] [PubMed]
105. Stashenko, P.; Teles, R. Periapical Inflammatory Responses and Their Modulation. *Crit. Rev. Oral Biol. Med.* **1998**, *9*, 498–521. [CrossRef] [PubMed]
106. Graves, D.T.; Chen, C.-P.; Douville, C.; Jiang, Y. Interleukin-1 Receptor Signalling Rather than That of Tumor Necrosis Factor Is Critical in Protecting the Host from the Severe Consquences of a Polymicrobial Anaerobic Infection. *Infect. Immun.* **2000**, *68*, 4746–4751. [CrossRef] [PubMed]
107. Kuchler, E.C.; Mazzi-Chaves, J.F.; Antunes, L.S.; Baratto-Filho, F.; Sousa-Neto, M.D. Current treens of genetics in apical periodontitis research. *Braz. Oral Res.* **2018**, *32*, 126–132. [CrossRef]
108. Garlet, G.P.; Cardoso, C.R.; Silva, T.A.; Ferreira, B.R.; Avila-Campos, M.J.; Cunha, F.Q.; Silva, J.S. Cytokine pattern determines the progression of experimental periodontal disease induced by Actinobacillus actinomycetemcomitans through the modulation of MMPs, RANKL, and their physiological inhibitors. *Oral Microbiol. Immunol.* **2006**, *21*, 12–20. [CrossRef]
109. Armitage, G.C. Periodontal diseases: Diagnosis. *Ann. Periodontol.* **1996**, *1*, 37–215. [CrossRef]
110. Ebersole, J.L.; Dawson, D.; Emecan-Huja, P.; Nagarajan, R.; Howard, K.; Grady, M.E.; Thompson, K.; Peyyala, R.; AL-Attar, A.; Lethbridge, K.; et al. The periodontal war: Microbes and immunity. *Periodontol. 2000* **2017**, *75*, 52–115. [CrossRef]

111. Van der Velden, U. Diagnosis of periodontitis. *J. Clin. Periodontol.* **2000**, *27*, 960–961.
112. Armitage, G.C. Comparison of the microbiological features of chronic and aggressive periodontitis. *Periodontol. 2000* **2010**, *53*, 70–88. [CrossRef] [PubMed]
113. Herrera, D.; Sanz, M.; Jepsen, S.; Needleman, I.; Roldan, S. A systematic review on the effect of systemic antimicrobials as an adjunct to scaling and root planing in periodontitis patients. *J. Clin. Periodontol.* **2002**, *29*, 136–159. [CrossRef] [PubMed]

© 2020 by the authors. Licensee MDPI, Basel, Switzerland. This article is an open access article distributed under the terms and conditions of the Creative Commons Attribution (CC BY) license (http://creativecommons.org/licenses/by/4.0/).

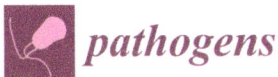

Review

Aggregatibacter Actinomycetemcomitans: Clinical Significance of a Pathobiont Subjected to Ample Changes in Classification and Nomenclature

Niels Nørskov-Lauritsen [1], Rolf Claesson [2], Anne Birkeholm Jensen [3], Carola Höglund Åberg [4] and Dorte Haubek [3],*

1. Department of Clinical Microbiology, Aarhus University Hospital, DK-8200 Aarhus N, Denmark; nielnoer@rm.dk
2. Department of Odontology, Division of Oral Microbiology, Umeå University, S-901 87 Umeå, Sweden; rolf.claesson@umu.se
3. Department of Dentistry and Oral Health, Aarhus University, DK-8000 Aarhus C, Denmark; abj@dent.au.dk
4. Department of Odontology, Division of Molecular Periodontology, Umeå University, S-901 87 Umeå, Sweden; carola.hoglund.aberg@umu.se
* Correspondence: dorte.haubek@dent.au.dk

Received: 2 October 2019; Accepted: 13 November 2019; Published: 18 November 2019

Abstract: *Aggregatibacter actinomycetemcomitans* is a Gram-negative bacterium that is part of the oral microbiota. The aggregative nature of this pathogen or pathobiont is crucial to its involvement in human disease. It has been cultured from non-oral infections for more than a century, while its portrayal as an aetiological agent in periodontitis has emerged more recently. *A. actinomycetemcomitans* is one species among a plethora of microorganisms that constitute the oral microbiota. Although *A. actinomycetemcomitans* encodes several putative toxins, the complex interplay with other partners of the oral microbiota and the suppression of host response may be central for inflammation and infection in the oral cavity. The aim of this review is to provide a comprehensive update on the clinical significance, classification, and characterisation of *A. actinomycetemcomitans*, which has exclusive or predominant host specificity for humans.

Keywords: adherence; endocarditis; fimbriae; JP2; leukotoxin; periodontitis

---

1. Introduction

Aggregatibacter actinomycetemcomitans is the type species of genus *Aggregatibacter*, which is part of bacterial family *Pasteurellaceae*. [*Bacterium actinomycetem comitans*] was cultured from actinomycotic lesions of humans in the early 20th century. The absence of related microorganisms rendered it difficult to classify this Gram-negative, fastidious rod, and isolates cultured from invasive infections were referred to national reference institutions. The expanding field of oral microbiology with a focus on periodontitis, particularly the localized, severe form that affects adolescents, caused a renewed interest in the bacterial species. In 2006, the current species name was adopted, and *A. actionmycetemcomtians* became type species of a new bacterial genus, *Aggregatibacter*. Influential events in the narrative of *A. actinomycetemcomitans* are listed in Table 1.

Table 1. Seminal events in the history of *Aggregatibacter actinomycetemcomitans*.

Year	Event	Reference
1912	Klinger describes [*Bacterium actinomycetem comitans*]	[1]
1929	Topley and Wilson relocate the species to genus *Actinobacillus*	[2]
1962	King and Tatum describe the close phenotypic similarity of [*Actinobacillus actinomycetemcomitans*] with [*Haemophilus aphrophilus*]	[3]
1976	[*Actinobacillus actinomycetemcomitans*] is associated with periodontitis in adolescents	[4,5]
1979	Extraction and partial characterisation of Ltx, a leukotoxin capable of specific lyse of human polymorphonuclear leukocytes	[6]
1982	The *Haemophilus*, *Aggregatibacter*, *Cardiobacterium*, *Eikenella*, and *Kingella* (HACEK) group of fastidious, Gram-negative bacteria causing infective endocarditis, is conceived	[7]
1982	Serum antibody levels link [*Actinobacillus actinomycetemcomitans*] with localized juvenile periodontitis	[8]
1983	Three distinct surface antigens are identified and a particularly high periodontopathogenic potential of serotype b is indicated	[9]
1994	The 530-bp deletion in the *ltx* promoter region is associated with enhanced expression of Ltx and becomes a marker for the so-called JP2 genotype of [*Actinobacillus actinomycetemcomitans*]	[10]
2006	A new bacterial genus, *Aggregatibacter* is created with *Aggregatibacter actinomycetemcomitans* being the type species	[11]
2008	Clinical follow-up studies unequivocally demonstrate that carriage of the JP2 clone of *Aggregatibacter actinomycetemcomitans* is linked with aggressive periodontitis	[12]

A. actinomycetemcomitans is one species among a plethora of microorganisms that constitute the oral microbiota. It has been estimated that at least 500 different bacterial species colonise the oral cavity [13–15], and half of these may have been cultivated and validly named because of vigorous efforts directed to the cultivation of oral bacteria. Analysis of a large number of 16S rRNA gene clones from studies of the oral microbiota increased the number of taxa to 619 [16], and the number is steadily increasing (www.homd.org). Bacterial species cannot be validly named in the absence of a cultured type strain [17]. Although "taxa", "phylotypes" or "operative taxonomic units" revealed by deep sequencing of polymerase chain reaction (PCR)-amplified 16S rRNA genes have relevance for recognition of microbial fluctuations in health and disease, only cultivable microbiota can be made subject to extensive characterisation, including adherence, animal experiments, antimicrobial susceptibility, co-culture, generation of mutants, and growth characteristics.

Carriage of *A. actinomycetemcomitans* appears to be highly host-specific. Although the spread and dissemination of bacterial clones occur, these are not frequent events; hosts tend to carry their strain from teething to edentulous old age [18]. Yet, the species encompasses properties that sometimes reveal its significance in human disease. Particularly, a single serotype b clonal lineage designated the JP2 clone is associated with a severe form of localised periodontitis and tooth loss in adolescents [12]. But rather than being the causative agent of aggressive periodontitis, *A. actinomycetemcomitans* may be necessary for the action of a consortium of bacterial partners by suppressing host defences [19]. It may be classified as a low abundance oral pathobiont, defined as a member of the microbiota that exerts specific effects on the host's mucosal immune system associated with the development of disease [20]. Although *A. actinomycetemcomitans* may accompany (*comitans*) *Actinomyces*, the narrative of a pathobiont is not valid for other invasive infections such as infectious endocarditis, where *A. actinomycetemcomitans*—when identified—is detected as the sole pathogen by culture and/or PCR on removed heart valves. Severe periodontitis and infective endocarditis are two prominent diseases of very different prevalence, symptoms, and outcome. Although they may share a causative microorganism, a number of conditions is still unknown, and host factors, oral hygiene, and incidental circumstances may be instrumental.

The aim of the present review is to provide a comprehensive update on the characterisation, classification and clinical significance of *A. actinomycetemcomitans* with a particular focus on selected clinical entities. Adhesion, persistence, and inactivation of immune cells are probably essential for the understanding of the intimate association with the host, and these factors are detailed for the purpose of the elucidation of pathogenicity. A number of relevant publications and reviews of other important biochemical mechanisms of this bacterial species are listed in the relevant sections.

2. Taxonomy, Classification, Serotype (St) and Population Structure

More than 100 years ago, [*Bacterium actinomycetem comitans*] was co-isolated with *Actinomyces* from actinomycotic lesions of humans [1] (*Actinomyces*, ray fungus, referring to the radial arrangement of filaments in *Actinomyces bovis* sulfur granules; actinomycosis, a chronic disease characterised by hard granulomatous masses). Ample changes have occurred in the classification and nomenclature of this species. Despite the limited similarity with *Actinobacillus lignieresii*, it was reclassified as [*Actinobacillus actinomycetemcomitans*] in a seminal textbook from 1929 [2]. According to Cowan [21], the bacterium was placed in this genus because 'neither Topley nor Wilson could think where to put it'. In 1962 the phenotypic resemblance of [*Actinobacillus actinomycetemcomitans*] with [*Haemophilus aphrophilus*] was described [3], and a subsequent relocation of [*Actinobacillus actinomycetemcomitans*] to genus *Haemophilus* occurred [22]. Nomenclatural classification as [*Haemophilus actinomycetemcomitans*] within the genus *Haemophilus* permitted antimicrobial susceptibility testing according to standards outlined by the US Clinical and Laboratory Standards Institute. Disk diffusion could be performed and interpreted on *Haemophilus* test medium (HTM) in 5% CO_2, and HTM broth microdilution testing was carried out in ambient air [23]. However, the nomenclatural relocation did not result in a satisfying classification, because neither [*Actinobacillus actinomycetemcomitans*] nor [*Haemophilus aphrophilus*] are adequately related to *Haemophilus influenzae*, the type species of the genus *Haemophilus*. Finally, in 2006 the new genus *Aggregatibacter* was created to accomodate *Aggregatibacter actinomycetemcomitans*, *Aggregatibacter aphrophilus* and *Aggregatibacter segnis* [11]. A fourth *Aggregatibacter* species, *Aggregatibacter kilianii*, has recently been named (Figure 1) [24].

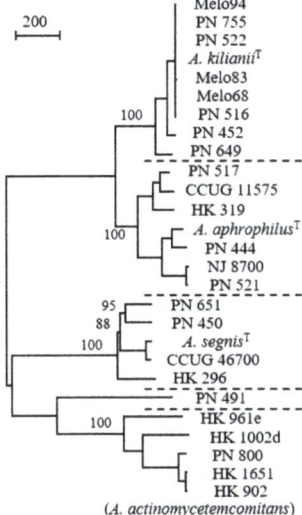

Figure 1. Comparison of *Aggregatibacter* strains by whole genome sequences; distinct species are separated by dotted lines (strain PN_491 is unclustered). A total of 3261 positions with single nucleotide polymorphism (SNP) are included in the dataset. Values at nodes are percentages of bootstrap replications supporting the node (500 replicates). Bar represents 200 SNPs. Reprinted from *Journal of Clinical Microbiology* [24] with permission.

In the early 1980s, three distinct surface antigens of *A. actinomycetemcomitans* were identified [9], while six serotypes (a through f) were recognised by 2001. The serological specificity is defined by structurally and antigenically distinct O-polysaccharide components of their respective lipopolysaccharide molecules. A seventh St, designated St(g), with a 1:1 ratio of 2,4-di-O-methyl-rhamnose and 2,3,6-tri-O-methyl-glucose, was recently added [25]. St(a), St(b), and St(c) are globally dominant [26], but the distribution may vary according to ethnicity and geography. In Scandinavia, the three dominant serotypes are equally prevalent, while predominance of St(c) is observed in Chinese, Japanese, Korean, Thai and Vietnamese populations [27–31]; a noticeable high prevalence of St(e) has been reported among Japanese periodontitis patients [32]. Assessment of serotype-specific antibodies supports these findings, as all early-onset periodontitis patients from Turkey and Brazil had elevated antibody levels to St(c) and St(a), while St(b) levels were higher in the US [33,34].

An initial characterisation of the population structure of the species was published in 1994, using multi-locus enzyme electrophoresis [35]. Two large and four small divisions were identified, with division I (St(a) and St(d)) and III (St(b) and St(c)) encompassing 34% and 58% of the 97 strains analysed, respectively. Two St(e) strains occupied separate divisions (II and VI), one St(c) strain constituted electrophoretic division IV, while division V was composed of two St(a) and one non-serotypable strain. Sequencing of a 16S rRNA gene fragment from 35 strains suggested a different structure with three major clusters [36]. RNA cluster I included 12 strains of four serotypes (a, d, e, and f), all 10 St(b) strains belonged to RNA cluster II, while RNA cluster III only included St(c) strains (N = 10). Strains of particular serotypes were not exclusively confined to specific RNA clusters; one St(a) strain belonged to the St(b) cluster (II), and two divergent RNA clusters were composed of single strains, namely a St(c) (RNA cluster IV) and a St(e) strain (RNA cluster V), respectively [36].

One study attempted to establish a multi-locus sequence typing (MLST) scheme for *A. actinomycetemcomitans* [37]. Six gene fragments from the *Haemophilus influenzae* MLST scheme were used. The investigation focused on the JP2 clone, which contributed 66 of 82 strains. MLST has insufficient power to reveal dissemination patterns of clonally related strains, and point mutations of two pseudogenes present in the JP2 clone were more versatile in this respect [37]. Moreover, a MLST web site was not organised and, therefore, the benefits of a portable typing scheme were not corroborated. But MLST of 16 non-JP2 strains carefully selected from the enzyme electrophoresis study [35] suggested the existence of four phylogenetic clusters, rooted by an outgroup consisting of an uncommon St(e) strain. Two related clusters were composed of St(b) and St(c) strains, respectively, while a more distinct cluster encompassed strains of St(a), St(d) and St(e) [37].

Restriction fragment length polymorphism using various restriction enzymes and arbitrarily-primed PCR has been used to differentiate types of *A. actinomycetemcomitans* cultured from patients with severe periodontitis and healthy controls [30,37–42]. The method is versatile and discriminative, but lacks portability and a common nomenclature; thus, it is of value for individual studies of specific strains, but lacks general applicability and descriptive significance.

Finally, whole genome sequencing has been introduced for characterisation of the species [43–45]. In the largest study, sequences from two human strains of *Aggregatibacter aphrophilus*, 30 human *A. actinomycetemcomitans* strains, and one St(b) strain isolated from a rhesus macaque Old World monkey were used for selection of 397 core genes which were concatenated and trimmed to produce a single alignment of 335,400 bp [45]. Five clades were recognised, designated clade b, clade c, clade e/f, clade a/d and clade e'. Although the analysis clearly separated six strains of serotype b from six strains of serotype c, a close similarity was observed between these two clades, as well as between clade a/d and e/f. In contrast, the clade designated e', encompassing four St(e) strains, was phylogenetically distinct. The open reading frames necessary for expression of St(e) antigen were highly conserved between clade e and clade e' strains, but e' strains were found to be missing the genomic island that carries genes encoding the cytolethal distending toxin. Moreover, the clade e' strains were more related to an Old World primate strain and carried the unusual 16S rRNA type V sequence (RNA types as defined by Kaplan et al. [36]). Although bacterial species are not defined by DNA sequence, average nucleotide identity (ANI) values locate whole genome sequences from this group/clade outside the species boundary [44]. Thus, strains belonging to the so-called clade e' (as well as the rhesus macaque monkey strain) may possibly be transferred to new species, and *A. actinomycetemcomitans* may be restricted to strains with exclusive host specificity for humans.

A recent study compared whole genome sequences of strains from blood stream infections supplemented with oral reference strains [46]. Exclusion of so-called clade e' strains increased the number of core genes present in all strains from 1146 to 1357. Strains of *A. actinomycetemcomitans* are basically divided into three lineages (numbering of lineages differs from reference [44]). Lineage I encompasses the type strain and consists of two groups (St(b) and St(c), respectively). Lineage II consists of St(a) plus St(d)-(g). In contrast to lineage I, many strains of different serotypes from this lineage are competent for natural transformation, and the average size of genomes is approximately 10% larger than in lineage I. Lineage III also expresses St(a) membrane O polysaccharide, and the genome size is comparable to lineage II. However, all six investigated strains were incompetent for transformation due to inactivation of multiple competence genes [46].

In conclusion, St designations are valuable for initial typing of clinical strains, but insufficient for characterisation. Recognition of a general MLST scheme could be helpful, and whole genome sequences could be used for MLST and in silico serotyping, as well as further characterisation and epidemiologic investigations. The species description consisting of three separate lineages is figurative, but more knowledge on the new lineage III is needed to disclose the relevance for phenotype, host specificity and pathogenicity.

3. General Characteristics

A. actinomycetemcomitans is a fastidious, facultatively anaerobic, non-motile, small Gram-negative rod, 0.4–0.5 µm × 1.0–1.5 µm in size. Microscopically, the cells may appear as cocci in broth and in clinical samples. It grows poorly in ambient air, but well in 5% CO_2 [47]. Colonies on chocolate agar are small, with a diameter of ≤0.5 mm after 24 h, but may exceed 1–2 mm after 48 h [48]. Primary colonies are rough-textured and adhere strongly to the surface of agar plates (Figure 2).

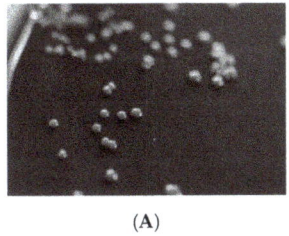
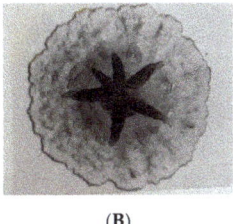

(A)   (B)

Figure 2. (**A**) Tenacious, rough-textured colonies of *A. actinomycetemcomitans* strain HK1651 on chocolate agar. Diameter of colonies did not reach 2 mm after 3 days incubation in 5% CO_2. (**B**) Clinical isolate incubated on TSBV (tryptic soy-serum-bacitracin-vancomycin) agar for 4 days in 5% CO_2. Expression of the distinctive "star-shaped" colony is facilitated by growth on TSBV agar. Pictures by courtesy of Jan Berg Gertsen and Rolf Claesson.

3.1. Recovery, Phenotype, and Molecular Detection

Relevant sites in the oral cavity for sampling of *A. actinomycetemcomitans* are periodontal pockets, the mucosa, and saliva. Sampling techniques include use of sterile paper points to be inserted in periodontal pockets, cotton swab for the mucosa, and chewing on a piece of paraffin for the collection of stimulated saliva. For transport of paper points, the VMGAIII-medium is recommended [49]; samples collected with cotton swab can be transported in a salt buffer or in TE-buffer [50]. Saliva can be transported in tubes without additives. For short-time transportation, saliva can be transported in tubes without additives. Otherwise, it can be frozen or stored at room temperature in a Saliva DNA Preservation Buffer. Proteomic analysis of gingival crevicular fluid and saliva is an expanding diagnostic field that may require improvements in standardised collection techniques and devices [51,52].

The selective medium TSBV (tryptic soy-serum-bacitracin-vancomycin) agar [53] is commonly used for culture. If *Enterobacterales* are present in significant amounts in the samples, a modified version of TSBV is recommended [54]. Detection of *A. actinomycetemcomitans* in clinical samples renders limited information on prediction, progression, and treatment planning of periodontal disease. For these purposes, the proportion of the bacterium at diseased sites is more relevant. This is in line with the ecological plaque hypothesis [55]. The detection level of *A. actinomycetemcomitans* is around 100 viable bacteria (colony-forming units) per mL. *Fusobacterium nucleatum* and other strict anaerobes will grow on TSBV in the absence of oxygen. The total concentration of viable bacteria is estimated by parallel cultivation on 5% blood agar plates, and the proportion of *A. actinomycetemcomitans* in the sample can be calculated.

A. actinomycetemcomitans is suspected when rough-textured, tenacious colonies appear on selective agar after one or two days (Figure 2). The species is distinguished from closely related bacteria by a positive catalase reaction and negative β-galactosidase reaction. Salient biochemical characters of *A. actinomycetemcomitans* have been published [56]. In addition, the bacterium is readily identified by MALDI-TOF mass spectrometry [57]; however, the current version of the Bruker database (v3.1) only includes mass spectra from a limited number of strains, and modest log-scores are not unusual when clinical strains are examined.

Leukotoxicity, i.e., the capacity of the bacterium to kill or inactivate immune cells, is properly determined in biological assays involving human cell lines [58], but a semi-quantitative method based on hemolysis on blood agar plates has been reported [42,59]. Quantification of the leukotoxin by enzyme-linked immunosorbent assay (ELISA) is also used; most studies have assessed the leukotoxin released from the surface of the bacterium, either during growth in broth [60], or by treatment of bacteria cultured in media that inhibit leukotoxin release with a hypertonic salt solution [42]. Leukotoxicity may also be estimated by determination of the total amount of leukotoxin produced by the strain. Bacterial suspensions are solubilized by SDS, and the leukotoxin is subsequently quantitated by Western blot–based methodology [60]. It is anticipated that the amount of leukotoxin released from the bacterial cell surface reflects the total amount of leukotoxin produced, but this relationship remains to be corroborated.

Polymerase chain reaction (PCR) is frequently used for identification and characterisation of *A. actinomycetemcomitans* in clinical samples. The leukotoxin promoter was an early focal point [59]. PCR amplification of the *ltx* promoter region and visualization on gel can discriminate the JP2 genotype from other strains of the species [61], but preferential amplification of smaller products characterised by a 530-bp deletion will overestimate the prevalence of the JP2 genotype. Recent improvements in PCR offer more precise quantification of periodontal pathogens in a complex plaque biofilm [62]. By real-time or quantitative PCR (qPCR), the instrument reports the cycling threshold (CT)-value, which can estimate the concentration of the target in the sample. qPCR has been used to separately quantitate JP2 and non-JP2 genotypes [63]. To approximate the total number of bacteria by qPCR, the 16S rRNA gene is generally targeted. The method can only provide a rough estimate, as primers and probes may preferentially bind to certain bacterial phyla, and because the number of copies of the gene varies substantially between different bacterial species [64].

Serotypes a through f can be identified by PCR as described [65,66]. A method for detecting St(g) has not yet been described.

3.2. Aggregative Properties and the Leukotoxin Gene Operon

A. actinomycetemcomitans expresses three potential toxins, fimbriae and a number of adhesins, plus a number of other gene products that may have significance for microbial interplay, persistence, transformation to planktonic state, and pathogenicity (Table 2).

Table 2. Genomic characteristics and putative virulence determinants of *A. actinomycetemcomitans*.

Genomic Characteristics and Putative Virulence Determinants of *A. actinomycetemcomitans*	References
Widespread colonization island or the *tad* locus	[67]
Autotransporter adhesins Aae, EmaA and Omp100/ApiA	[68–70]
A leukotoxin of the repeats in toxin (RTX) family with specificity for leukocytes	[71]
Growth-inhibitory factor cytolethal distending toxin	[72,73]
CagE, capable of inducing apoptosis	[74]
Dispersin B, a biofilm-releasing beta-hexosaminidase	[75]
Vesicle-independent extracellular release of proinflammatory lipoprotein	[76]

The distinct growth in broth as small granules adhering to the walls of the test tube was included in the initial description of [*Bacterium actinomycetem comitans*] [1]. Fresh isolates of *A. actinomycetemcomitans* invariably form colonies that are rough-textured with an opaque, star-shaped internal structure (Figure 2B). Subculture in broth yields clumps of autoaggregated cells that attach tightly to the glass, leaving a clear broth. *A. actinomycetemcomitans* possesses fimbriae, and these appendages can be irreversibly lost after prolonged subculture in the laboratory [77]. Antibodies to synthetic fimbrial peptide significantly reduce the binding of *A. actinomycetemcomitans* to saliva-coated hydroxyapatite beads, buccal epithelial cells and a fibroblast cell line, indicating a decisive role of these structures for adherence to multiple surfaces [78]. Moreover, autoaggregation (spontaneous formation of aggregates with rapid settling in un-agitated suspensions) was completely lost by a smooth-colony, isogenic variant [79]. Fimbriae are assembled as bundles of 5- to 7-nm-diameter pili composed of a 6.5 kDa protein designated Flp (fimbrial low-molecular-weight protein) [80,81]. The RcpA/B (rough colony proteins) were the first outer membrane proteins identified that were associated with rough colony variants [82], and they are encoded by a 14-gene locus designated the *tad* locus. The Tad (tight adherence) macromolecular transport system is a subtype of type II secretion. The *tad* locus is composed of nine *tad*, three *rcp* and two *flp* genes [67]. Mutation analysis of the naturally competent strain D7S revealed *flp-1*, *rcpA*, *rcpB*, *tadB*, *tadD*, *tadE* and *tadF* to be indispensable for expression of fimbriae, while mutants of five other genes expressed reduced levels of fimbriae, or fimbriae that had different gross appearance [83,84]. In a rat model, the *tad* locus was critical for colonizing the oral cavity and for pathogenesis, measured as maxillae bone loss and *A. actinomycetemcomitans*-specific IgG levels [85].

Many pathogenic bacteria can undergo phase variation, but smooth-to-rough conversion has not been substantiated for *A. actinomycetemcomitans*. Rather, the rough-to-smooth conversion is typically caused by mutations in the *flp* promoter region, and replacement with wild-type promoter can restore the rough phenotype [86]. However, one study indicated that smooth strains could re-express the fimbriae in low humidity environments [87].

In addition to expression of fimbriae decisive for autoaggregation and adherence to a wide range of solid surfaces (biofilm formation), *A. actinomycetemcomitans* encodes a spectrum of autotransporter adhesins, proteins that promote their own transport from the periplasm to the exterior surface, where they may be decisive for adhesion to specific human cellular epitopes. A homologue with similarity to the monomeric *H. influenzae* autotransporter, Hap, was designated Aae. Inactivation of *aae* in two naturally transformable strains caused a 70% reduction in adhesion to cultured epithelial cells [68]. Aae exhibits specificity for buccal epithelial cells from humans and Old World primates, and does not bind to human pharyngeal or cervical epithelial cells [88]. Two trimeric autotransporters with homology to the YadA adhesin/invasin family were identified. Omp100 has also been designated Api (*Aggregatibacter* putative invasin). *Escherichia coli* expressing ApiA bound to various types of human collagen plus fibronectin. Adhesion to human cells was specific to buccal epithelial cells from humans and Old-World primates, although the specificity was not as prominent as observed for AaE [70,89]. Screening of a large number of insertion transposon mutants identified the extracellular matrix adhesin A encoded by *emaA*, which is involved in collagen adhesion [90]. Collagen prevail in the supporting tissue of cardiac valves, and EmaA (extracellular matrix adhesin) may play a role in the pathogenesis of infective endocarditis [91].

Iron is an essential transition metal for nearly all forms of life. The host limits the availability of iron through a process termed nutritional immunity [92]. Haemolysis can be an initial step for release of iron from heme by Gram-negative bacteria. The RTX (repeats in toxin) family is an important group of toxins, whose name refers to glycine- and apartate-rich, calcium-binding repeats in the carboxy terminus of the toxin proteins [93]. RTX toxins are produced by many Gram-negative bacteria including members of family *Pasteurellaceae* – it has, indeed, been proposed that these toxins may originate in *Pasteurellaceae* [94].

In 1977, it was shown that polymorphonuclear leukocytes exposed to gingival bacterial plaque in vitro released lysosomal constituents [95], and the leukotoxin (Ltx) of *A. actinomycetemcomitans* was extracted and partially characterised in 1979 [6]. Ltx is a RTX cytolysin. By 1989, the gene was cloned and analysed [96,97], and the 530-bp deletion in the *ltx* promoter associated with enhanced expression of Ltx characterising the JP2 genotype was subsequently described [10]. The difference between minimally toxic and highly toxic strains were convincingly illustrated in clinical studies from Northern Africa [12]. The significance of the 530-bp deletion may reside in a potential transcriptional terminator spanning 100 bp [60]. The leukotoxin of *A. actinomycetemcomitans* is highly specific for human and primate white blood cells and is capable of neutralising local mucosal immune responses. However, purified leukotoxin can lyse sheep and human erythrocytes in vitro, and beta-haemolysis can be demonstrated on certain media [98].

In addition to the JP2 genotype characterised by the 530-bp promoter deletion, two other leukotoxin promoter variants have been reported. One genotype is characterised by a slightly enlarged (640-bp) deletion [99], while the other promoter variant carries an 886-bp insertion sequence [100]. Both these variants produce levels of leukotoxin similar to the JP2 genotype of *A. actinomycetemcomitans*.

3.3. Geographic Dissemination of Specific Genotypes

The JP2 clone of *A. actinomycetemcomitans* is suggested to have arisen 2400 years ago in the northern Mediterranean part of Africa [37]. The bacterial clone is endemically present in Moroccan and Ghanaian populations [12,101] and almost exclusively detected among individuals of African origin [37,102]. However, among 17 JP2 clone carriers, living in Sweden and identified during 2000–2014, ten were of Scandinavian heritage [31]. Among six of the identified JP2 clone carriers, three were of Swedish origin. Detection of the JP2 clone of *A. actinomycetemcomitans* has not been reported in Asian populations [30,100,103,104]. The occurrence of the JP2 clone of *A. actinomycetemcomitans* in Caucasians may be caused by horizontal transmission, and may weaken the theory of racial tropism of the clone [59]. More data and research are needed to explain the dissemination of the leukotoxic JP2 clone of *A. actinomycetemcomitans*.

Other genotypes characterised by an increased leukotoxic potential comprise a 640-bp deletion cultured from a host of Ethiopian origin [99], an 886-bp insertion sequence from a host of Japanese origin [100], and two strains of serotype c, originating from Thailand with a JP2-like deletion in the promoter region of *ltx*, and with virulence of similar magnitude to the JP2 genotype strains [105]. All these genotypes were collected from individuals with severe periodontitis.

4. Prevalence and Clinical Significance

Cultivable *A. actinomycetemcomitans* is present in at least 10% of periodontally healthy children with primary dentition [106]. An influential publication found carrier rates of 20% for normal juveniles, 36% for normal adults, 50% for adult periodontitis patients, and 90% for young periodontitis patients [107]. Early studies failed to culture the species from edentulous infants [108,109], but molecular studies using PCR on unstimulated saliva samples have challenged this association: 37 of 59 completely edentulous infants were positive for *A. actinomycetemcomitans*, reaching 100% at 12 months of age [110]. Vertical transmission is common. Two studies reported detection rates by culture of 30–60% in children of adult periodontitis patient, and the genotypes of the strains were always identical [111,112]. A smaller study from Brazil of women with severe chronic periodontitis did not corroborate this finding, as the two culture-positive children carried genotypes that were different from those of their mothers [113]. Horizontal transmission of *A. actinomycetemcomitans* can occur, and transmission rates between 14% and 60% between spouses have been estimated [18,114]. However, members of most families with aggressive periodontitis also harbour additional clonal types of *A. actinomycetemcomitans* [115].

Once colonized, *A. actinomycetemcomitans* remains detectable in patients with periodontitis. Irrespective of periodontal treatment, colonisation by the same strain is remarkably stable within subjects for periods of 5 to 12 years, as revealed by restriction fragment length polymorphism [40], serotyping combined with arbitrarily primed PCR [116], or JP2 clone-specific PCR [117]. Genomic stability during persistent oral infections has been demonstrated by genome sequencing of strains cultured from the same individual 10 years later [118].

The natural habitat of *A. actinomycetemcomitans* is the oral cavity, but *A. actinomycetemcomitans* can be isolated from a variety of oral as well as non-oral infectious diseases, including arthritis, bacteraemia, endocarditis, osteomyelitis, skin infections, urinary tract infections and various types of abscesses [119]. Characterisation of 52 non-oral strains showed similarity to oral strains [120], and the portal of entry for systemic infections is usually the oral cavity [121].

4.1. Infective Endocarditis

The oral cavity is the only known habitat of *A. actinomycetemcomitans*, but only a few layers of crevicular epithelial cells separate the gingival location from the parenteral space of the host. Entry into the blood stream has not been quantitated, but incidental introductions may occur during tooth brushing, injuries, chewing of granular matters etc., and this may be accelerated by the presence of periodontitis. *A. actinomycetemcomitans* was originally co-isolated with *Actinomyces* from actinomycotic lesions [1], and the association with *Actinomyces* has been confirmed by case reports of infections in a variety of anatomical localizations. Among *Actinomyces* species, co-isolation of *A. actinomycetemcomitans* appears restricted to *Actinomyces israelii* [122,123].

Infective endocarditis is an infection of the endocardium, the lining of the interior surfaces of the chambers of the heart. It usually affects the heart valves (Figure 3A), where corrosion and incidental exposure of sub-endothelium tissue during the extensive motion of the valves may serve as a starting point for bacterial adhesion.

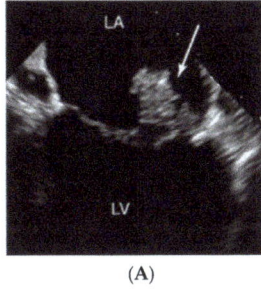 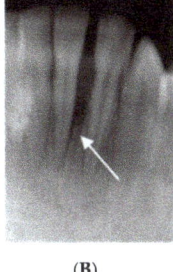

(A) (B)

Figure 3. Imaging signs of infections and inflammation that may be associated with *A. actinomycetemcomitans*. (**A**) Transesophageal echocardiography of a heart with mitral valve infective endocarditis. The arrow marks a large vegetation on the posterior leaflet between left atrium (LA) and left ventricle (LV); usually, vegetations caused by *A. actinomycetemcomitans* are of smaller size. (**B**) 14-year old girl of African ethnicity. The radiograph shows an extensive and apparently rapid loss of the periodontal support of the lower incisor 31. Pictures by courtesy of close clinical collaborators of the authors.

A. actinomycetemcomitans is part of the *Haemophilus, Aggregatibacter, Cardiobacterium, Eikenella,* and *Kingella* (HACEK) group of fastidious Gram-negative bacteria that is responsible for 1.4–3% of cases infective endocarditis [124,125]. The group originally included *Haemophilus* species, *Actinobacillus actinomycetemcomitans, Cardiobacterium hominis, Eikenella corrodens,* and *Kingella kingae* [7]. The HACEK acronym is still valid, but currently denotes non-*influenzae Haemophilus* sp., *Aggregatibacter* sp., *Cardiobacterium* sp., *E. corrodens*, and *Kingella* sp. [126]. *A. actinomycetemcomitans* is the HACEK organism most strongly associated with infective endocarditis [121,125], and bacteraemia with *A. actinomycetemcomitans* necessitates clarification of this putative focus of infection. In a retrospective study of 87 cases of HACEK bacteraemia from New Zealand, the association between HACEK bacteraemia and infective endocarditis varied among bacterial species ranging from 0% (*E. corrodens*) to 100% (*A. actinomycetemcomitans*) [127]. Specific features of infective endocarditis caused by *A. actinomycetemcomitans* have been reviewed [121].

4.2. The Complex Interplay with Periodontitis

Periodontitis is an inflammatory disease associated with loss of connective tissue and bone around teeth (Figure 3B). The bacterial tooth biofilm initiates the gingival inflammation, and further progression of the periodontal lesion depends on dysbiotic ecological changes within the gingival sulcus area. Unfavourable lifestyles and hygiene contribute to the development and progression of periodontitis, which has been designated as one of mankind's most common chronic inflammatory diseases [48].

The complexity of the periodontal microbiota and the variety of clinical symptoms delayed the identification of specific microbial aetiological agents. In 1996, *A. actinomycetemcomitans, Porphyromonas gingivalis,* and *Tannerella forsythia* were officially designated as aetiological agents of periodontitis [128]. *A. actinomycetemcomitans* was targeted based on prevalence studies in health and disease, serum antibody levels, and presence of virulence determinants (Tables 1 and 2). More recently, attention has been directed to the complex interplay between other cultivable and other non-cultivable bacteria in the oral microbiota, as well as to the interplay with the host [16,48,129,130]. Indeed, it has been suggested that *A. actinomycetemcomitans* conducts its business by concealing itself from the scrutiny of the host immune system, or even being a community activist that suppresses host responses to allow overgrowth of its collaborators [19].

The earlier classification of aggressive periodontitis was based mainly on the clinical presentation and the rapid loss of periodontal tissue [131]. A new classification scheme has been adopted, in which chronic and aggressive forms of the disease are now merged into a single category, which is characterised by a multi-dimensional staging and grading system [132,133]. Staging assesses severity and extent of disease at presentation, and attempts to include the complexity of disease management. The grading provides an evaluation of the risk of progression, and attempts to predict response to standard periodontal therapy [132].

5. Therapy

Treatment of periodontitis aims to stop the progression of the periodontal lesion and to maximise periodontal health [134]. Mechanical debridement of biofilm is considered the most effective therapy, but must be combined with a detailed oral hygiene. If periodontal lesions persist after 3–6 months, a second phase of therapy is planned. A favourable healing potential has been documented for lesions associated with the rapidly progressive, localised periodontitis that affects adolescents [135]. Systemic antibiotics should only be administered as adjunctive therapy in selected cases.

Access surgery with regenerative techniques have been used for periodontitis stages III–IV [132,134]. Notable risk factors are non-compliance, smoking, elevated gingival bleeding index, and inadequate plaque control [136].

Very different amoxicillin resistance rates have been reported, ranging from 0% in Switzerland [137], over 33% in Spain [138] to 84% in the United Kingdom [139]. The mechanisms of resistance were not reported. Production of β-lactamase is the most common cause of β-lactam resistance in Gram-negative bacteria, but these enzymes have not been detected in *A. actinomycetemcomitans*. The fastidious nature of the bacterium is a challenge for antimicrobial susceptibility testing, and methodology as well as interpretative criteria must be addressed when reports of resistance are evaluated. A recent investigation using different methods could not confirm the emergence of resistance to β-lactams in *A. actinomycetemcomitans*; the study included strains that had previously been reported as resistant [140]. Thus, there is currently no convincing evidence for replacement of oral amoxicillin when antimicrobial agents are indicated for treatment of *A. actinomycetemcomitans*-associated periodontitis.

Gram-negative bacteria are generally more susceptible to the cephalosporin-class than the penicillin-class of β-lactams. For infective endocarditis, an intravenous course of at least four weeks with a third-generation cephalosporin, or a combination of ampicillin and an aminoglycoside, is recommended [121]. Recently, a well-designed randomised study reported favourable outcomes for oral antimicrobial follow up regimens given to patients with infective endocarditis deemed clinically stable and without complications [141]. *A. actinomycetemcomitans* could be a candidate microorganism for use of partial oral antimicrobial treatment of infective endocarditis, but the relative rare occurrence of HACEK bacteraemia poses difficulties for additional clinical studies.

6. Conclusions

A. actinomycetemcomitans is part of the human microbiota. It can be cultured from one-third of healthy adults, while PCR-based methods suggest a more ubiquitous presence. The bacterium's tenacious, aggregative character is instrumental for the remarkable genotype stability in colonised hosts, and for progression to persistent, distant infections after incidental entry into the parental space. *A. actinomycetemcomitans* are commonly detected if adolescents present with periodontitis. Chronically inflamed gingival crevices may spark the repeated, intermittent entry into the blood stream. Its participation in the disease process of periodontitis is beyond reasonable doubt, but its orchestration of severe periodontitis continues to be fascinating and disputed. Adhesion and leukotoxic features are well-described, but interplay with other members of the oral microbiota is more difficult to elucidate, as is the interchangeable position of eliciting antibody response and "staying under the radar". The recent division into three subspecies or lineages has not been investigated by clinical studies linking disease and lineage. Disease-specific treatment options are currently widely accepted.

Author Contributions: All authors made a substantial, direct, and intellectual contribution to the work. N.N.-L. compiled the contributions and made the first draft of the manuscript. All authors approved it for publication.

Funding: This research received no external funding.

Acknowledgments: Mogens Kilian is thanked for profound inspiration. Furthermore, we thank the members of the European Network for *Aggregatibacter actinomycetemcomitans* Research (ENAaR; https://projects.au.dk/aggregatibacter/) for valuable discussions.

Conflicts of Interest: The authors declare no conflict of interest.

Abbreviations

aae, *Aggregatibacter* autotransporter adhesin; Api, *Aggregatibacter* putative invasion; CT, cycling threshold; emaA, extracellular matrix adhesin A; HACEK, *Haemophilus, Aggregatibacter, Cardiobacterium, Eikenella,* and *Kingella*; JP2 clone, a specific juvenile periodontitis-related bacterial clone; Ltx, leukotoxin; MLST, multilocus sequence type; Omp, outer membrane protein; PCR, polymerase chain reaction; RTX, repeats in toxin; St, serotype; SNP, single nucleotide polymorphism; YadA, *Yersinia* adhesin A.

References

1. Klinger, R. Untersuchungen über menschliche Aktinomykose. *Zentralbl. Bakteriol.* **1912**, *62*, 191–200. (In German)
2. Topley, W.W.C.; Wilson, G.S. *The Principles of Bacteriology and Immunity*; Edward Arnold: London, UK, 1929; pp. 1–587.
3. King, E.O.; Tatum, H.W. Actinobacillus actinomycetemcomitans and Hemophilus aphrophilus. *J. Infect. Dis.* **1962**, *111*, 85–94. [CrossRef] [PubMed]
4. Slots, J. The predominant cultivable organisms in juvenile periodontitis. *Scand. J. Dent. Res.* **1976**, *84*, 1–10. [CrossRef] [PubMed]

5. Newman, M.G.; Socransky, S.S.; Savitt, E.D.; Propas, D.A.; Crawford, A. Studies of the microbiology of periodontosis. *J. Periodontol.* **1976**, *47*, 373–379. [CrossRef] [PubMed]
6. Tsai, C.C.; McArthur, W.P.; Baehni, P.C.; Hammond, B.F.; Taichman, N.S. Extraction and partial characterization of a leukotoxin from a plaque-derived Gram-negative microorganism. *Infect. Immun.* **1979**, *25*, 427–439. [PubMed]
7. Geraci, J.E.; Wilson, W.R. Symposium on infective endocarditis. III. Endocarditis due to gram-negative bacteria. Report of 56 cases. *Mayo Clin. Proc.* **1982**, *57*, 145–148.
8. Ebersole, J.L.; Taubman, M.A.; Smith, D.J.; Genco, R.J.; Frey, D.E. Human immune responses to oral micro-organisms. I. Association of localized juvenile periodontitis (LJP) with serum antibody responses to *Actinobacillus actinomycetemcomitans*. *Clin. Exp. Immunol.* **1982**, *47*, 43–52.
9. Zambon, J.J.; Slots, J.; Genco, R.J. Serology of oral *Actinobacillus actinomycetemcomitans* and serotype distribution in human periodontal disease. *Infect. Immun.* **1983**, *41*, 19–27.
10. Brogan, J.M.; Lally, E.T.; Poulsen, K.; Kilian, M.; Demuth, D.R. Regulation of *Actinobacillus actinomycetemcomitans* leukotoxin expression: Analysis of the promoter regions of leukotoxic and minimally leukotoxic strains. *Infect. Immun.* **1994**, *62*, 501–508.
11. Nørskov-Lauritsen, N.; Kilian, M. Reclassification of *Actinobacillus actinomycetemcomitans*, *Haemophilus aphrophilus*, *Haemophilus paraphrophilus* and *Haemophilus segnis* as *Aggregatibacter actinomycetemcomitans* gen. nov., comb. nov., *Aggregatibacter aphrophilus* comb. nov. and *Aggregatibacter segnis* comb. nov., and emended description of *Aggregatibacter aphrophilus* to include V factor-dependent and V factor-independent isolates. *Int. J. Syst. Evol. Microbiol.* **2006**, *56*, 2135–2146.
12. Haubek, D.; Ennibi, O.K.; Poulsen, K.; Vaeth, M.; Poulsen, S.; Kilian, M. Risk of aggressive periodontitis in adolescent carriers of the JP2 clone of *Aggregatibacter* (*Actinobacillus*) *actinomycetemcomitans* in Morocco: A prospective longitudinal cohort study. *Lancet* **2008**, *371*, 237–242. [CrossRef]
13. Moore, W.E.; Moore, L.V. The bacteria of periodontal diseases. *Periodontology 2000* **1994**, *5*, 66–77. [CrossRef] [PubMed]
14. Socransky, S.S.; Haffajee, A.D. Evidence of bacterial etiology: A historical perspective. *Periodontology 2000* **1994**, *5*, 7–25. [CrossRef] [PubMed]
15. Wilson, M.J.; Weightman, A.J.; Wade, W.G. Applications of molecular ecology in the characterisation of uncultured microorganisms associated with human disease. *Rev. Med. Microbiol.* **1997**, *8*, 91–101. [CrossRef]
16. Dewhirst, F.E.; Chen, T.; Izard, J.; Paster, B.J.; Tanner, A.C.; Yu, W.H.; Lakshmanan, A.; Wade, W.G. The human oral microbiome. *J. Bacteriol.* **2010**, *192*, 5002–5017.
17. Bisgaard, M.; Christensen, H.; Clermont, D.; Dijkshoorn, L.; Janda, J.M.; Moore, E.R.B.; Nemec, A.; Nørskov-Lauritsen, N.; Overmann, J.; Reubsaet, F.A.G. The use of genomic DNA sequences as type material for valid publication of bacterial species names will have severe implications for clinical microbiology and related disciplines. *Diagn. Microbiol. Infect. Dis.* **2019**, *95*, 102–103. [CrossRef] [PubMed]
18. Asikainen, S.; Chen, C. Oral ecology and person-to-person transmission of *Actinobacillus actinomycetemcomitans* and *Porphyromonas gingivalis*. *Periodontol 2000* **1999**, *20*, 65–81.
19. Fine, D.H.; Pati, A.G.; Velusamy, S.K. *Aggregatibacter actinomycetemcomitans* (Aa) Under the Radar: Myths and Misunderstandings of Aa and Its Role in Aggressive Periodontitis. *Front. Immunol.* **2019**, *10*, 728. [CrossRef]
20. Hornef, M. Pathogens, commensal symbionts, and pathobionts: Discovery and functional effects on the host. *ILAR J.* **2015**, *56*, 159–162. [CrossRef]
21. Cowan, S.T. *Cowan and Steel's Manual for the Identification of Medical Bacteria*, 2nd ed.; Cambridge University Press: Cambridge, UK, 1974; p. 95.
22. Potts, T.V.; Mitra, T.; O'Keefe, T.; Zambon, J.J.; Genco, R.J. Relationships among isolates of oral haemophili as determined by DNA-DNA hybridization. *Arch. Microbiol.* **1986**, *145*, 136–141. [CrossRef]
23. Munson, E.; Carroll, K.C. What's in a name? New bacterial species and changes to taxonomic status from 2012 through 2015. *J. Clin. Microbiol.* **2017**, *55*, 24–42. [PubMed]
24. Murra, M.; Lützen, L.; Barut, A.; Zbinden, R.; Lund, M.; Villesen, P.; Nørskov-Lauritsen, N. Whole-genome sequencing of *aggregatibacter* species isolated from human clinical specimens and description of *aggregatibacter kilianii* sp. nov. *J. Clin. Microbiol.* **2018**, *56*, e00053-18. [PubMed]
25. Takada, K.; Saito, M.; Tsuzukibashi, O.; Kawashima, Y.; Ishida, S.; Hirasawa, M. Characterization of a new serotype g isolate of *Aggregatibacter actinomycetemcomitans*. *Mol. Oral Microbiol.* **2010**, *25*, 200–206. [CrossRef] [PubMed]

26. Brígido, J.A.; da Silveira, V.R.; Rego, R.O.; Nogueira, N.A. Serotypes of *Aggregatibacter actinomycetemcomitans* in relation to periodontal status and geographic origin of individuals—A review of the literature. *Med. Oral Patol. Oral Cir. Bucal* **2014**, *19*, e184–e191. [CrossRef]
27. Saarela, M.; Asikainen, S.; Alaluusua, S.; Pyhälä, L.; Lai, C.H.; Jousimies-Somer, H. Frequency and stability of mono-or poly-infection by *Actinobacillus actinomycetemcomitans* serotypes a, b, c, d or e. *Oral Microbiol. Immunol.* **1992**, *7*, 277–279. [CrossRef]
28. Thiha, K.; Takeuchi, Y.; Umeda, M.; Huang, Y.; Ohnishi, M.; Ishikawa, I. Identification of periodontopathic bacteria in gingival tissue of Japanese periodontitis patients. *Oral Microbiol. Immunol.* **2007**, *22*, 201–207. [CrossRef]
29. Rylev, M.; Kilian, M. Prevalence and distribution of principal periodontal pathogens worldwide. *J. Clin. Periodontol.* **2011**, *3*, 346–361. [CrossRef]
30. Bandhaya, P.; Saraithong, P.; Likittanasombat, K.; Hengprasith, B.; Torrungruang, K. Aggregatibacter actinomycetemcomitans serotypes, the JP2 clone and cytolethal distending toxin genes in a Thai population. *J. Clin. Periodontol.* **2012**, *39*, 519–525.
31. Claesson, R.; Höglund Åberg, C.; Haubek, D.; Johansson, A. Age-related prevalence and characteristics of *Aggregatibacter actinomycetemcomitans* in periodontitis patients living in Sweden. *J. Oral Microbiol.* **2017**, *9*, 1334504. [CrossRef]
32. Yamamoto, M.; Nishihara, T.; Koseki, T.; He, T.; Yamato, K.; Zhang, Y.J.; Nakashima, K.; Oda, S.; Ishikawa, I. Prevalence of *Actinobacillus actinomycetemcomitans* serotypes in Japanese patients with periodontitis. *J. Periodontal Res.* **1997**, *32*, 676–681. [CrossRef]
33. Celenligil, H.; Ebersole, J.L. Analysis of serum antibody responses to periodontopathogens in early-onset periodontitis patients from different geographical locations. *J. Clin. Periodontol.* **1998**, *25*, 994–1002. [CrossRef] [PubMed]
34. Saraiva, L.; Rebeis, E.S.; Martins Ede, S.; Sekiguchi, R.T.; Ando-Suguimoto, E.S.; Mafra, C.E.; Holzhausen, M.; Romito, G.A.; Mayer, M.P. IgG sera levels against a subset of periodontopathogens and severity of disease in aggressive periodontitis patients: A cross-sectional study of selected pocket sites. *J. Clin. Periodontol.* **2014**, *41*, 943–951. [CrossRef] [PubMed]
35. Poulsen, K.; Theilade, E.; Lally, E.T.; Demuth, D.R.; Kilian, M. Population structure of *Actinobacillus actinomycetemcomitans*: A framework for studies of disease-associated properties. *Microbiology* **1994**, *140*, 2049–2060. [CrossRef] [PubMed]
36. Kaplan, J.B.; Schreiner, H.C.; Furgang, D.; Fine, D.H. Population structure and genetic diversity of *Actinobacillus actinomycetemcomitans* strains isolated from localized juvenile periodontitis patients. *J. Clin. Microbiol.* **2002**, *40*, 1181–1187. [CrossRef]
37. Haubek, D.; Poulsen, K.; Kilian, M. Microevolution and patterns of dissemination of the JP2 clone of *Aggregatibacter (Actinobacillus) Actinomycetemcomitans*. *Infect. Immun.* **2007**, *75*, 3080–3088. [CrossRef]
38. DiRienzo, J.M.; Slots, J. Genetic approach to the study of epidemiology and pathogenesis of *Actinobacillus actinomycetemcomitans* in localized juvenile periodontitis. *Arch. Oral Biol.* **1990**, *35*, S79–S84. [CrossRef]
39. Zambon, J.J.; Sunday, G.J.; Smutko, J.S. Molecular genetic analysis of *Actinobacillus actinomycetemcomitans* epidemiology. *J. Periodontol.* **1990**, *61*, 75–80. [CrossRef]
40. DiRienzo, J.M.; Slots, J.; Sixou, M.; Sol, M.A.; Harmon, R.; McKay, T.L. Specific genetic variants of *Actinobacillus actinomycetemcomitans* correlate with disease and health in a regional population of families with localized juvenile periodontitis. *Infect. Immun.* **1994**, *62*, 3058–3065.
41. Eriksen, K.T.; Haubek, D.; Poulsen, K. Intragenomic recombination in the highly leukotoxic JP2 clone of *Actinobacillus actinomycetemcomitans*. *Microbiology* **2005**, *151*, 3371–3379. [CrossRef]
42. Höglund Åberg, C.; Haubek, D.; Kwamin, F.; Johansson, A.; Claesson, R. Leukotoxic activity of *Aggregatibacter actinomycetemcomitans* and periodontal attachment loss. *PLoS ONE* **2014**, *9*, e104095. [CrossRef]
43. Kittichotirat, W.; Bumgarner, R.E.; Asikainen, S.; Chen, C. Identification of the pangenome and its components in 14 distinct *Aggregatibacter actinomycetemcomitans* strains by comparative genomic analysis. *PLoS ONE* **2011**, *6*, e22420. [CrossRef]
44. Jorth, P.; Whiteley, M. An evolutionary link between natural transformation and CRISPR adaptive immunity. *MBio* **2012**, *3*, e00309-12. [CrossRef] [PubMed]
45. Kittichotirat, W.; Bumgarner, R.E.; Chen, C. Evolutionary divergence of *Aggregatibacter actinomycetemcomitans*. *J. Dent. Res.* **2016**, *95*, 94–101. [CrossRef]

46. Nedergaard, S.; Kobel, C.M.; Nielsen, M.B.; Møller, R.T.; Jensen, A.B.; Nørskov-Lauritsen, N.; The Danish HACEK Study Group. Whole genome sequencing of *Aggregatibacter actinomycetemcomitans* cultured from blood stream infections reveals three major phylogenetic groups including a novel lineage expressing serotype a membrane O polysaccharide. *Pathogens*. submitted.
47. Holm, P. The influence of carbon dioxide on the growth of *Actinobacillus actinomycetemcomitans* (Bacterium actinomycetem comitans Klinger 1912). *Acta. Pathol. Microbiol. Scand.* **1954**, *34*, 235–248. [CrossRef] [PubMed]
48. Henderson, B.; Ward, J.M.; Ready, D. *Aggregatibacter (Actinobacillus) actinomycetemcomitans*: A triple A* periodontopathogen? *Periodontology 2000* **2010**, *54*, 78–105. [CrossRef] [PubMed]
49. Möller, Å.J.R. Microbiological examination of root canals and periapical tissues of human teeth. *Scand. Dent. J.* **1966**, *74*, 5–6.
50. Johansson, E.; Claesson, R.; van Dijken, J.W.V. Antibacterial effect of ozone on cariogenic bacterial species. *J. Dent.* **2009**, *37*, 449–453. [CrossRef] [PubMed]
51. Khurshid, Z.; Zohaib, S.; Najeeb, S.; Zafar, M.S.; Slowey, P.D.; Almas, K. Human saliva collection devices for proteomics: An update. *Int. J. Mol. Sci.* **2016**, *17*, 846. [CrossRef] [PubMed]
52. Khurshid, Z.; Mali, M.; Naseem, M.; Najeeb, S.; Zafar, M.S. Human gingival crevicular fluids (GCF) proteomics: An overview. *Dent. J.* **2017**, *5*, 12. [CrossRef]
53. Slots, J. Selective medium for isolation of *Actinobacillus actinomycetemcomitans*. *J. Clin. Microbiol.* **1982**, *15*, 606–609. [PubMed]
54. Höglund Åberg, C.; Kwamin, F.; Claesson, R.; Johansson, A.; Haubek, D. Presence of JP2 and non-JP2 genotypes of *Aggregatibacter actinomycetemcomitans* and periodontal attachment loss in adolescents in Ghana. *J. Periodontol.* **2012**, *83*, 1520–1528. [CrossRef] [PubMed]
55. Marsh, P. Microbial ecology of dental plaque and its significance in health and disease. *Adv. Dent. Res.* **1994**, *8*, 263–271. [CrossRef] [PubMed]
56. Slots, J. Salient Biochemical Characters of *Actinobacillus actinomycetemcomitans*. *Arch. Microbiol.* **1982**, *131*, 60–67. [CrossRef] [PubMed]
57. Couturier, M.R.; Mehinovic, E.; Croft, A.C.; Mark, A.; Fisher, M.A. Identification of HACEK clinical isolates by matrix-assisted laser desorption ionization—Time of flight mass spectrometry. *J. Clin. Microbiol.* **2011**, *49*, 1104–1106. [CrossRef] [PubMed]
58. Zambon, J.J.; DeLuca, C.; Slots, J.; Genco, R.J. Studies of leukotoxin from *Actinobacillus actinomycetemcomitans* using the promyelocytic HL-60 cell line. *Infect. Immun.* **1983**, *40*, 205–212.
59. Haubek, D.; DiRienzo, J.J.; Tinoco, E.M.; Westergaard, J.; Lopez, N.J.; Chung, C.P.; Poulsen, K.; Kilian, M. Racial tropism of a highly toxic clone of *Actinbacillus actinomycetemcomitans* associated with juvenile periodontitis. *J. Clin. Microbiol.* **1997**, *35*, 3037–3042.
60. Sampathkumar, V.; Velusamy, S.K.; Godboley, D.; Fine, D.H. Increased leukotoxin production: Characterization of 100 base pairs within the 530 base pair leukotoxin promoter region of *Aggregatibacter actinomycetemcomitans*. *Sci. Rep.* **2017**, *7*, 1887. [CrossRef]
61. Poulsen, K.; Ennibi, O.K.; Haubek, D. Improved PCR for detection of the highly leukotoxic JP2 clone of *Actinobacillus actinomycetemcomitans* in subgingival plaque samples. *J. Clin. Microbiol.* **2003**, *41*, 4829–4832. [CrossRef]
62. Kirakodu, S.S.; Govindaswami, M.; Novak, M.J.; Ebersole, J.L.; Novak, K.F. Optimizing qPCR for the quantification of periodontal pathogens in a complex plaque biofilm. *Open Dent. J.* **2008**, *2*, 49–55. [CrossRef]
63. Yoshida, A.; Ennibi, O.K.; Miyazaki, H.; Hoshino, T.; Hayashida, H.; Nishihara, T.; Awano, S.; Ansai, T. Quantitative discrimination of *Aggregatibacter actinomycetemcomitans* highly leukotoxic JP2 clone from non-JP2 clones in diagnosis of aggressive periodontitis. *BMC Inf. Dis.* **2012**, *12*, 253. [CrossRef] [PubMed]
64. Větrovský, T.; Baldrian, P. The variability of the 16S rRNA gene in bacterial genomes and its consequences for bacterial community analyses. *PLoS ONE* **2013**, *8*, e57923. [CrossRef] [PubMed]
65. Suzuki, N.; Nakano, Y.; Yoshida, Y.; Ikeda, D.; Koga, T. Identification of *Actinobacillus actinomycetemcomitans* serotypes by multiplex PCR. *J. Clin. Microbiol.* **2001**, *9*, 2002–2005. [CrossRef] [PubMed]
66. Kaplan, J.B.; Perry, M.B.; MacLean, L.L.; Furgang, D.; Wilson, M.E.; Fine, D.H. Structural and genetic analyses of O polysaccharide from *Actinobacillus actinomycetemcomitans* serotype f. *Infect. Immun.* **2001**, *69*, 5375–5384. [CrossRef]

67. Tomich, M.; Planet, P.J.; Figurski, D.H. The *tad* locus: Postcards from the widespread colonization island. *Nat. Rev. Microbiol.* **2007**, *5*, 363–375. [CrossRef]
68. Rose, J.E.; Meyer, D.H.; Fives-Taylor, P.M. Aae, an autotransporter involved in adhesion of *Actinobacillus actinomycetemcomitans* to epithelial cells. *Infect. Immun.* **2003**, *71*, 2384–2393. [CrossRef]
69. Danforth, D.R.; Tang-Siegel, G.; Ruiz, T.; Mintz, K.P. A nonfimbrial adhesin of *Aggregatibacter actinomycetemcomitans* mediates biofilm biogenesis. *Infect. Immun.* **2018**, *87*, e00704-18. [CrossRef]
70. Yue, G.; Kaplan, J.B.; Furgang, D.; Mansfield, K.G.; Fine, D.H. A second *Aggregatibacter actinomycetemcomitans* autotransporter adhesin exhibits specificity for buccal epithelial cells in humans and Old World primates. *Infect. Immun.* **2007**, *75*, 4440–4448. [CrossRef]
71. Vega, B.A.; Belinka, B.A.; Kachlany, S.C. *Aggregatibacter actinomycetemcomitans* Leukotoxin (LtxA; Leukothera®): Mechanisms of Action and Therapeutic Applications. *Toxins* **2019**, *11*, 489. [CrossRef]
72. Sugai, M.; Kawamoto, T.; Pérès, S.Y.; Ueno, Y.; Komatsuzawa, H.; Fujiwara, T.; Kurihara, H.; Suginaka, H.; Oswald, E. The cell cycle-specific growth-inhibitory factor produced by *Actinobacillus actinomycetemcomitans* is a cytolethal distending toxin. *Infect. Immun.* **1998**, *66*, 5008–5019.
73. Boesze-Battaglia, K.; Alexander, D.; Dlakić, M.; Shenker, B.J. A Journey of cytolethal distending toxins through cell membranes. *Front. Cell. Infect. Microbiol.* **2016**, *6*, 81. [CrossRef] [PubMed]
74. Teng, Y.T.; Hu, W. Expression cloning of a periodontitis-associated apoptotic effector, cagE homologue, in *Actinobacillus actinomycetemcomitans*. *Biochem. Biophys. Res. Commun.* **2003**, *303*, 1086–1094. [CrossRef]
75. Ramasubbu, N.; Thomas, L.M.; Ragunath, C.; Kaplan, J.B. Structural analysis of dispersin B, a biofilm-releasing glycoside hydrolase from the periodontopathogen *Actinobacillus actinomycetemcomitans*. *J. Mol. Biol.* **2005**, *349*, 475–486. [CrossRef] [PubMed]
76. Karched, M.; Ihalin, R.; Eneslätt, K.; Zhong, D.; Oscarsson, J.; Wai, S.N.; Chen, C.; Asikainen, S.E. Vesicle-independent extracellular release of a proinflammatory outer membrane lipoprotein in free-soluble form. *BMC Microbiol.* **2008**, *8*, 18. [CrossRef] [PubMed]
77. Rosan, B.; Slots, J.; Lamont, R.J.; Listgarten, M.A.; Nelson, G.M. *Actinobacillus actinomycetemcomitans* fimbriae. *Oral. Microbiol. Immunol.* **1988**, *3*, 58–63. [CrossRef]
78. Harano, K.; Yamanaka, A.; Okuda, K. An antiserum to a synthetic fimbrial peptide of *Actinobacillus actinomycetemcomitans* blocked adhesion of the microorganism. *FEMS Microbiol. Lett.* **1995**, *130*, 279–285. [CrossRef]
79. Fine, D.H.; Furgang, D.; Schreiner, H.C.; Goncharoff, P.; Charlesworth, J.; Ghazwan, G.; Fitzgerald-Bocarsly, P.; Figurski, D.H. Phenotypic variation in *Actinobacillus actinomycetemcomitans* during laboratory growth: Implications for virulence. *Microbiology* **1999**, *145*, 1335–1347. [CrossRef]
80. Inoue, T.; Tanimoto, I.; Ohta, H.; Kato, K.; Murayama, Y.; Fukui, K. Molecular characterization of low-molecular-weight component protein, Flp, in *Actinobacillus actinomycetemcomitans* fimbriae. *Microbiol. Immunol.* **1998**, *42*, 253–258. [CrossRef]
81. Kachlany, S.C.; Planet, P.J.; Desalle, R.; Fine, D.H.; Figurski, D.H.; Kaplan, J.B. *flp-1*, the first representative of a new pilin gene subfamily, is required for non-specific adherence of *Actinobacillus actinomycetemcomitans*. *Mol. Microbiol.* **2001**, *40*, 542–554. [CrossRef]
82. Haase, E.M.; Zmuda, J.L.; Scannapieco, F.A. Identification and molecular analysis of rough-colony-specific outer membrane proteins of *Actinobacillus actinomycetemcomitans*. *Infect. Immun.* **1999**, *67*, 2901–2908.
83. Wang, Y.; Chen, C. Mutation analysis of the flp operon in *Actinobacillus actinomycetemcomitans*. *Gene* **2005**, *351*, 61–71. [CrossRef] [PubMed]
84. Perez, B.A.; Planet, P.J.; Kachlany, S.C.; Tomich, M.; Fine, D.H.; Figurski, D.H. Genetic analysis of the requirement for flp-2, tadV, and rcpB in *Actinobacillus actinomycetemcomitans* biofilm formation. *J. Bacteriol.* **2006**, *188*, 6361–6375. [CrossRef] [PubMed]
85. Schreiner, H.C.; Sinatra, K.; Kaplan, J.B.; Furgang, D.; Kachlany, S.C.; Planet, P.J.; Perez, B.A.; Figurski, D.H.; Fine, D.H. Tight-adherence genes of *Actinobacillus actinomycetemcomitans* are required for virulence in a rat model. *Proc. Natl. Acad. Sci. USA* **2003**, *100*, 7295–7300. [CrossRef] [PubMed]
86. Wang, Y.; Liu, A.; Chen, C. Genetic basis for conversion of rough-to-smooth colony morphology in *Actinobacillus actinomycetemcomitans*. *Infect. Immun.* **2005**, *73*, 3749–3753. [CrossRef] [PubMed]
87. Pei, Z.; Niu, Z.; Shi, S.; Shi, L.; Tang, C. Phenotypic changes in nonfimbriated smooth strains of *Aggregatibacter actinomycetemcomitans* grown in low-humidity solid medium. *Ultrastruct. Pathol.* **2013**, *37*, 121–126. [CrossRef]

88. Fine, D.H.; Velliyagounder, K.; Furgang, D.; Kaplan, J.B. The *Actinobacillus actinomycetemcomitans* autotransporter adhesin Aae exhibits specificity for buccal epithelial cells from humans and old world primates. *Infect. Immun.* **2005**, *73*, 1947–1953. [CrossRef]
89. Li, L.; Matevski, D.; Aspiras, M.; Ellen, R.P.; Lépine, G. Two epithelial cell invasion-related loci of the oral pathogen *Actinobacillus actinomycetemcomitans*. *Oral. Microbiol. Immunol.* **2004**, *19*, 16–25. [CrossRef]
90. Mintz, K.P. Identification of an extracellular matrix protein adhesin, EmaA, which mediates the adhesion of *Actinobacillus actinomycetemcomitans* to collagen. *Microbiology* **2004**, *150*, 2677–2688. [CrossRef]
91. Tang, G.; Kitten, T.; Munro, C.L.; Wellman, G.C.; Mintz, K.P. EmaA, a potential virulence determinant of *Aggregatibacter actinomycetemcomitans* in infective endocarditis. *Infect. Immun.* **2008**, *76*, 2316–2324. [CrossRef]
92. Cornelissen, C.N. Subversion of nutritional immunity by the pathogenic Neisseriae. *Pathog. Dis.* **2018**, *76*, ftx112. [CrossRef]
93. Benz, R. Channel formation by RTX-toxins of pathogenic bacteria: Basis of their biological activity. *Biochim. Biophys. Acta* **2016**, *1858*, 526–537. [CrossRef] [PubMed]
94. Frey, J.; Kuhnert, P. RTX toxins in *Pasteurellaceae*. *Int. J. Med. Microbiol.* **2002**, *292*, 149–158. [CrossRef] [PubMed]
95. Taichman, N.S.; Tsai, C.C.; Baehni, P.C.; Stoller, N.; McArthur, W.P. Interaction of inflammatory cells and oral microorganisms. IV. In vitro release of lysosomal constituents from polymorphonuclear leukocytes exposed to supragingival and subgingival bacterial plaque. *Infect. Immun.* **1977**, *16*, 1013–1023. [PubMed]
96. Lally, E.T.; Golub, E.E.; Kieba, I.R.; Taichman, N.S.; Rosenbloom, J.; Rosenbloom, J.C.; Gibson, C.W.; Demuth, D.R. Analysis of the *Actinobacillus actinomycetemcomitans* leukotoxin gene. Delineation of unique features and comparison to homologous toxins. *J. Biol. Chem.* **1989**, *264*, 15451–15456. [PubMed]
97. Kolodrubetz, D.; Dailey, T.; Ebersole, J.; Kraig, E. Cloning and expression of the leukotoxin gene from *Actinobacillus actinomycetemcomitans*. *Infect. Immun.* **1989**, *57*, 1465–1469. [PubMed]
98. Balashova, N.V.; Crosby, J.A.; Al Ghofaily, L.; Kachlany, S.C. Leukotoxin confers beta-hemolytic activity to *Actinobacillus actinomycetemcomitans*. *Infect. Immun.* **2006**, *74*, 2015–2021. [CrossRef] [PubMed]
99. Claesson, R.; Gudmundson, J.; Åberg, C.H.; Haubek, D.; Johansson, A. Detection of 640-bp deletion in *Aggregatibacter actinomycetemcomitans* leukotoxin promoter region in isolates from an adolescent of Ethiopian origin. *J. Oral Microbiol.* **2015**, *7*, 26974. [CrossRef]
100. He, T.; Nishihara, T.; Demuth, D.R.; Ishikawa, I. A novel insertion sequence increases the expression of leukotoxicity in *Actinobacillus actinomycetemcomitans* clinical isolates. *J. Periodontol.* **1999**, *70*, 1261–1268. [CrossRef]
101. Höglund Åberg, C.; Kwamin, F.; Claesson, R.; Dáhlen, G.; Johansson, A.; Haubek, D. Progression of attachment loss is strongly associated with presence of the JP2 genotype of *Aggregatibacter actinomycetemcomitans*: A prospective cohort study of a young adolescent population. *J. Clin. Periodontol.* **2014**, *41*, 232–241. [CrossRef]
102. Burgess, D.; Huang, H.; Harrison, P.; Aukhil, I.; Shaddox, L. *Aggregatibacter actinomycetemcomitans* in African Americans with localized aggressive periodontitis. *JDR Clin. Trans. Res.* **2017**, *2*, 249–257. [CrossRef]
103. Leung, W.K.; Ngai, V.K.; Yau, J.Y.; Cheung, B.P.; Tsang, P.W.; Corbet, E.F. Characterization of *Actinobacillus actinomycetemcomitans* isolated from young Chinese aggressive periodontitis patients. *J. Periodontal Res.* **2005**, *40*, 258–268. [CrossRef] [PubMed]
104. van der Reijden, W.A.; Bosch-Tijhof, C.J.; van der Velden, U.; van Winkelhoff, A.J. Java project on periodontal diseases: Serotype distribution of *Aggregatibacter actinomycetemcomitans* and serotype dynamics over an 8-year period. *J. Clin. Periodontol.* **2008**, *35*, 407–492. [CrossRef] [PubMed]
105. Pahumunto, N.; Ruangsri, P.; Wongsuwanlert, M.; Piwat, S.; Dahlen, G.; Teanpaisan, R. *Aggregatibacter actinomycetemcomitans* serotypes and DGGE subtypes in Thai adults with chronic periodontitis. *Arch. Oral Biol.* **2015**, *60*, 1789–1796. [CrossRef] [PubMed]
106. Alaluusua, S.; Asikainen, S. Detection and distribution of *Actinobacillus actinomycetemcomitans* in the primary dentition. *J. Periodontol.* **1988**, *59*, 504–507. [CrossRef] [PubMed]
107. Slots, J.; Reynolds, H.S.; Genco, R.J. *Actinobacillus actinomycetemcomitans* in human periodontal disease: A cross-sectional microbiological investigation. *Infect. Immun.* **1980**, *29*, 1013–1020. [PubMed]
108. Frisken, W.; Higgins, T.; Palmer, J.M. The incidence of periodontopathic microorganisms in young children. *Oral Microbiol. Immunol.* **1990**, *5*, 43–45. [CrossRef]
109. Kononen, E.; Asikainen, S.; Jousimies-Somer, H. The early colonization of gram-negative anaerobic bacteria in edentulous infants. *Oral Microbiol. Immunol.* **1992**, *7*, 28–31. [CrossRef]

110. Merglova, V.; Polenik, P. Early colonization of the oral cavity in 6-and 12-month-old infants by cariogenic and periodontal pathogens: A case-control study. *Folia Microbiol.* **2016**, *61*, 423–429. [CrossRef]
111. Preus, H.R.; Zambon, J.J.; Dunford, R.G.; Genco, R.J. The distribution and transmission of *Actinobacillus actinomycetemcomitans* in families with established adult periodontitis. *J. Periodontol.* **1994**, *65*, 2–7. [CrossRef]
112. Asikainen, S.; Chen, C.; Slots, J. Likelihood of transmitting *Actinobacillus actinomycetemcomitans* and *Porplyromonna gingivalis* in families with periodontitis. *Oral Microbiol. Immunol.* **1996**, *11*, 387–394. [CrossRef]
113. Rêgo, R.O.; Spolidorio, D.M.; Salvador, S.L.; Cirelli, J.A. Transmission of *Aggregatibacter actinomycetemcomitans* between Brazilian women with severe chronic periodontitis and their children. *Braz. Dent. J.* **2007**, *18*, 220–224. [CrossRef]
114. Van Winkelhoff, A.J.; Boutaga, K. Transmission of periodontal bacteria and models of infection. *J. Clin. Periodontol.* **2005**, *32*, 16–27. [CrossRef] [PubMed]
115. Doğan, B.; Kipalev, A.S.; Okte, E.; Sultan, N.; Asikainen, S.E. Consistent intrafamilial transmission of *Actinobacillus actinomycetemcomitans* despite clonal diversity. *J. Periodontol.* **2008**, *79*, 307–315. [CrossRef] [PubMed]
116. Saarela, M.H.; Doğan, B.; Alaluusua, S.; Asikainen, S. Persistence of oral colonization by the same *Actinobacillus actinomycetemcomitans* strain(s). *J. Periodontol.* **1999**, *70*, 504–509. [CrossRef] [PubMed]
117. Haubek, D.; Ennibi, O.K.; Vaeth, M.; Poulsen, S.; Poulsen, K. Stability of the JP2 clone of *Aggregatibacter actinomycetemcomitans*. *J. Dent. Res.* **2009**, *88*, 856–860. [CrossRef] [PubMed]
118. Sun, R.; Kittichotirat, W.; Wang, J.; Jan, M.; Chen, W.; Asikainen, S.; Bumgarner, R.; Chen, C. Genomic stability of *Aggregatibacter actinomycetemcomitans* during persistent oral infection in human. *PLoS ONE* **2013**, *8*, e66472. [CrossRef]
119. van Winkelhoff, A.J.; Slots, J. Actinobacillus actinomycetemcomitans and Porphyromonas gingivalis in nonoral infections. *Periodontology 2000* **1999**, *20*, 122–135. [CrossRef]
120. Paju, S.; Carlson, P.; Jousimies-Somer, H.; Asikainen, S. Heterogeneity of *Actinobacillus actinomycetemcomitans* strains in various human infections and relationships between serotype, genotype, and antimicrobial susceptibility. *J. Clin. Microbiol.* **2000**, *38*, 79–84.
121. Paturel, L.; Casalta, J.P.; Habib, G.; Nezri, M.; Raoult, D. *Actinobacillus actinomycetemcomitans* endocarditis. *Clin. Microbiol. Infect.* **2004**, *10*, 98–118. [CrossRef]
122. Clarridge, J.E.; Zhang, Q. Genotypic diversity of clinical *Actinomyces* species: Phenotype, source, and disease correlation among genospecies. *J. Clin. Microbiol.* **2002**, *40*, 3442–3448. [CrossRef]
123. Kaplan, A.H.; Weber, D.J.; Oddone, E.Z.; Perfect, J.R. Infection due to *Actinobacillus actinomycetemcomitans*: 15 cases and review. *Rev. Infect. Dis.* **1989**, *11*, 46–63. [CrossRef] [PubMed]
124. Brouqui, P.; Raoult, D. Endocarditis due to rare and fastidious bacteria. *Clin. Microbiol. Rev.* **2001**, *14*, 177–207. [CrossRef] [PubMed]
125. Nørskov-Lauritsen, N. Classification, identification, and clinical significance of *Haemophilus* and *Aggregatibacter* species with host specificity for humans. *Clin. Microbiol. Rev.* **2014**, *27*, 214–240. [CrossRef] [PubMed]
126. Lützen, L.; Olesen, B.; Voldstedlund, M.; Christensen, J.J.; Moser, C.; Knudsen, J.D.; Fuursted, K.; Hartmeyer, G.N.; Chen, M.; Søndergaard, T.S.; et al. Incidence of HACEK bacteraemia in Denmark: A 6-year population-based study. *Int. J. Infect. Dis.* **2018**, *68*, 83–87. [CrossRef] [PubMed]
127. Yew, H.S.; Chambers, S.T.; Roberts, S.A.; Holland, D.J.; Julian, K.A.; Raymond, N.J.; Beardsley, J.; Read, K.M.; Murdoch, D.R. Association between HACEK bacteraemia and endocarditis. *J. Med. Microbiol.* **2014**, *63*, 892–895. [PubMed]
128. Armitage, G.C.; Offenbacher, S. Consensus Report. Periodontal diseases: Epidemiology and diagnosis. *Ann. Periodontol.* **1996**, *1*, 16–22. [CrossRef]
129. Fine, D.H.; Markowitz, K.; Fairlie, K.; Tischio-Bereski, D.; Ferrendiz, J.; Furgang, D.; Paster, B.J.; Dewhirst, F.E. A consortium of *Aggregatibacter actinomycetemcomitans*, *Streptococcus parasanguinis*, and *Filifactor alocis* is present in sites prior to bone loss in a longitudinal study of localized aggressive periodontitis. *J. Clin. Microbiol.* **2013**, *51*, 2850–2861. [CrossRef]
130. Ebbers, M.; Lübcke, P.M.; Volzke, J.; Kriebel, K.; Hieke, C.; Engelmann, R.; Lang, H.; Kreikemeyer, B.; Müller-Hilke, B. Interplay between *P. gingivalis*, *F. nucleatum* and *A. actinomycetemcomitans* in murine alveolar bone loss, arthritis onset and progression. *Sci. Rep.* **2018**, *8*, 15129. [CrossRef]

131. Armitage, G.C. Development of a classification system for periodontal diseases and conditions. *Northwest Dent.* **2000**, *79*, 31–35. [CrossRef]
132. Tonetti, M.S.; Greenwell, H.; Kornman, K.S. Staging and grading of periodontitis: Framework and proposal of a new classification and case definition. *J. Clin. Periodontal.* **2018**, *45*, S149–S161. [CrossRef]
133. Fine, D.H.; Patil, A.G.; Loos, B.G. Classification and diagnosis of aggressive periodontitis. *J. Periodontol.* **2018**, *89*, s103–s119. [CrossRef] [PubMed]
134. Teughels, W.; Dhondt, R.; Dekeyser, D.; Quirynen, M. Treatment of aggressive periodontitis. *Periodontology 2000* **2014**, *65*, 107–133. [CrossRef] [PubMed]
135. Hamad, C.; Haller, B.; Hoffmann, T.; Lorenz, K. Five-year results of nonsurgical generalized aggressive periodontitis. *Quintessence Int.* **2019**, *50*, 104–113. [PubMed]
136. Dopico, J.; Nibali, L.; Donos, N. Disease progression in aggressive periodontitis patients. A restrspective study. *J. Clin. Periodontol.* **2016**, *43*, 531–537. [CrossRef] [PubMed]
137. Kulik, E.M.; Lenkeit, K.; Chenaux, S.; Meyer, J. Antimicrobial susceptibility of periodontopathogenic bacteria. *J. Antimicrob. Chemother.* **2008**, *61*, 1087–1091. [CrossRef] [PubMed]
138. van Winkelhoff, A.J.; Herrera, D.; Oteo, A.; Sanz, M. Antimicrobial profiles of periodontal pathogens isolated from periodontitis patients in the Netherlands and Spain. *J. Clin. Periodontol.* **2005**, *32*, 893–898. [CrossRef] [PubMed]
139. Akrivopoulou, C.; Green, I.M.; Donos, N.; Nair, S.P.; Ready, D. *Aggregatibacter actinomycetemcomitans* serotype prevalence and antibiotic resistance in a UK population with periodontitis. *J. Glob. Antimicrob. Resist.* **2017**, *10*, 54–58. [CrossRef]
140. Jensen, A.B.; Haubek, D.; Claesson, R.; Johansson, A.; Nørskov-Lauritsen, N. Comprehensive antimicrobial susceptibility testing of a large collection of clinical strains of *Aggregatibacter actinomycetemcomitans* does not identify resistance to amoxicillin. *J. Clin. Periodontol.* **2019**, *46*, 846–854. [CrossRef]
141. Iversen, K.; Ihlemann, N.; Gill, S.U.; Madsen, T.; Elming, H.; Jensen, K.T.; Bruun, N.E.; Høfsten, D.E.; Fursted, K.; Christensen, J.J.; et al. Partial oral versus intravenous antibiotic treatment of endocarditis. *N. Engl. J. Med.* **2019**, *380*, 415–424. [CrossRef]

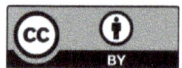

© 2019 by the authors. Licensee MDPI, Basel, Switzerland. This article is an open access article distributed under the terms and conditions of the Creative Commons Attribution (CC BY) license (http://creativecommons.org/licenses/by/4.0/).

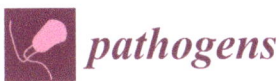

Review

Virulence and Pathogenicity Properties of *Aggregatibacter actinomycetemcomitans*

Georgios N. Belibasakis [1], Terhi Maula [2], Kai Bao [1], Mark Lindholm [3], Nagihan Bostanci [1], Jan Oscarsson [3], Riikka Ihalin [2] and Anders Johansson [3,*]

[1] Division of Oral Diseases, Department of Dental Medicine, Karolinska Institutet, S-141 04 Huddinge, Sweden; george.belibasakis@ki.se (G.N.B.); kai.bao@ki.se (K.B.); nagihan.bostanci@ki.se (N.B.)
[2] Department of Biochemistry, University of Turku, FI-20014 Turku, Finland; terhi.maula@utu.fi (T.M.); riikka.ihalin@utu.fi (R.I.)
[3] Department of Odontology, Umeå University, S-901 87 Umeå, Sweden; mark.lindholm@umu.se (M.L.); jan.oscarsson@umu.se (J.O.)
* Correspondence: anders.p.johansson@umu.se; Tel.: +46-90-7856291

Received: 27 September 2019; Accepted: 4 November 2019; Published: 6 November 2019

Abstract: *Aggregatibacter actinomycetemcomitans* is a periodontal pathogen colonizing the oral cavity of a large proportion of the human population. It is equipped with several potent virulence factors that can cause cell death and induce or evade inflammation. Because of the large genetic diversity within the species, both harmless and highly virulent genotypes of the bacterium have emerged. The oral condition and age, as well as the geographic origin of the individual, influence the risk to be colonized by a virulent genotype of the bacterium. In the present review, the virulence and pathogenicity properties of *A. actinomycetemcomitans* will be addressed.

Keywords: *Aggregatibacter actinomycetemcomitans*; leukotoxin; cytolethal distending toxin; lipopolysaccharides; cytokine binding factors; horizontal gene transfer; outer membrane vesicles; biofilm; proteomic

1. Introduction

Aggregatibacter actinomycetemcomitans is a facultative anaerobic Gram-negative bacterium that expresses several virulence factors, which activates a host response that could be associated to the pathogenesis of periodontitis [1]. This review will elaborate in more detail the virulence properties of *A. actinomycetemcomitans* that contribute to the increased pathogenicity of this species, particularly with regard to early and rapidly progressive forms of periodontal disease [2,3], such as localized aggressive periodontitis, where it is frequently a predominant find (Figure 1). The "crown jewel" of the virulence factors of *A. actinomycetemcomitans* has long been its leukotoxin [4,5]. However, a cytolethal distending toxin (CDT) has also been identified, making this species the only member of the oral microbiome to produce these two, or any of the two, protein exotoxins [6]. Its lipopolysaccharide is quite special in that the immunological responses elicited by the host can be used in classifying (serotyping) the virulence identity of each one of its strains [7]. More recently identified cytokine-binding molecules add to its potential virulence factors, suggesting additional pathogenicity mechanisms by which it can manipulate the host [8]. *A. actinomycetemcomitans* is also equipped with a wealth of outer membrane vesicles, like all Gram-negative species, which might confer special virulence properties to this species [9]. There is a great genetic diversity within this species, with base composition biases in the genomic islands suggesting their acquisitions via horizontal gene transfer [10]. Recent advances in biofilm modeling and proteomic technologies have helped define the localization of *A. actinomycetemcomitans* within biofilms, characterize the full range of its protein components, and define how these are regulated by other species, and vice versa, when growing within complex polymicrobial communities [11].

Increased knowledge about bacterial virulence markers in periodontal disease may be important tools in future strategies for personalized dentistry [12].

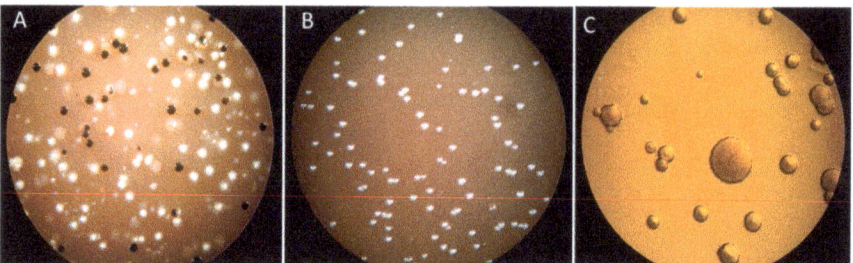

Figure 1. Subgingival biofilm samples from pathological periodontal pockets cultivated on blood agar plates for 48 h at 37 °C in an anaerobic atmosphere. (**A**) Sample obtained from a periodontal pocket of a middle-aged patient diagnosed with generalized chronic periodontitis. The macroscopical observation of the plated sample showed occurrence of a variety of colonies corresponding to different bacterial species. (**B**) Sample obtained from a periodontal pocket of a 25-year-old patient diagnosed with localized aggressive periodontitis. The macroscopical observation of the plated sample showed predominantly the occurrence a single colony type. (**C**) Microscopical (50× magnification) examination indicated that all colonies belonged to the *A. actinomycetemcomitans* species, which was confirmed in assays based on genetic characterization.

2. Leukotoxin (LtxA)

The leukotoxin (LtxA) of *A. actinomycetemcomitans* affects the different leukocyte populations with various death mechanisms [4]. It activates neutrophil degranulation causing a massive release of lysosomal enzymes, net-like structures, and matrix metallo proteinases (MMPs) and induces apoptosis in lymphocytes [13–15]. Interestingly, net-like structures can also be released from the LtxA-exposed neutrophils under anaerobic conditions and contain citrullinated proteins with sequence homology to proteins found in inflamed joints [16,17]. In the monocytes/macrophages, the toxin activates the inflammasome complex including the cysteine proteinase caspase-1, which induces an activation and secretion of the pro-inflammatory cytokines IL-1β and IL-18 [2,18,19]. These cellular and molecular mechanisms have been previously described in detail [20] (Figure 2). Taken together, several of the mechanisms by which LtxA affects leukocytes are also involved in the pathogenic mechanisms of many inflammatory disorders, such as periodontitis [21]. LtxA show a high target cell specificity expressed and affect only cells of hematopoetic origin from humans and some other primates [5]. This species-specificity of LtxA is reported to act through a unique target cell receptor and a specific region in the toxin that recognizes and interacts with this receptor [22,23]. A region of LtxA contains a series of 14 tandemly repeated amino acid sequences in the repeat region of the toxin and are shown to be responsible for the receptor binding to Lymphocyte function–associated antigen 1 (LFA-1) [4,23]. The LFA-1 molecule is a heterodimer consisting of the αL (CD11a) and β2 (CD18) subunits and is suggested to help the toxin to have a correct orientation on the target cell membrane [24–27].

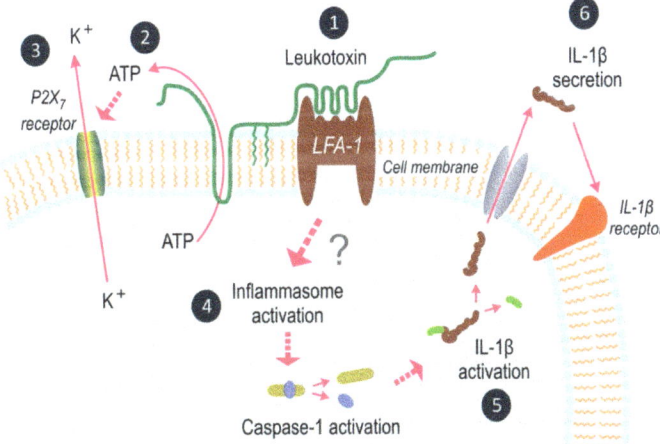

Figure 2. Leukotoxin (LtxA) induces a rapid inflammatory cell death in human macrophages. Briefly, LtxA binds to the LFA-1 receptor (1) and induces an extracellular release of ATP (2), which act as a ligand for the P2X7-receptor and result in an efflux of potassium (3). These processes promote the formation of an inflammasome multimer (4) that activates the cysteine proteinase caspase-1, resulting in a rapid activation (5) and secretion of IL-1β (6). Courtesy of Haubek and Johansson [20].

2.1. LtxA Production

The LtxA operon belongs to the core genome of *A. actinomycetemcomitans* and is so far present in all examined strains [28]. The operon consists of four coding genes named *ltxC*, *ltxA*, *ltxB*, and *ltxD* and an upstream promoter region [29]. The gene *ltxA* encodes the LtxA protein, *ltxC* a protein required for the posttranslational acylation of LtxA, and *ltxB* and *ltxD* proteins needed for the transport of the LtxA to the bacterial outer membrane. For regulation of the LtxA expression, there is a promoter region located upstream of the *ltxC* gene, and genetic differences within this region result in different genotypes with various LtxA expression [10].

Zambon [30] reported that leukotoxicity of *A. actinomycetemcomitans* isolated from individuals with periodontitis was enhanced compared with isolates from individuals without periodontitis. Later, it was discovered that many of the isolates with enhanced leukotoxicity have been shown to have a different type of promoter in the leukotoxin operon [29]. A specific genotype (JP2) of *A. actinomycetemcomitans* with enhanced leukotoxicity has been shown to significantly correlate to disease onset in infected individuals [31,32]. The JP2 genotype was first identified by Brogan and co-workers [33] and was a serotype b isolate with a 530 base pair (bp) deletion in the *ltxCABD* promoter. Based on this finding, isolates with such a deletion in the promoter are named JP2 genotype, and those lacking this deletion are non-JP2 genotype [20,34]. The discovery of the JP2 genotype introduced a new terminology of high and low leukotoxic *A. actinomycetemcomitans* based only on the *ltx* promoter type [33,35]. The presence of the JP2 genotype is highly associated to adolescents of North and West African origin [31,36]. However, the JP2 genotype has recently been shown to also colonize individuals of other geographic origin, as confirmed by genotyping [37,38]. Alterations in the *ltx* promoter region are the most studied genotypes associated with enhanced LtxA expression. In addition to the JP2 genotype, an insertion of 886 bp, as well as a 640 bp deletion in the *ltx* promoter, has been discovered in *A. actinomycetemcomitans* isolates [39,40]. These three different genotypes are all associated with high virulence due to enhanced production of LtxA. Whether the deletions or insertions per se are causing the increased leukotoxin production is not entirely clear.

Enhanced leukotoxicity has been reported from serotype b isolates with an intact *ltx* promoter region, indicating a high production of the toxin [41]. These isolates represent a subgroup of serotype b with a high association with disease progression in the infected individual. Genetic characterization of this subgroup showed a genetic pattern with similarities to that of the JP2 genotype, and such strains are frequently carried by young individuals with periodontitis [2,38,42]. A specific genetic marker (*cagE*) correlates to *A. actinomycetemcomitans* with enhanced leukotoxicity, including the JP2 genotype and other virulent serotype b isolates [42,43]. Interestingly, the activity of LtxA has been reported to be involved in induction of systemic autoantibodies to citrulline, which are risk markers for rheumatoid arthritis [17,44]. In addition, LtxA has a crucial role in sepsis induced by bacteremia in an animal model [45].

2.2. Leukotoxin Secretion

The secretion of LtxA is mediated by a Type I secretion system in line with other proteins of the repeat in toxin (RTX family) expressed by several Gram-negative pathogens [46–48]. A unique property for LtxA among the RTX proteins is that the secreted toxin is reported to be associated to the bacterial outer membrane [47]. The export of the toxin to the bacterial outer membrane has been shown to require expression of three proteins—LtxB, LtxD, and TdeA—for export of the toxin to the bacterial outer membrane, and a fourth—LtxC—for the acylation [49]. In addition, the inner membrane protein MorC, which affects the outer membrane structure, has been reported to be necessary for efficient export of the toxin [50]. The localization of LtxA was found to be on the outside of the bacterial membrane and on vesicles associated to the outer membrane [51,52]. The responsible mechanisms for the association of LtxA to the membrane are still not fully clarified, and whether the secreted LtxA remains associated to the bacterial outer membrane or is released to the environment is a topic of controversy. A suggestion is that the hydrophobic domain of LtxA mediates the association to the bacterial membrane [27]. Ohta and co-workers [53,54] reported that LtxA could be released from the bacterial membrane by DNase or RNase treatment, which indicates involvement of electrostatic forces between the negatively charged nucleic acid and the positively charged LtxA. This phenomenon was later supported by the observation that LtxA on the bacterial membrane and on vesicles was released in hypertonic NaCl solutions [55]. LtxA was also released from the bacterial membrane in presence of serum proteins, which indicates involvement of competitive mechanisms [56]. Differences in the culture media have been shown to determine the distribution of the produced LtxA between the bacterial outer membrane and the culture supernatant [56–58]. Whether LtxA is associated with the bacterial membrane or released to the environment at the infected site in vivo is still not known. However, the serum mediated release of the LtxA [56], as well as the activation of a systemic immunogenic response [59,60], indicates a release of LtxA from bacteria growing in an in vivo oral biofilm.

The secreted LtxA has been shown to be efficiently inactivated by proteases and superoxide radicals [55,61,62]. In 1981, McArthur and co-workers reported that the activity of LtxA in interaction with polymorphonuclear leukocytes (PMNs) was enhanced in the presence of human serum [63]. This phenomenon could later be explained by the protective effect of the serum protease inhibitors on the proteolytic enzymes released from LtxA challenged PMNs that degrades the toxin [56,64].

2.3. Quantification of LtxA Production

The great genetic diversity of *A. actinomycetemcomitans* has resulted in various genotypes with substantially different virulence properties, i.e., LtxA production [10,28]. The expression of LtxA is also influenced by environmental factors, such as growth conditions and substrates [46]. Notably, an anaerobic culture condition enhances substantially the production of LtxA, which mirrors the condition in the periodontal pocket [65].

Due to the complex regulation of *ltxA* expression, the balance between membrane-associated and secreted toxin, as well as its sensitivity to proteolytic degradation, a gold standard for quantification of LtxA production, is still not available. The first attempt to quantify LtxA activity was to add bacteria to isolated leukocytes and determine cell death by trypan blue exclusion [66]. In a study by Zambon and co-workers [67], the leukocyte lysis method was used to discriminate between leukotoxic and non-leukotoxic strains. This study showed that the prevalence of more leukotoxic variants of *A. actinomycetemcomitans* was higher in young individuals with periodontitis than in older individuals with the disease or in periodontally healthy individuals.

Except for examining the leukotoxicity of the isolates, methods targeting gene expression or immunodetection have been developed [58,68]. These methods have been employed on a limited number of *A. actinomycetemcomitans* isolates and support findings from previous leukotoxicity determinations, with enhanced expression in the JP2 genotype [69,70]. To obtain a gold standard for quantification of leukotoxicity of isolated *A. actinomycetemcomitans* is one of several challenges for future research.

3. Cytolethal Distending Toxin (CDT)

The CDT family comprises a number of bacterial protein exotoxins that is expressed by several Gram-negative species. Due to its deleterious effects on the host, as revealed in various experimental models, CDTs are likely to be involved in the etiopathogenesis of the associated human infections. They can be described as genotoxins, as their main action is to elicit DNA damage upon the intoxicated host cells [71]. The CDT holotoxin consists of subunits CdtA, CdtB, and CdtC. While CdtA and CdtC subunits mediate the internalization of the CdtB into the cell, the latter is translocated to the nucleus, causing its deleterious effects on the host cells. This subunit is functionally homologous to deoxyribonuclease I, hence it can cause DNA damage. It is postulated that CdtB internalization occurs via a mechanism involving the recognition of cell membrane cholesterol by both CdtC and CdtB [72,73].

A. actinomycetemcomitans expresses a CDT and is the only known oral species with this property. An estimated 66% to 86% of its strains express a CDT, and its presence has been associated with the occurrence of periodontal disease [74]. It is very plausible that its pathogenic effects are related to its capacity to cause DNA damage, cell cycle arrest, and eventually apoptosis to the intoxicated cells. This has been shown in structural cells like gingival fibroblasts and periodontal ligament cells [75,76], gingival epithelial cells [77–80], or gingival tissue explants [79], denoting that it can compromise the structural integrity and homeostatic capacity of the tissues. The capacity of CDT to affect the gingival epithelium has also been shown in human gingival explants [81], as well as in vivo upon inoculation of the toxin on rat gingival tissue [82]. Cells of the immune system are also highly susceptible to the cell cycle–arresting and apoptotic action of CDT, as has been demonstrated in human T cell [83], B-cells [84], and mononuclear cells [85]. CDT may also subvert the phagocytic capacity of macrophages and subvert their cytokine producing capacity [85]. The deleterious effects of CDT on cells of the immune system denote an impairment of the local immunity, which may compromise the capacity of the periodontium to recognize and eliminate the bacterial challenge, be it *A. actinomycetemcomitans* or other microbial constituents of the biofilm community.

Another potentially pathogenic mechanisms activated by CDT is the stimulation of pro-inflammatory and osteolytic cytokine production by the intoxicated host cells [86]. It has been shown that CDT can stimulate the production of pro-inflammatory cytokines by peripheral blood mononuclear cells, such as interferon (IFN)-γ, Interleukin (IL)-1β, IL-6, and IL-8, a virulence property potentially independent of the toxin's deoxyribonuclease I activity [85]. However, *A. actinomycetemcomitans* can stimulate the production of several pro-inflammatory cytokines and regulate inflammasome expression irrespective of its CDT, as demonstrated by the use of the *CDT*-deletion strains [87,88]. An important virulence property of CDT is revealed by its capacity to induce the major osteolytic factor receptor activator of nuclear factor kappa-B ligand (RANKL). This is a crucial molecule that stimulates the differentiation of osteoclasts and, consequently, bone resorption in periodontitis [89]. It has been shown that CDT induces RANKL expression and production in periodontal connective tissue cells, such as gingival fibroblasts and periodontal ligament cells [90,91], as well as T-cells [92]. This implies that the CDT may increase the levels RANKL in the periodontal tissues and therefore potentiate bone destruction by this action. The induction of inflammatory and bone-destructive molecular cascades in the periodontium by CDT may well constitute an additional mechanism through which *A. actinomycetemcomitans* is involved in the etiopathogenesis of periodontitis. On the other side of the bone remodeling equilibrium, when CDT acts directly on pre-osteoclasts, it may also induce apoptosis and hinder their differentiation to osteoclastic cells, thereby contributing a dysbalanced bone remodeling equilibrium that leads to periodontal breakdown [93].

4. Lipopolysaccharide and Cytokine-Binding Factors

4.1. The Virulence Properties of A. actinomycetemcomitans Lipopolysaccharide

Like other Gram-negative species, *A. actinomycetemcomitans* surface is covered by lipopolysaccharide (LPS), a potent pro-inflammatory molecule. *A. actinomycetemcomitans* LPS comprises a group of structurally related molecules in which the O-specific polysaccharide chain (O-antigen), formed by oligosaccharide repeating units, is the most variable portion (Figure 3).

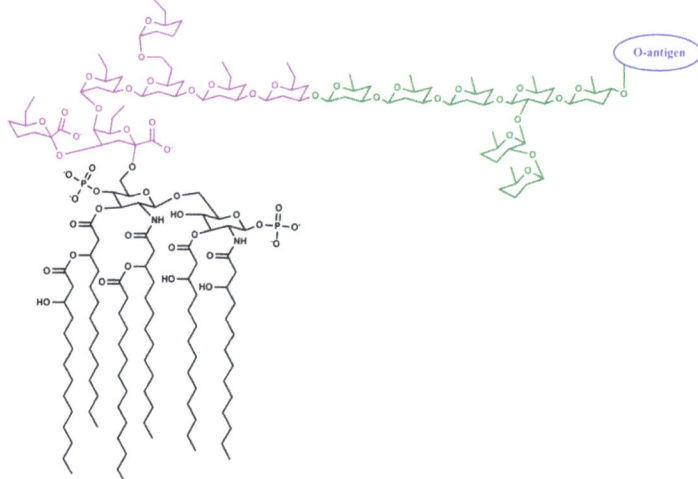

Figure 3. Schematic representation of a putative structure of the lipid A and the core oligosaccharides of *A. actinomycetemcomitans* lipopolysaccharide (LPS). The lipid A (black) of *A. actinomycetemcomitans* LPS is formed by four primary fatty acyl chains (myristic or 3-hydroxymyristic acid) linked by ester and amide linkages to a disaccharide of glucosamine. Two of the primary fatty acyl chains are esterified by secondary fatty acids. The acylation pattern of lipid A is asymmetric with four fatty acyl chains on the non-reducing glucosamine and two on the reducing glucosamine. The inner core (purple) is linked to lipid A by a ketosidic bond and is formed by 3-deoxy-D-*manno*-oct-2-ulosonic acid (Kdo) together with heptose residues such as *glycero-manno*-heptose. The outer core (green) usually consists of hexoses such as glucose and galactose. Functional groups such as hydroxyl and phosphate groups are common substituents in the lipid A and the core oligosaccharides. The O-specific polysaccharide chain (O-antigen) is the most variable portion in the LPS. The O-antigen consists of a large variety of sugar residues in many combinations and glycosidic linkages. For simplicity, substituents such as hydroxyl and phosphate groups (other than those in lipid A), conformational details of the monosaccharide residues, and the stereochemistry of the glycosidic bonds are not presented.

The serotyping of *A. actinomycetemcomitans* to seven different serotypes from a to f, as well as to non-serotypeable, is based on the structural differences in the O-antigen part of LPS. Commonly found monosaccharide residues in the *A. actinomycetemcomitans* O-antigen include the hexoses glucose, galactose, mannose, and talose; the hexosamines glucosamine and galactosamine; and the deoxyhexoses rhamnose and fucose. However, between different *A. actinomycetemcomitans* strains, there appears to be significant variation in the final architecture of the oligosaccharide repeating units, which may be either di-, tri-, or tetrasaccharide moieties [94–97]. Thus, variation in the gene clusters involved in the synthesis of the highly variable polysaccharide moieties serves as the basis for PCR serotyping of *A. actinomycetemcomitans* strains [94,98].

The structures of the core oligosaccharide and the lipid A in *A. actinomycetemcomitans* LPS have a lower degree of structural freedom than the O-antigenic polysaccharides. The core oligosaccharide consists of 3-deoxy-D-*manno*-oct-2-ulosonic acid (Kdo), *glycero-manno*-heptose, glucose, and galactose, and appears conserved among different serotypes [96,97]. The lipid A consists of two phosphorylated glucosamine residues [96,97] and primarily myristic and 3-hydroxymyristic acid as the fatty acyl chains [97,99–102]. Amino compounds such as ethanolamine and glycine are found associated with *A. actinomycetemcomitans* lipid A and core oligosaccharides but in fewer numbers than the commonly found hydroxyl and phosphate group substituents [97]. *A. actinomycetemcomitans* growth is favoured in slightly alkaline environments [103,104] in which the phosphate groups and the Kdo occur in deprotonated form. The phosphate groups and the Kdo interact with positively charged ions and participate in hydrogen bonding, and thus contribute to the stabilization of the bacterial outer membrane.

The fatty acyl composition of lipid A generally varies between different Gram-negative species. For example, in lipid A of *Escherichia coli* and *Salmonella typhimurium* LPS the relative amount of myristic acid is lower than in *A. actinomycetemcomitans* LPS, while lauric acid and palmitic acid are more frequently found [100]. The lipid A composition of closely related species may not always be specific enough to allow taxonomic differentiation, as demonstrated by the similar composition of *A. actinomycetemcomitans* and *Aggregatibacter aphrophilus* lipid A [100]. Closely related species may, however, be differentiated by the composition of their (core) oligosaccharides. A distinct feature of the oligosaccharides of *A. actinomycetemcomitans* is the presence of both D- and L-*glycero*-D-*manno*-heptose, whereas *A. aphrophilus* LPS only contains the L-enantiomer of this aldoheptose [105,106]. By contrast, galactose appeared twice as abundant in LPS from *A. aphrophilus* as in LPS from *A. actinomycetemcomitans* [99,105,106].

Although there are several studies that indicate a distinct effect of *A. actinomycetemcomitans* LPS on rodent cells [107–111], we will focus here on describing how *A. actinomycetemcomitans* LPS stimulates human cells. This outlining is done due to the known differences between the murine/rat and human immune systems [112]. The various virulence-related effects of *A. actinomycetemcomitans* LPS are summarized in Table 1. The first cells encountered by detached *A. actinomycetemcomitans* LPS in junctional epithelium (JE) of a tooth are the epithelial cells. These human epithelial cells have been shown to respond to *A. actinomycetemcomitans* LPS by expressing IL-15 which results in enhanced IFN-γ production and proliferation of human T cells [113]. Moreover, *A. actinomycetemcomitans* LPS causes widening of the intercellular spaces in primary tissue cultures mimicking the JE, a phenomenon not observed with *Porphyromonas gingivalis* LPS [113]. Various direct effects of *A. actinomycetemcomitans* LPS on the other main human gingival cell type, fibroblasts, have also been reported. Collagen is ingested and digested by gingival fibroblasts in balanced conditions of healthy gingiva. *A. actinomycetemcomitans* LPS is able to enhance the phagocytosis of collagen by fibroblasts which may result in imbalance in regeneration of the gingival tissue [114]. In addition to changes in cellular functions, *A. actinomycetemcomitans* LPS stimulate the production of IL-6 and IL-8 [114], tissue plasminogen activator (t-PA), and plasminogen activator inhibitor 2 (PAI-2) by human gingival fibroblasts [115]. The plasminogen/plasmin system is involved in the complex process of extracellular matrix degradation and renewal in the gingival tissue, a step that most likely precedes the collagen phagocytosis by the gingival fibroblasts.

Gingival tissue contains various resident immune cells, of which macrophages play a central role in periodontitis. *A. actinomycetemcomitans* LPS has shown to stimulate the expression of microRNA miR-146a [116], which downregulates the expression of TNF receptor–associated factor 6 and IL-1 receptor–associated kinase 1, which serves as a negative feedback loop in cytokine signaling [117].

On the contrary, high doses of *A. actinomycetemcomitans* LPS downregulated the expression of miR-32 and miR-29b, which target the pro-apoptotic factor Bim of acute myeloid leukemia cells [118] and IL-6 receptor α [117], respectively. Another human cell type that originates from mesenchymal stem cells is osteoblast which plays a significant role in bone formation. *A. actinomycetemcomitans* LPS has capacity to increase the inducible nitric oxide synthase (iNOS) activity and induce the nitric oxide (NO) production by human osteoblast-like cell line [119]. If osteoblasts produce NO rapidly, when responding to bacterial infection, it may lead to bone resorption [120].

Table 1. Virulence-related properties of *A. actinomycetemcomitans* LPS.

Target	Effect	Reference
Epithelial cells	IL-15 expression, widening of the intercellular spaces	[113,121]
Gingival fibroblasts	Enhancement of collagen phagocytosis, increase the production of IL-8, IL-6, t-PA, PAI-2	[114–116,122]
Macrophages	Upregulation of miR-146a and downregulation of miR-32 and miR-29b microRNAs	
Osteoblasts	Increases iNOS activity and induce NO production	[119,123,124]
Dendritic cells	Production of IL-12, IFN-γ, TNF-α, IL-1β, IL-6, and IL-23	
PMN	Induce ROS production, stimulate IL-1β, TNF-α, and IL-6 production, downregulate surface expression of L-selectin, upregulate the expression of β2-integrins	[125–128]
Human hemoglobin	Binding	[129]
Human IL-8	Binding	[130]

Another type of resident immune cells in periodontium is dendritic cells (DCs), which are involved in antigen presenting to T cells. Conventional DCs originate from monocytes, like macrophages, and are called mDCs. Monocytes originating from localized aggressive periodontitis (LagP) patients, recently renamed molar-incisor pattern periodontitis with rapid progression [131], spontaneously give rise to mDCs [132]. *A. actinomycetemcomitans* LPS enhances the IL-12 production by mDCs leading to stimulation of IFN-γ expression of natural killer cells and undetectable levels of IL-4, which together may cause the polarization of naïve T cells toward the Th1 type response [123]. There are differences of DCs stimulation potential of *A. actinomycetemcomitans* LPS originating from different serotypes, serotype b LPS inducing the strongest production of IL-12, IFN-γ, TNF-α, IL-1β, IL-6, and IL-23 [124]. The differences in the response of DCs to serotype b *A. actinomycetemcomitans* LPS compared to the response to other serotype LPS most likely causes Th1/Th17 type of T cell response in serotype b related infection [133].

PMNs are innate immune cells which may play both defensive and destructive role in periodontitis [134]. Neutrophils produce reactive oxygen species (ROS) when responding to whole bacteria or their components. *A. actinomycetemcomitans* LPS has been shown to be more potent inducer of neutrophil ROS production than, for example, *P. gingivalis* or *Prevotella intermedia* LPS [125]. Moreover, *A. actinomycetemcomitans* LPS stimulate the production of inflammatory cytokines IL-1β and TNF-α by PMN more efficiently than *P. gingivalis* LPS [126], and in human whole blood, *A. actinomycetemcomitans* LPS causes higher production of the above mentioned cytokines as well as IL-6 than *E. coli* LPS [127]. *A. actinomycetemcomitans* LPS can shift the movement of monocytes and granulocytes from rolling to the passaging through the vascular wall by downregulating the surface expression of L-selectin and increasing the expression of β2 integrins, respectively [128].

Despite the vast literature concerning the inflammatory related functions of *A. actinomycetemcomitans* LPS, this outer membrane linked polysaccharide has also functions related to bacterial physiology. The serotype specific O-antigen part of *A. actinomycetemcomitans* LPS takes part in the secretion of leukotoxin, since a serotype b mutant with inactive *rmlC* and altered

O-antigen sugar composition, contained more cytoplasmic and membrane-bound leukotoxin, and secreted less leukotoxin than the wild-type serotype b strain [135]. Moreover, the O-antigen part of *A. actinomycetemcomitans* LPS may mediate direct adhesion to abiotic surfaces [7]. Besides abiotic surfaces, *A. actinomycetemcomitans* LPS interacts with host molecules, such as human hemoglobin [129] and IL-8 [136], which may facilitate the iron acquisition and disturbance of host defense, respectively.

4.2. Sensing of Host Signal Molecules

A. actinomycetemcomitans is one of the human pathogens that is able to bind host cytokines, such as IL-1β, IL-8, and IL-6 [137,138], and internalize them [138,139], which leads to changes in the properties of biofilm, decreasing the metabolic activity [139], and changing the composition of the extracellular matrix [136,138]. Several potential bacterial proteins that may interact with human cytokines have been identified in *A. actinomyctemcomitans*, including intracellular ATP synthase subunit β [139], histone like DNA binding protein HU [139], and outer membrane proteins bacterial interleukin receptor I (BilRI) [138,140] and secretin channel HofQ [136]. The majority of these proteins have other functions in the bacterial cell related to metabolism, gene regulation, and uptake of nutrients and DNA for horizontal gene transfer, a character of so called "moonlighting" bacterial proteins [1]. Interactions with the above mentioned proteins may result in the observed uptake of cytokines, decreased metabolic activity and potentially, although not yet proved, also changes in the gene expression profile of *A. actinomycetemcomitans*. Both Gram-positive *Staphylococcus aureus* [141] and Gram-negatives *Pseudomonas aeruginosa* [142] and *Neisseria meningitidis* [143] are able to respond to cytokines, such as IL-1β, IFN-γ, IL-8, and TNF-α, by changing their virulence gene expression pattern.

Human cytokines are not the only host signalling molecules that *A. actinomyctemcomitans* is able to bind and sense. *A. actinomyctemcomitans* harbours the two-component system QseCB, which has originally been detected from enterohemorrhagic *Escherichia coli* EHEC [144]. In EHEC, QseCB senses either endogenous autoinducer-3 or host catecholamine hormones epinephrine/norepinephrine and induces the expression of Locus of Enterocyte Effacement (LEE) vital for the virulence of EHEC [145]. However, *A. actinomycetemcomitans* needs also iron, in addition to catecholamine hormone, to activate the QseC sensor kinase [146]. The QseCB signalling changes the gene expression pattern of *A. actinomycetemcomitans*, and especially the genes needed for anaerobic metabolisms are upregulated [146]. Moreover, QseC plays role in the biofilm formation in a flow cell in vitro model, since ΔqseC mutant strain forms significantly less biofilm in flow cells than the corresponding *A. actinomyctemcomitans* wild type and the complemented strains [147]. It is not known whether this impaired capacity to form biofilms also affects the virulence potential of *A. actinomyctemcomitans* in vivo. Yet, ΔqseC mutant strain causes less bone loss in murine model of periodontitis than the wild-type strain, suggesting a strong link between *A. actinomycetemcomitans* QseC and virulence [147].

5. Outer Membrane Vesicles

During the latest decades it has become apparent that membrane vesicles (MVs) are naturally shed during growth by many bacteria, archaea, and eukaryotes. Membrane vesicles, also known as "Type Zero secretion", or referred to as outer membrane vesicles (OMVs) in Gram-negative organisms, serve as a general but relevant mechanism of antigen delivery, and are discharged by both commensal and pathogenic organisms in vivo and when infecting host cells in vitro [148,149]. Biologically active virulence factors such as CDT and OmpA can be transported into HeLa cells and human gingival fibroblasts via *A. actinomycetemcomitans* OMVs [150]. OMVs are also involved in the export of leukotoxin, peptidoglycan-associated lipoprotein (Pal), and the chaperonin GroEL to host cells [52,151–153]. Characterization of the OMV proteome of one *A. actinomycetemcomitans* clinical isolate using Matrix-Assisted Laser Desorption/Ionization Time of Flight-Mass Spectrometry (MALDI-TOF MS) revealed an array of additional tentative virulence-related proteins, including BilRI, Omp100, TdeA, and a ferritin-like protein [154,155]. This is in line with an OMV proteome exhibiting multiple offensive and defensive functions, such as drug targeting, iron acquisition, and immune evasion. A role of *A. actinomycetemcomitans* OMVs in serum resistance can be hypothesized based on observations that the vesicles could bind to the complement system regulator C4-binding protein in an OmpA-dependent manner [156]. Moreover, it has been shown that *A. actinomycetemcomitans* OMVs can transport small molecules such as those contributing to bone resorption, including LPS [157] and lipid A-associated proteins [158]. *A. actinomycetemcomitans* OMVs carry NOD1- and NOD2-active peptidoglycan, and upon vesicle internalization into non-phagocytic human cells such as gingival fibroblasts, the OMVs can act as an innate immunity trigger [9]. *A. actinomycetemcomitans* OMVs contain in addition nucleic acids [53], and recent evidence supports the concept that the OMVs can carry microRNA-sized small RNAs (msRNAs). These small RNAs might represent novel bacterial signaling molecules, which by means of OMVs can be transported into host cells to modulate the immune response [159]. *A. actinomycetemcomitans* OMVs appear to mainly internalize into host cells via clathrin-dependent endocytosis [9,160] but can also fuse with host cell membranes in a cholesterol-dependent manner [150]. Toxins associated with OMVs can function as adhesins in receptor-mediated endocytosis of vesicles [161], but such a role of CDT or leukotoxin appears less likely, as neither of the toxins are required for the uptake of OMVs into host cells [150,151]. Additionally, despite the evident localization of leukotoxin on the surface of *A. actinomycetemcomitans* OMVs, there is no requirement of the toxin receptor LFA1 for vesicle-mediated trafficking of LtxA into host cells [162].

6. Biofilm Interactions and Proteomic Regulations

6.1. Localization in Pocket and Tissue

As a microaerophic organism, *A. actinomycetemcomitans* is able to grow both supragingivally and subgingivally, corresponding to aerobic and anaerobic growth, respectively. As it can be detected at both locations, it has been postulated that the environment of supragingival plaque harbouring *A. actinomycetemcomitans* can act as a reservoir for the spread or reinfection of this bacterium of subgingivally [163]. When growing subgingivally, *A. actinomycetemcomitans* is reported to be detected in the loosely attached unattached plaque area in the middle pocket zone [164]. Earlier histopathological studies determined the prevalence and gingival localization of *A. actinomycetemcomitans* in periodontal lesions of juvenile periodontitis patients (earlier classification), using culture techniques on disrupted tissue or immunofluorescence microscopy on intact tissue. The former demonstrated the presence of *A. actinomycetemcomitans* in almost all diseased tissues examined, with evidence of microcolonies and single bacterial cells within the gingival connective tissue, as well as inside the phagocytic cells within the tissue [165]. The latter demonstrated an increase in *A. actinomycetemcomitans* colony-forming units, which correlated with its presence in the tissue and in the periodontal pocket [165]. In situ hybridization studies have detected *A. actinomycetemcomitans* in epithelial cells from the lining gingival crevice [166] or in close relationship with the polymorphonuclear infiltrate of the pocket [167]. By quantitative real-time PCR of gingival tissue lysates, it was shown that *A. actinomycetemcomitans* is present at a higher prevalence in tissues of younger patients with aggressive periodontitis as compared to chronic periodontitis or health [168].

6.2. Localization in Biofilms and Proteomic Interactions with Other Species

Studies on the localization of *A. actimomycetemcomitans* in biofilms largely comes from in vitro models. In supragingival and subgingival biofilms, *A. actinomycetemcomitans* does not appear to affect the number of the other species present and appears to form small, dense, and secluded cell clusters of its own species throughout the biofilm mass [169,170]. Yet, the lack of numeric changes on other species of the biofilm does exclude the possibility that *A. actinomycetemcomitans* exerts regulatory proteomic and metabolic changes in the biofilm, as discussed further.

The development of mass spectrometry (MS) technology made it possible to identify multiple proteins in a single run. Therefore, it is a useful tool to study how *A. actinomycetemcomitans* orchestrates proteomic changes in the context of biofilms. Using 2D gels, Llama-Palacios et al. discovered 87 protein spots differently expressed (1.5-fold, $p < 0.05$) between planktonic and mono-species biofilm cultures of *A. actinomycetemcomitans* [171]. Then, using MALDI-TOF MS, 13 upregulated proteins (from 24 proteins spots) and 37 downregulated proteins (from 50 spots) were identified. The upregulated proteins were mainly outer membrane proteins involved the immunologic process, whereas downregulated proteins were related to the metabolism, biosynthesis, and transport. This is consistent with the finding that mature biofilms display increased virulence [172] despite lower metabolic activity [173] as compared to planktonic culture.

Because oral biofilms occur as complex polymicrobial communities, the study of *A. actinomycetemcomitans* within multispecies biofilms is highly relevant. When integrated within a 10-species subgingival biofilm model, *A. actinomycetemcomitans* did not significantly impact the abundance of the other bacterial species, nor did it affect the biofilm structure, which is consistent with findings in a supragingival biofilm model. Using liquid chromatography–tandem mass spectrometry (LC-MS/MS), 3225 and 3352 microbial proteins were identified in multi-species biofilms in the absence or presence of *A. actinomycetemcomitans*, respectively [170]. Further investigations with label-free quantification (LFQ) method displayed 728 bacterial proteins and found 483 of them to be differentially regulated (2-fold, $p < 0.05$) among these two kinds of biofilms. Interestingly, the regulation trend for individual species was highly individual. For *Prevotella intermedia*, all quantified proteins were upregulated in the presence of *A. actinomycetemcomitans*, whereas the majority of the proteins were downregulated for *Campylobacter rectus*, *Streptococcus anginosus*, and *P. gingivalis*. These findings are well in line with the competing growth between *P. gingivalis* and *A. actinomycetemcomitans*, shown in a dual-species biofilm [174]. Furthermore, based on the GO analysis, *A. actinomycetemcomitans* appears to downregulate proteins with ferric iron binding functions and alter the metabolic rate for the overall biofilm.

To understand the effects of this *A. actinomycetemcomitans*-containing biofilms on host tissues, the biofilm model was introduced into a bioreactor-supervised 3D cell culture system, which consisted of epithelial and connective tissue structures to mimic the periodontium, as well as monocytes to stimulate the immune response [173]. As a result, *S. anginosus*, *A. oris*, *V. dispar*, *C. rectus*, and *P. gingivalis* were suppressed when present with the host tissue, while the tissue itself exhibited morphological, immunological, and proteomic changes. The numbers of *A. actinomycetemcomitans* in the biofilm were not reduced, but more of its proteins were expressed when co-cultured with the 3D (21 proteins) than the biofilm stand-alone (15 proteins) [173]. Yet, *A. actinomycetemcomitans* proteins only comprised a small fraction of all identified proteins in biofilm lysates (21 of 3363) and supernatants (one of 896).

Attachment to biotic surfaces or other biofilms enhances *A. actinomyctemcomitans* virulence properties. We have found that deletion of the gene *hns*, encoding a histone-like family of DNA-binding, nucleoid-structuring protein (H-NS), a global gene silencer [179], leads to a less piliated phenotype of *A. actinomycetemcomitans* and decreases its biofilm formation ability when cultured as mono-species biofilms [11]. LFQ showed that the majority (29) of the differentially expressed proteins (2-fold, $p < 0.05$) were upregulated in the *hns* mutant biofilm, supporting the role of H-NS as gene suppressor in *A. actinomyctemcomitans*. Notably, the affected proteins included virulence factors such as leukotoxin A and D (LtxA and LtxD). A similar repression activity of H-NS for virulence factors from other microbes was observed on hemolysin operons *hlyCABD* [180] and *ehxCABD* [181] in *E. coli* and *rtxACBD* in *Vibrio cholerae* [182]. Within multi-species biofilms, using the *hns* mutant there was a significant reduction of *A. actinomycetemcomitans* numbers, without affecting the number of other species. On the protein level, LFQ data suggested that many *Fusobacterium nucleatum* and *Streptococcus oralis* proteins were downregulated in biofilm harbouring the wild-type *A. actinomyctemcomitans* strain, as compared to its *hns* mutant counterpart, and these proteomic regulations may occur long before the corresponding bacterial growth is affected. Most of the regulated proteins were associated with peptide metabolic process and regulation of translation, supporting a protein-orchestrating role of H-NS in *A. actinomycetemcomitans*.

A literature summary of the proteomic findings on *A. actinomycetemcomitans* in single-species biofilms and multi-species biofilms is provided in Tables 2 and 3, respectively.

Table 2. Proteomic studies on single species *A. actinomycetemcomitans*.

Author	Year (Ref)	Brief Description	Identified Proteins *	Proteomic Application, Label Free Quantification	Cutoff	PMID
Llama-Palacios et al.	2017 [171]	A.a planktonic and mono-species biofilm cultures	50	2DE, MALDI-TOF MS	N/A	28707473
Kieselbach T et al.	2016 [155]	A.a outer membrane vesicles dataset	501	In solution digestion, LC-MS/MS	protein FDR < 1%	28050585
Kieselbach T et al.	2015 [154]	A.a outer membrane vesicles	151	In solution digestion, LC-MS/MS	protein FDR < 1%	26381655
Smith KP et al.	2015 [175]	A.a membrane proteins related to morphogenesis protein C	613	Stable-isotope dimethyl labeling, nanoscale LC-MS	FP < 1%	25684173
Smith KP et al.	2015 [176]	A.a membrane proteins	648	Stable-isotope dimethyl labeling, nanoscale LC-MS	FP < 1%	25055881
Zijnge V et al.	2012 [177]	A.a secreted proteins from mono-species biofilm	179	2DE, HCT-Ultra ETD II IT-MS	Peptide ion score > 30	22848560
Rylev M et al.	2011 [178]	A.a JP2 strain HK1651	114	2DE, MALDI-TOF MS	N/A	21867783

Ion trap: IT, False positive: FP, False-discovery rate: FDR, Matrix assisted laser desorption ionization: MALDI, Time of flight mass spectrometry: TOF MS, Mass spectrometer: MS. * Maximum identified/quantified proteins were report base on the following rules: (1) Only maximum identified protein number was reported if the experiment was done under different conditions. (2) Total protein numbers were reported if the experiment has replicates. (3) The number of identified and quantified proteins were reported if only regulated protein were reported.

Table 3. Proteomic studies on multi-species biofilms including *A. actinomycetemcomitans*.

Author	Year (Ref)	Brief Description	Identified Proteins *	Proteomic Application	Peptide Cutoff	PMID
Bao et al.	2018 [169]	A. a hns + 10 species biofilms **	3352	Orbitrap Fusion, LFQ	2≥	25483866
Bao et al.	2015 [183]	10-species biofilm model * Vs 3D culture **	3363	Q-Exactive MS, LFQ	2≥	26525412
Bao et al.	2015 [170]	A. a + 10 species biofilms **	3352	Q-Exactive MS, LFQ	2≥	25756960

A.a: *A. actinomycetemcomitans*, Label free quantification: LFQ, Matrix-assisted laser desorption ionization- time of flight mass spectrometry: MALDI-TOF MS, Two-Dimensional Differential Gel Electrophoresis: 2DE, * Maxium identified/quantified proteins were report base on the following rules: (1) Only maximum identified protein number was reported if the experiment was done under different conditions. (2) Total protein numbers were reported if the experiment has replicates. (3) The number of identified and quantified proteins were reported if only regulated protein were reported. ** 10-species biofilm model (consisting of *Campylobacter rectus, Fusobacterium nucleatum, Porphyromonas gingivalis, Prevotella intermedia, Tannerella forsythia, Treponema denticola, Veillonella dispar, Actinomyces oris, Streptococcus anginosous, Streptococcus oralis*).

7. Horizontal Gene Transfer

A. actinomycetemcomitans strains can be divided into competent and non-competent ones, which refer to their ability to acquire new genes from up-taken extracellular DNA (eDNA) using homologous recombination. Competent strains may have some advantage of being able to uptake eDNA, which could be related to additional means to repair DNA damage, obtain nucleotides and possibly also novel genes [184]. Approximately 30% of clinical *A. actinomycetemcomitans* strains are naturally competent [185], leading to greater genetic diversity, whereas noncompetent strains are genetically stable and need to use other mechanisms, such as conjugative plasmids, for horizontal gene transfer (HGT) [186]. It is thought that the ancestral Pasteurellacean was naturally competent and that noncompetent lineages lost their ability to take up DNA due to various mutations in the competence gene locus [187]. This may explain the findings that noncompetent strains are more common among some serotype groups, such as serotype b and c [185]. The competence gene locus consists of regulatory *sxy*, DNA uptake–related *comABCDE*, *pilABCD*, *comEAFE1*, *rec2*, and transformation-related *comM* and *urpA* [186,188,189]. Noncompetent strains may contain nonsense mutations, or insertions in one or several of these genes, which makes the strain either unable to uptake eDNA and/or to incorporate it into the genome [186]. In addition to the above described gene locus, the CRISPR-*cas* system is also closely involved in natural competence, since the loss of CRISPR-*cas* system is connected to the loss of competence [186]. Thus, non-competent *A. actinomycetemcomitans* strains are more prone to HGT caused by plasmids and phages. However, in the non-competent strains, the maintained CRISPRs contains few spacers that most likely are used for chromosomal gene regulation, since they possess specificity for endogenous genes [186].

The expression on genes of competence locus are regulated by *sxy* (*tfoX*), of which levels in the cell is affected by various environmental factors, such as extracellular calcium ions [190] and the biofilm mode of growth [190]. Moreover, in addition to competence locus and CRISPR-*cas* system, the development of competence and expression levels of *sxy* are stimulated by cyclic AMP [191] and affected by the *pga* gene cluster [190], respectively. The genes in *pga* cluster are needed in the production of most abundant extracellular polysaccharide, N-acetyl-D-glucosamine, in *A. actinomycetemcomitans* biofilms.

Naturally competent *A. actinomycetemcomitans* strains recognize related eDNA, which is suitable to be taken up, using uptake signal sequence (USS). The *Pasteurellaceae* family has two types of USS, *Hin* and *ApI*, which contain distinctive consensus sequences of nine base pairs. *A. actinomycetemcomitans* has *Hin* type USS, consisting of *A. actinomycetemcomitans* GTGCGGT consensus sequence followed by AT-rich repeats [187,191]. This sequence is most likely recognized by the outer membrane proteins involved in the eDNA uptake. However, the recognizing protein has not yet been identified.

8. Conclusions

Aggregatibacter actinomycetemcomitans is a facultative anaerobic Gram-negative bacterium with the capacity to employ many virulence mechanisms closely associated to the pathogenesis of periodontitis. The variety of virulence properties of this bacterium contribute to the pathogenicity of this species, particularly with regard to early and rapidly progressive forms of periodontal disease. *A. actinomycetemcomitans* can be found in a large proportion of the human population, and due to the large genetic diversity of this species, several different genotypes or phenotypes with various virulence properties have emerged. Without doubt, individuals carrying *A. actinomycetemcomitans* genotypes with a proven enhanced leukotoxin production have a significantly increased risk to develop disease. More recent studies have identified suitable genes of this species, which can potentially be traced as markers for epidemiological population monitoring and utilization in individual risk assessment programs. Such bacterial virulence markers in periodontal disease may prove to be important tools in future strategies for personalized dentistry.

Author Contributions: Conceptualization, A.J., G.N.B., N.B., J.O., K.B., M.L., R.I., and T.M; Leukotoxin, A.J.; Cytolethal distending toxin, G.N.B.; Outer membrane vesicles, M.L. and J.O.; Lipopolysaccharides, cytokine binding and horizontal gene transfer, R.I. and T.M.; Proteomic N.B. and K.B.; Data Curation, A.J., R.I., and J.O.; Writing—Original Draft Preparation, A.J. and G.N.B.; Writing—Review & Editing, A.J., G.N.B., N.B., J.O., K.B., M.L., R.I., and T.M.

Funding: This work was supported by institutional funds and by funds from the Swedish Research Council (N.B.; 2017-01198), TUA grants from the County Council of Västerbotten, Sweden (A.J.; 7003193), and the Academy of Finland (R.I.; 265609, 303781).

Acknowledgments: We thank the European Network for *A. actinomycetemcomitans* Research (https://projects.au.dk/aggregatibacter/) for encouraging us to prepare this review. In addition, we thank Rolf Claesson for the nice photos for Figure 1 and Sotirios Kalfas for excellent artwork in Figure 2.

Conflicts of Interest: The authors declare no conflict of interest.

References

1. Henderson, B.; Ward, J.M.; Ready, D. *Aggregatibacter (Actinobacillus) actinomycetemcomitans*: A triple A* periodontopathogen? *Periodontology 2000* **2010**, *54*, 78–105. [CrossRef] [PubMed]
2. Åberg, C.H.; Kelk, P.; Johansson, A. *Aggregatibacter actinomycetemcomitans*: Virulence of its leukotoxin and association with aggressive periodontitis. *Virulence* **2015**, *6*, 188–195. [CrossRef] [PubMed]
3. Fine, D.H.; Patil, A.G.; Velusamy, S.K. *Aggregatibacter actinomycetemcomitans* (Aa) Under the Radar: Myths and Misunderstandings of Aa and Its Role in Aggressive Periodontitis. *Front. Immunol.* **2019**, *10*, 728. [CrossRef] [PubMed]
4. Johansson, A. *Aggregatibacter actinomycetemcomitans leukotoxin*: A powerful tool with capacity to cause imbalance in the host inflammatory response. *Toxins* **2011**, *3*, 242–259. [CrossRef] [PubMed]
5. Vega, B.A.; Belinka, B.A., Jr.; Kachlany, S.C. *Aggregatibacter actinomycetemcomitans* Leukotoxin (LtxA.; Leukothera((R))): Mechanisms of Action and Therapeutic Applications. *Toxins* **2019**, *11*, 489. [CrossRef]
6. DiRienzo, J.M. Breaking the Gingival Epithelial Barrier: Role of the *Aggregatibacter actinomycetemcomitans* Cytolethal Distending Toxin in Oral Infectious Disease. *Cells* **2014**, *3*, 476–499. [CrossRef]
7. Fujise, O.; Wang, Y.; Chen, W.; Chen, C. Adherence of *Aggregatibacter actinomycetemcomitans* via serotype-specific polysaccharide antigens in lipopolysaccharides. *Oral Microbiol. Immunol.* **2008**, *23*, 226–233. [CrossRef]
8. Oscarsson, J.; Claesson, R.; Lindholm, M.; Höglund Åberg, C.; Johansson, A. Tools of *Aggregatibacter actinomycetemcomitans* to Evade the Host Response. *J. Clin. Med.* **2019**, *8*, 1079. [CrossRef]
9. Thay, B.; Damm, A.; Kufer, T.A.; Wai, S.N.; Oscarsson, J. *Aggregatibacter actinomycetemcomitans* outer membrane vesicles are internalized in human host cells and trigger NOD1- and NOD2-dependent NF-kappaB activation. *Infect. Immun.* **2014**, *82*, 4034–4046. [CrossRef]
10. Kittichotirat, W.; Bumgarner, R.E.; Chen, C. Evolutionary Divergence of *Aggregatibacter actinomycetemcomitans*. *J. Dent. Res.* **2016**, *95*, 94–101. [CrossRef]
11. Bao, K.; Bostanci, N.; Thurnheer, T.; Grossmann, J.; Wolski, W.E.; Thay, B.; Belibasakis, G.N.; Oscarsson, J. *Aggregatibacter actinomycetemcomitans* H-NS promotes biofilm formation and alters protein dynamics of other species within a polymicrobial oral biofilm. *NPJ Biofilms Microbiomes* **2018**, *4*, 12. [CrossRef] [PubMed]
12. Belibasakis, G.N.; Bostanci, N.; Marsh, P.D.; Zaura, E. Applications of the oral microbiome in personalized dentistry. *Arch. Oral Biol.* **2019**, *104*, 7–12. [CrossRef] [PubMed]
13. Claesson, R.; Johansson, A.; Belibasakis, G.; Hanstrom, L.; Kalfas, S. Release and activation of matrix metalloproteinase 8 from human neutrophils triggered by the leukotoxin of *Actinobacillus actinomycetemcomitans*. *J. Periodontal Res.* **2002**, *37*, 353–359. [CrossRef] [PubMed]
14. Johansson, A.; Claesson, R.; Hanstrom, L.; Sandstrom, G.; Kalfas, S. Polymorphonuclear leukocyte degranulation induced by leukotoxin from *Actinobacillus actinomycetemcomitans*. *J. Periodontal Res.* **2000**, *35*, 85–92. [CrossRef]
15. Hirschfeld, J.; Roberts, H.M.; Chapple, I.L.; Parcina, M.; Jepsen, S.; Johansson, A.; Claesson, R. Effects of *Aggregatibacter actinomycetemcomitans* leukotoxin on neutrophil migration and extracellular trap formation. *J. Oral Microbiol.* **2016**, *8*, 33070. [CrossRef]
16. Lopes, J.P.; Stylianou, M.; Backman, E.; Holmberg, S.; Jass, J.; Claesson, R.; Urban, C.F. Evasion of Immune Surveillance in Low Oxygen Environments Enhances *Candida albicans* Virulence. *mBio* **2018**, *9*. [CrossRef]
17. Konig, M.F.; Abusleme, L.; Reinholdt, J.; Palmer, R.J.; Teles, R.P.; Sampson, K.; Rosen, A.; Nigrovic, P.A.; Sokolove, J.; Giles, J.T.; et al. *Aggregatibacter actinomycetemcomitans*-induced hypercitrullination links periodontal infection to autoimmunity in rheumatoid arthritis. *Sci. Transl. Med.* **2016**, *8*, 369ra176. [CrossRef]
18. DiFranco, K.M.; Gupta, A.; Galusha, L.E.; Perez, J.; Nguyen, T.V.; Fineza, C.D.; Kachlany, S.C. Leukotoxin (Leukothera(R)) targets active leukocyte function antigen-1 (LFA-1) protein and triggers a lysosomal mediated cell death pathway. *J. Biol. Chem.* **2012**, *287*, 17618–17627. [CrossRef]
19. Kelk, P.; Abd, H.; Claesson, R.; Sandstrom, G.; Sjostedt, A.; Johansson, A. Cellular and molecular response of human macrophages exposed to *Aggregatibacter actinomycetemcomitans* leukotoxin. *Cell Death Dis.* **2011**, *2*, e126. [CrossRef]
20. Haubek, D.; Johansson, A. Pathogenicity of the highly leukotoxic JP2 clone of *Aggregatibacter actinomycetemcomitans* and its geographic dissemination and role in aggressive periodontitis. *J. Oral Microbiol.* **2014**, *6*. [CrossRef]

21. Kononen, E.; Gursoy, M.; Gursoy, U.K. Periodontitis: A Multifaceted Disease of Tooth-Supporting Tissues. *J. Clin. Med.* **2019**, *8*, 1135. [CrossRef]
22. Lally, E.T.; Golub, E.E.; Kieba, I.R. Identification and immunological characterization of the domain of *Actinobacillus actinomycetemcomitans* leukotoxin that determines its specificity for human target cells. *J. Biol. Chem.* **1994**, *269*, 31289–31295.
23. Lally, E.T.; Kieba, I.R.; Sato, A.; Green, C.L.; Rosenbloom, J.; Korostoff, J.; Wang, J.F.; Shenker, B.J.; Ortlepp, S.; Robinson, M.K.; et al. RTX toxins recognize a beta2 integrin on the surface of human target cells. *J. Biol. Chem.* **1997**, *272*, 30463–30469. [CrossRef]
24. Dileepan, T.; Kachlany, S.C.; Balashova, N.V.; Patel, J.; Maheswaran, S.K. Human CD18 is the functional receptor for *Aggregatibacter actinomycetemcomitans* leukotoxin. *Infect. Immun.* **2007**, *75*, 4851–4856. [CrossRef]
25. Kieba, I.R.; Fong, K.P.; Tang, H.Y.; Hoffman, K.E.; Speicher, D.W.; Klickstein, L.B.; Lally, E.T. *Aggregatibacter actinomycetemcomitans* leukotoxin requires beta-sheets 1 and 2 of the human CD11a beta-propeller for cytotoxicity. *Cell. Microbiol.* **2007**, *9*, 2689–2699. [CrossRef]
26. Ristow, L.C.; Tran, V.; Schwartz, K.J.; Pankratz, L.; Mehle, A.; Sauer, J.D.; Welch, R.A. The Extracellular Domain of the beta2 Integrin beta Subunit (CD18) Is Sufficient for *Escherichia coli* Hemolysin and *Aggregatibacter actinomycetemcomitans* Leukotoxin Cytotoxic Activity. *mBio* **2019**, *10*. [CrossRef]
27. Lally, E.T.; Hill, R.B.; Kieba, I.R.; Korostoff, J. The interaction between RTX toxins and target cells. *Trends Microbiol.* **1999**, *7*, 356–361. [CrossRef]
28. Kittichotirat, W.; Bumgarner, R.E.; Asikainen, S.; Chen, C. Identification of the pangenome and its components in 14 distinct *Aggregatibacter actinomycetemcomitans* strains by comparative genomic analysis. *PLoS ONE* **2011**, *6*, e22420. [CrossRef]
29. Haubek, D. The highly leukotoxic JP2 clone of *Aggregatibacter actinomycetemcomitans*: Evolutionary aspects, epidemiology and etiological role in aggressive periodontitis. *APMIS Suppl.* **2010**, 1–53. [CrossRef]
30. Zambon, J.J. *Actinobacillus actinomycetemcomitans* in adult periodontitis. *J. Periodontol.* **1994**, *65*, 892–893. [CrossRef]
31. Haubek, D.; Ennibi, O.K.; Poulsen, K.; Vaeth, M.; Poulsen, S.; Kilian, M. Risk of aggressive periodontitis in adolescent carriers of the JP2 clone of *Aggregatibacter (Actinobacillus) actinomycetemcomitans* in Morocco: A prospective longitudinal cohort study. *Lancet* **2008**, *371*, 237–242. [CrossRef]
32. Höglund Åberg, C.; Kwamin, F.; Claesson, R.; Dahlen, G.; Johansson, A.; Haubek, D. Progression of attachment loss is strongly associated with presence of the JP2 genotype of *Aggregatibacter actinomycetemcomitans*: A prospective cohort study of a young adolescent population. *J. Clin. Periodontol.* **2014**, *41*, 232–241. [CrossRef]
33. Brogan, J.M.; Lally, E.T.; Poulsen, K.; Kilian, M.; Demuth, D.R. Regulation of *Actinobacillus actinomycetemcomitans* leukotoxin expression: Analysis of the promoter regions of leukotoxic and minimally leukotoxic strains. *Infect. Immun.* **1994**, *62*, 501–508.
34. Tsai, C.C.; Ho, Y.P.; Chou, Y.S.; Ho, K.Y.; Wu, Y.M.; Lin, Y.C. *Aggregatibacter (Actinobacillus) actimycetemcomitans* leukotoxin and human periodontitis—A historic review with emphasis on JP2. *Kaohsiung J. Med. Sci.* **2018**, *34*, 186–193. [CrossRef]
35. Zambon, J.J.; Haraszthy, V.I.; Hariharan, G.; Lally, E.T.; Demuth, D.R. The Microbiology of Early-Onset Periodontitis: Association of Highly Toxic *Actinobacillus actinomycetemcomitans* Strains with Localized Juvenile Periodontitis. *J. Periodontol.* **1996**, *67* (Suppl. 3S), 282–290. [CrossRef]
36. Aberg, C.H.; Kwamin, F.; Claesson, R.; Johansson, A.; Haubek, D. Presence of JP2 and Non-JP2 Genotypes of *Aggregatibacter actinomycetemcomitans* and attachment loss in adolescents in Ghana. *J. Periodontol.* **2012**, *83*, 1520–1528. [CrossRef]
37. Claesson, R.; Lagervall, M.; Hoglund-Aberg, C.; Johansson, A.; Haubek, D. Detection of the highly leucotoxic JP2 clone of *Aggregatibacter actinomycetemcomitans* in members of a Caucasian family living in Sweden. *J. Clin. Periodontol.* **2011**, *38*, 115–121. [CrossRef]
38. Claesson, R.; Höglund-Åberg, C.; Haubek, D.; Johansson, A. Age-related prevalence and characteristics of *Aggregatibacter actinomycetemcomitans* in periodontitis patients living in Sweden. *J. Oral Microbiol.* **2017**, *9*, 1334504. [CrossRef]
39. He, T.; Nishihara, T.; Demuth, D.R.; Ishikawa, I. A novel insertion sequence increases the expression of leukotoxicity in *Actinobacillus actinomycetemcomitans* clinical isolates. *J. Periodontol.* **1999**, *70*, 1261–1268. [CrossRef]

40. Claesson, R.; Gudmundson, J.; Åberg, C.H.; Haubek, D.; Johansson, A. Detection of a 640-bp deletion in the *Aggregatibacter actinomycetemcomitans* leukotoxin promoter region in isolates from an adolescent of Ethiopian origin. *J. Oral Microbiol.* **2015**, *7*, 26974. [CrossRef]
41. Höglund Åberg, C.; Haubek, D.; Kwamin, F.; Johansson, A.; Claesson, R. Leukotoxic activity of *Aggregatibacter actinomycetemcomitans* and periodontal attachment loss. *PLoS ONE* **2014**, *9*, e104095. [CrossRef] [PubMed]
42. Johansson, A.; Claesson, R.; Höglund Åberg, C.; Haubek, D.; Lindholm, M.; Jasim, S.; Oscarsson, J. Genetic Profiling of *Aggregatibacter actinomycetemcomitans* Serotype B Isolated from Periodontitis Patients Living in Sweden. *Pathogenes* **2019**, *8*, 153. [CrossRef] [PubMed]
43. Johansson, A.; Claesson, R.; Höglund Åberg, C.; Haubek, D.; Oscarsson, J. The cagE gene sequence as a diagnostic marker to identify JP2 and non-JP2 highly leukotoxic *Aggregatibacter actinomycetemcomitans* serotype b strains. *J. Periodontal Res.* **2017**, *52*, 903–912. [CrossRef] [PubMed]
44. Gomez-Banuelos, E.; Mukherjee, A.; Darrah, E.; Andrade, F. Rheumatoid Arthritis-Associated Mechanisms of *Porphyromonas gingivalis* and *Aggregatibacter actinomycetemcomitans*. *J. Clin. Med.* **2019**, *8*, 1309. [CrossRef]
45. Skals, M.; Greve, A.S.; Fagerberg, S.K.; Johnsen, N.; Christensen, M.G.; Praetorius, H.A. P2X1 receptor blockers reduce the number of circulating thrombocytes and the overall survival of urosepsis with haemolysin-producing *Escherichia coli*. *Purinergic Signal.* **2019**, *15*, 265–276. [CrossRef] [PubMed]
46. Kachlany, S.C. *Aggregatibacter actinomycetemcomitans* leukotoxin: From threat to therapy. *J. Dent. Res.* **2010**, *89*, 561–570. [CrossRef]
47. Linhartova, I.; Bumba, L.; Masin, J.; Basler, M.; Osicka, R.; Kamanova, J.; Prochazkova, K.; Adkins, I.; Hejnova-Holubova, J.; Sadilkova, L.; et al. RTX proteins: A highly diverse family secreted by a common mechanism. *FEMS Microbiol. Rev.* **2010**, *34*, 1076–1112. [CrossRef]
48. Harding, C.M.; Pulido, M.R.; Di Venanzio, G.; Kinsella, R.L.; Webb, A.I.; Scott, N.E.; Pachon, J.; Feldman, M.F. Pathogenic Acinetobacter species have a functional type I secretion system and contact-dependent inhibition systems. *J. Biol. Chem.* **2017**, *292*, 9075–9087. [CrossRef]
49. Crosby, J.A.; Kachlany, S.C. TdeA, a TolC-like protein required for toxin and drug export in *Aggregatibacter (Actinobacillus) actinomycetemcomitans*. *Gene* **2007**, *388*, 83–92. [CrossRef]
50. Gallant, C.V.; Sedic, M.; Chicoine, E.A.; Ruiz, T.; Mintz, K.P. Membrane morphology and leukotoxin secretion are associated with a novel membrane protein of *Aggregatibacter actinomycetemcomitans*. *J. Bacteriol.* **2008**, *190*, 5972–5980. [CrossRef]
51. Berthold, P.; Forti, D.; Kieba, I.R.; Rosenbloom, J.; Taichman, N.S.; Lally, E.T. Electron immunocytochemical localization of *Actinobacillus actinomycetemcomitans* leukotoxin. *Oral Microbiol. Immunol.* **1992**, *7*, 24–27. [CrossRef] [PubMed]
52. Kato, S.; Kowashi, Y.; Demuth, D.R. Outer membrane-like vesicles secreted by *Actinobacillus actinomycetemcomitans* are enriched in leukotoxin. *Microb. Pathog.* **2002**, *32*, 1–13. [CrossRef] [PubMed]
53. Ohta, H.; Kato, K.; Kokeguchi, S.; Hara, H.; Fukui, K.; Murayama, Y. Nuclease-sensitive binding of an *Actinobacillus actinomycetemcomitans* leukotoxin to the bacterial cell surface. *Infect. Immun.* **1991**, *59*, 4599–4605. [PubMed]
54. Ohta, H.; Hara, H.; Fukui, K.; Kurihara, H.; Murayama, Y.; Kato, K. Association of *Actinobacillus actinomycetemcomitans* leukotoxin with nucleic acids on the bacterial cell surface. *Infect. Immun.* **1993**, *61*, 4878–4884.
55. Johansson, A.; Hanstrom, L.; Kalfas, S. Inhibition of *Actinobacillus actinomycetemcomitans* leukotoxicity by bacteria from the subgingival flora. *Oral Microbiol. Immunol.* **2000**, *15*, 218–225. [CrossRef]
56. Johansson, A.; Claesson, R.; Hanstrom, L.; Kalfas, S. Serum-mediated release of leukotoxin from the cell surface of the periodontal pathogen *Actinobacillus actinomycetemcomitans*. *Eur. J. Oral Sci.* **2003**, *111*, 209–215. [CrossRef]
57. Balashova, N.V.; Diaz, R.; Balashov, S.V.; Crosby, J.A.; Kachlany, S.C. Regulation of *Aggregatibacter (Actinobacillus) actinomycetemcomitans* leukotoxin secretion by iron. *J. Bacteriol.* **2006**, *188*, 8658–8661. [CrossRef]
58. Reinholdt, J.; Poulsen, K.; Brinkmann, C.R.; Hoffmann, S.V.; Stapulionis, R.; Enghild, J.J.; Jensen, U.B.; Boesen, T.; Vorup-Jensen, T. Monodisperse and LPS-free *Aggregatibacter actinomycetemcomitans* leukotoxin: Interactions with human beta2 integrins and erythrocytes. *Biochim. Biophys. Acta* **2013**, *1834*, 546–558. [CrossRef]

59. Brage, M.; Holmlund, A.; Johansson, A. Humoral immune response to *Aggregatibacter actinomycetemcomitans* leukotoxin. *J. Periodontal Res.* **2011**, *46*, 170–175. [CrossRef]
60. Johansson, A.; Buhlin, K.; Sorsa, T.; Pussinen, P.J. Systemic *Aggregatibacter actinomycetemcomitans* Leukotoxin-Neutralizing Antibodies in Periodontitis. *J. Periodontol.* **2017**, *88*, 122–129. [CrossRef]
61. Johansson, A.; Claesson, R.; Belibasakis, G.; Makoveichuk, E.; Hanstrom, L.; Olivecrona, G.; Sandstrom, G.; Kalfas, S. Protease inhibitors, the responsible components for the serum-dependent enhancement of *Actinobacillus actinomycetemcomitans* leukotoxicity. *Eur. J. Oral Sci.* **2001**, *109*, 335–341. [CrossRef] [PubMed]
62. Balashova, N.V.; Park, D.H.; Patel, J.K.; Figurski, D.H.; Kachlany, S.C. Interaction between leukotoxin and Cu, Zn superoxide dismutase in *Aggregatibacter actinomycetemcomitans*. *Infect. Immun.* **2007**, *75*, 4490–4497. [CrossRef] [PubMed]
63. McArthur, W.P.; Tsai, C.C.; Baehni, P.C.; Genco, R.J.; Taichman, N.S. Leukotoxic effects of *Actinobacillus actinomycetemcomitans*. Modulation by serum components. *J. Periodontal Res.* **1981**, *16*, 159–170. [CrossRef] [PubMed]
64. Johansson, A.; Claesson, R.; Belibasakis, G.; Makoveichuk, E.; Hanstrom, L.; Olivecrona, G.; Kalfas, S. Lack of lipoprotein-dependent effects on the cytotoxic interactions of *Actinobacillus actinomycetemcomitans* leukotoxin with human neutrophils. *APMIS* **2002**, *110*, 857–862. [CrossRef]
65. Hritz, M.; Fisher, E.; Demuth, D.R. Differential regulation of the leukotoxin operon in highly leukotoxic and minimally leukotoxic strains of *Actinobacillus actinomycetemcomitans*. *Infect. Immun.* **1996**, *64*, 2724–2729.
66. Tsai, C.C.; McArthur, W.P.; Baehni, P.C.; Hammond, B.F.; Taichman, N.S. Extraction and partial characterization of a leukotoxin from a plaque-derived Gram-negative microorganism. *Infect. Immun.* **1979**, *25*, 427–439.
67. Zambon, J.J.; DeLuca, C.; Slots, J.; Genco, R.J. Studies of leukotoxin from *Actinobacillus actinomycetemcomitans* using the promyelocytic HL-60 cell line. *Infect. Immun.* **1983**, *40*, 205–212.
68. Sampathkumar, V.; Velusamy, S.K.; Godboley, D.; Fine, D.H. Increased leukotoxin production: Characterization of 100 base pairs within the 530 base pair leukotoxin promoter region of *Aggregatibacter actinomycetemcomitans*. *Sci. Rep.* **2017**, *7*, 1887. [CrossRef]
69. Kelk, P.; Claesson, R.; Chen, C.; Sjostedt, A.; Johansson, A. IL-1beta secretion induced by *Aggregatibacter (Actinobacillus) actinomycetemcomitans* is mainly caused by the leukotoxin. *Int. J. Med. Microbiol. IJMM* **2008**, *298*, 529–541. [CrossRef]
70. Umeda, J.E.; Longo, P.L.; Simionato, M.R.; Mayer, M.P. Differential transcription of virulence genes in *Aggregatibacter actinomycetemcomitans* serotypes. *J. Oral Microbiol.* **2013**, *5*. [CrossRef]
71. Lara-Tejero, M.; Galan, J.E. A bacterial toxin that controls cell cycle progression as a deoxyribonuclease I-like protein. *Science* **2000**, *290*, 354–357. [CrossRef] [PubMed]
72. Boesze-Battaglia, K.; Besack, D.; McKay, T.; Zekavat, A.; Otis, L.; Jordan-Sciutto, K.; Shenker, B.J. Cholesterol-rich membrane microdomains mediate cell cycle arrest induced by *Actinobacillus actinomycetemcomitans* cytolethal-distending toxin. *Cell Microbiol.* **2006**, *8*, 823–836. [CrossRef] [PubMed]
73. Boesze-Battaglia, K.; Alexander, D.; Dlakic, M.; Shenker, B.J. A Journey of Cytolethal Distending Toxins through Cell Membranes. *Front. Cell. Infect. Microbiol.* **2016**, *6*, 81. [CrossRef] [PubMed]
74. Fais, T.; Delmas, J.; Serres, A.; Bonnet, R.; Dalmasso, G. Impact of CDT Toxin on Human Diseases. *Toxins* **2016**, *8*, 220. [CrossRef] [PubMed]
75. Belibasakis, G.; Johansson, A.; Wang, Y.; Claesson, R.; Chen, C.; Asikainen, S.; Kalfas, S. Inhibited proliferation of human periodontal ligament cells and gingival fibroblasts by *Actinobacillus actinomycetemcomitans*: Involvement of the cytolethal distending toxin. *Eur. J. Oral Sci.* **2002**, *110*, 366–373. [CrossRef]
76. Belibasakis, G.N.; Mattsson, A.; Wang, Y.; Chen, C.; Johansson, A. Cell cycle arrest of human gingival fibroblasts and periodontal ligament cells by *Actinobacillus actinomycetemcomitans*: Involvement of the cytolethal distending toxin. *APMIS* **2004**, *112*, 674–685. [CrossRef]
77. Kang, P.; Korostoff, J.; Volgina, A.; Grzesik, W.; DiRienzo, J.M. Differential effect of the cytolethal distending toxin of *Actinobacillus actinomycetemcomitans* on co-cultures of human oral cells. *J. Med. Microbiol.* **2005**, *54*, 785–794. [CrossRef]
78. Alaoui-El-Azher, M.; Mans, J.J.; Baker, H.V.; Chen, C.; Progulske-Fox, A.; Lamont, R.J.; Handfield, M. Role of the ATM-checkpoint kinase 2 pathway in CDT-mediated apoptosis of gingival epithelial cells. *PLoS ONE* **2010**, *5*, e11714. [CrossRef]
79. Damek-Poprawa, M.; Haris, M.; Volgina, A.; Korostoff, J.; DiRienzo, J.M. Cytolethal distending toxin damages the oral epithelium of gingival explants. *J. Dent. Res.* **2011**, *90*, 874–879. [CrossRef]

80. Kanno, F.; Korostoff, J.; Volgina, A.; DiRienzo, J.M. Resistance of human periodontal ligament fibroblasts to the cytolethal distending toxin of *Actinobacillus actinomycetemcomitans*. *J. Periodontol.* **2005**, *76*, 1189–1201. [CrossRef]
81. Damek-Poprawa, M.; Korostoff, J.; Gill, R.; DiRienzo, J.M. Cell junction remodeling in gingival tissue exposed to a microbial toxin. *J. Dent. Res.* **2013**, *92*, 518–523. [CrossRef] [PubMed]
82. Ohara, M.; Miyauchi, M.; Tsuruda, K.; Takata, T.; Sugai, M. Topical application of *Aggregatibacter actinomycetemcomitans* cytolethal distending toxin induces cell cycle arrest in the rat gingival epithelium in vivo. *J. Periodontal Res.* **2011**, *46*, 389–395. [CrossRef] [PubMed]
83. Shenker, B.J.; McKay, T.; Datar, S.; Miller, M.; Chowhan, R.; Demuth, D. *Actinobacillus actinomycetemcomitans* immunosuppressive protein is a member of the family of cytolethal distending toxins capable of causing a G2 arrest in human T cells. *J. Immunol.* **1999**, *162*, 4773–4780. [PubMed]
84. Sato, T.; Koseki, T.; Yamato, K.; Saiki, K.; Konishi, K.; Yoshikawa, M.; Ishikawa, I.; Nishihara, T. p53-independent expression of p21(CIP1/WAF1) in plasmacytic cells during G(2) cell cycle arrest induced by *Actinobacillus actinomycetemcomitans* cytolethal distending toxin. *Infect. Immun.* **2002**, *70*, 528–534. [CrossRef] [PubMed]
85. Akifusa, S.; Poole, S.; Lewthwaite, J.; Henderson, B.; Nair, S.P. Recombinant *Actinobacillus actinomycetemcomitans* cytolethal distending toxin proteins are required to interact to inhibit human cell cycle progression and to stimulate human leukocyte cytokine synthesis. *Infect. Immun.* **2001**, *69*, 5925–5930. [CrossRef] [PubMed]
86. Belibasakis, G.N.; Bostanci, N. Inflammatory and bone remodeling responses to the cytolethal distending toxins. *Cells* **2014**, *3*, 236–246. [CrossRef]
87. Oscarsson, J.; Karched, M.; Thay, B.; Chen, C.; Asikainen, S. Proinflammatory effect in whole blood by free soluble bacterial components released from planktonic and biofilm cells. *BMC Microbiol.* **2008**, *8*, 206. [CrossRef]
88. Belibasakis, G.N.; Johansson, A. *Aggregatibacter actinomycetemcomitans* targets NLRP3 and NLRP6 inflammasome expression in human mononuclear leukocytes. *Cytokine* **2012**, *59*, 124–130. [CrossRef]
89. Belibasakis, G.N.; Bostanci, N. The RANKL-OPG system in clinical periodontology. *J. Clin. Periodontol.* **2012**, *39*, 239–248. [CrossRef]
90. Belibasakis, G.N.; Johansson, A.; Wang, Y.; Chen, C.; Kalfas, S.; Lerner, U.H. The cytolethal distending toxin induces receptor activator of NF-kappaB ligand expression in human gingival fibroblasts and periodontal ligament cells. *Infect. Immun.* **2005**, *73*, 342–351. [CrossRef]
91. Belibasakis, G.N.; Johansson, A.; Wang, Y.; Chen, C.; Lagergård, T.; Kalfas, S.; Lerner, U.H. Cytokine responses of human gingival fibroblasts to *Actinobacillus actinomycetemcomitans* cytolethal distending toxin. *Cytokine* **2005**, *30*, 56–63. [CrossRef] [PubMed]
92. Belibasakis, G.N.; Brage, M.; Lagergard, T.; Johansson, A. Cytolethal distending toxin upregulates RANKL expression in Jurkat T-cells. *APMIS* **2008**, *116*, 499–506. [CrossRef] [PubMed]
93. Kawamoto, D.; Ando-Suguimoto, E.S.; Bueno-Silva, B.; DiRienzo, J.M.; Mayer, M.P. Alteration of Homeostasis in Pre-osteoclasts Induced by *Aggregatibacter actinomycetemcomitans* CDT. *Front. Cell. Infect. Microbiol.* **2016**, *6*, 33. [CrossRef] [PubMed]
94. Kaplan, J.B.; Perry, M.B.; MacLean, L.L.; Furgang, D.; Wilson, M.E.; Fine, D.H. Structural and genetic analyses of O polysaccharide from *Actinobacillus actinomycetemcomitans* serotype f. *Infect. Immun.* **2001**, *69*, 5375–5384. [CrossRef]
95. Perry, M.B.; MacLean, L.M.; Brisson, J.R.; Wilson, M.E. Structures of the antigenic O-polysaccharides of lipopolysaccharides produced by *Actinobacillus actinomycetemcomitans* serotypes a, c, d and e. *Eur. J. Biochem.* **1996**, *242*, 682–688. [CrossRef]
96. Perry, M.B.; MacLean, L.L.; Gmur, R.; Wilson, M.E. Characterization of the O-polysaccharide structure of lipopolysaccharide from *Actinobacillus actinomycetemcomitans* serotype b. *Infect. Immun.* **1996**, *64*, 1215–1219.
97. Masoud, H.; Weintraub, S.T.; Wang, R.; Cotter, R.; Holt, S.C. Investigation of the structure of lipid A from *Actinobacillus actinomycetemcomitans* strain Y4 and human clinical isolate PO 1021-7. *Eur. J. Biochem.* **1991**, *200*, 775–781. [CrossRef]
98. Suzuki, N.; Nakano, Y.; Yoshida, Y.; Ikeda, D.; Koga, T. Identification of *Actinobacillus actinomycetemcomitans* serotypes by multiplex PCR. *J. Clin. Microbiol.* **2001**, *39*, 2002–2005. [CrossRef]

99. Brondz, I.; Olsen, I. Chemical differences in lipopolysaccharides from *Actinobacillus (Haemophilus) actinomycetemcomitans* and *Haemophilus aphrophilus*: Clues to differences in periodontopathogenic potential and taxonomic distinction. *Infect. Immun.* **1989**, *57*, 3106–3109.
100. Brondz, I.; Olsen, I. Determination of acids in whole lipopolysaccharide and in free lipid A from *Actinobacillus actinomycetemcomitans* and *Haemophilus aphrophilus*. *J. Chromatogr.* **1984**, *308*, 19–29. [CrossRef]
101. Bryn, K.; Jantzen, E. Analysis of lipopolysaccharides by methanolysis, trifluoroacetylation, and gas chromatography on a fused-silica capillary column. *J. Chromatogr.* **1982**, *240*, 405–413. [CrossRef]
102. Kiley, P.; Holt, S.C. Characterization of the lipopolysaccharide from *Actinobacillus actinomycetemcomitans* Y4 and N27. *Infect. Immun.* **1980**, *30*, 862–873. [PubMed]
103. Schneider, B.; Weigel, W.; Sztukowska, M.; Demuth, D.R. Identification and functional characterization of type II toxin/antitoxin systems in *Aggregatibacter actinomycetemcomitans*. *Mol. Oral Microbiol.* **2018**, *33*, 224–233. [CrossRef] [PubMed]
104. Sreenivasan, P.K.; Meyer, D.H.; Fives-Taylor, P.M. Factors influencing the growth and viability of *Actinobacillus actinomycetemcomitans*. *Oral Microbiol. Immunol.* **1993**, *8*, 361–369. [CrossRef] [PubMed]
105. Brondz, I.; Olsen, I. Differentiation between *Actinobacillus actinomycetemcomitans* and *Haemophilus aphrophilus* based on carbohydrates in lipopolysaccharide. *J. Chromatogr.* **1984**, *310*, 261–272. [CrossRef]
106. Brondz, I.; Olsen, I. Multivariate analyses of carbohydrate data from lipopolysaccharides of Actinobacillus (Haemophilus) actinomycetemcomitans, Haemophilus aphrophilus, and Haemophilus paraphrophilus. *Int. J. Syst. Bacteriol.* **1990**, *40*, 405–408. [CrossRef]
107. Patil, C.; Rossa, C., Jr.; Kirkwood, K.L. *Actinobacillus actinomycetemcomitans* lipopolysaccharide induces interleukin-6 expression through multiple mitogen-activated protein kinase pathways in periodontal ligament fibroblasts. *Oral Microbiol. Immunol.* **2006**, *21*, 392–398. [CrossRef]
108. Rogers, J.E.; Li, F.; Coatney, D.D.; Rossa, C.; Bronson, P.; Krieder, J.M.; Giannobile, W.V.; Kirkwood, K.L. *Actinobacillus actinomycetemcomitans* lipopolysaccharide-mediated experimental bone loss model for aggressive periodontitis. *J. Periodontol.* **2007**, *78*, 550–558. [CrossRef]
109. Morishita, M.; Ariyoshi, W.; Okinaga, T.; Usui, M.; Nakashima, K.; Nishihara, T. *A. actinomycetemcomitans* LPS enhances foam cell formation induced by LDL. *J. Dent. Res.* **2013**, *92*, 241–246. [CrossRef]
110. Park, O.J.; Cho, M.K.; Yun, C.H.; Han, S.H. Lipopolysaccharide of *Aggregatibacter actinomycetemcomitans* induces the expression of chemokines MCP-1, MIP-1alpha, and IP-10 via similar but distinct signaling pathways in murine macrophages. *Immunobiology* **2015**, *220*, 1067–1074. [CrossRef]
111. Valerio, M.S.; Herbert, B.A.; Basilakos, D.S.; Browne, C.; Yu, H.; Kirkwood, K.L. Critical role of MKP-1 in lipopolysaccharide-induced osteoclast formation through CXCL1 and CXCL2. *Cytokine* **2015**, *71*, 71–80. [CrossRef] [PubMed]
112. Tao, L.; Reese, T.A. Making Mouse Models That Reflect Human Immune Responses. *Trends Immunol.* **2017**, *38*, 181–193. [CrossRef] [PubMed]
113. Suga, T.; Mitani, A.; Mogi, M.; Kikuchi, T.; Fujimura, T.; Takeda, H.; Hishikawa, T.; Yamamoto, G.; Hayashi, J.; Ishihara, Y.; et al. *Aggregatibacter actinomycetemcomitans* lipopolysaccharide stimulated epithelial cells produce interleukin-15 that regulates T cell activation. *Arch. Oral Biol.* **2013**, *58*, 1541–1548. [CrossRef]
114. Takahashi, N.; Kobayashi, M.; Takaki, T.; Takano, K.; Miyata, M.; Okamatsu, Y.; Hasegawa, K.; Nishihara, T.; Yamamoto, M. *Actinobacillus actinomycetemcomitans* lipopolysaccharide stimulates collagen phagocytosis by human gingival fibroblasts. *Oral Microbiol. Immunol.* **2008**, *23*, 259–264. [CrossRef]
115. Xiao, Y.; Bunn, C.L.; Bartold, P.M. Effect of lipopolysaccharide from periodontal pathogens on the production of tissue plasminogen activator and plasminogen activator inhibitor 2 by human gingival fibroblasts. *J. Periodontal Res.* **2001**, *36*, 25–31. [CrossRef] [PubMed]
116. Naqvi, A.R.; Fordham, J.B.; Khan, A.; Nares, S. MicroRNAs responsive to *Aggregatibacter actinomycetemcomitans* and *Porphyromonas gingivalis* LPS modulate expression of genes regulating innate immunity in human macrophages. *Innate Immun.* **2014**, *20*, 540–551. [CrossRef] [PubMed]
117. Taganov, K.D.; Boldin, M.P.; Chang, K.J.; Baltimore, D. NF-kappaB-dependent induction of microRNA miR-146, an inhibitor targeted to signaling proteins of innate immune responses. *Proc. Natl. Acad. Sci. USA* **2006**, *103*, 12481–12486. [CrossRef]
118. Gocek, E.; Wang, X.; Liu, X.; Liu, C.G.; Studzinski, G.P. MicroRNA-32 upregulation by 1,25-dihydroxyvitamin D3 in human myeloid leukemia cells leads to Bim targeting and inhibition of AraC-induced apoptosis. *Cancer Res.* **2011**, *71*, 6230–6239. [CrossRef]

119. Sosroseno, W.; Bird, P.S.; Seymour, G.J. Nitric oxide production by a human osteoblast cell line stimulated with *Aggregatibacter actinomycetemcomitans* lipopolysaccharide. *Oral Microbiol. Immunol.* **2009**, *24*, 50–55. [CrossRef]
120. Ralston, S.H.; Grabowski, P.S. Mechanisms of cytokine induced bone resorption: Role of nitric oxide, cyclic guanosine monophosphate, and prostaglandins. *Bone* **1996**, *19*, 29–33. [CrossRef]
121. Pollanen, M.T.; Salonen, J.I.; Grenier, D.; Uitto, V.J. Epithelial cell response to challenge of bacterial lipoteichoic acids and lipopolysaccharides in vitro. *J. Med. Microbiol.* **2000**, *49*, 245–252. [CrossRef] [PubMed]
122. Ohguchi, Y.; Ishihara, Y.; Ohguchi, M.; Koide, M.; Shirozu, N.; Naganawa, T.; Nishihara, T.; Noguchi, T. Capsular polysaccharide from *Actinobacillus actinomycetemcomitans* inhibits IL-6 and IL-8 production in human gingival fibroblast. *J. Periodontal Res.* **2003**, *38*, 191–197. [CrossRef] [PubMed]
123. Kikuchi, T.; Hahn, C.L.; Tanaka, S.; Barbour, S.E.; Schenkein, H.A.; Tew, J.G. Dendritic cells stimulated with *Actinobacillus actinomycetemcomitans* elicit rapid gamma interferon responses by natural killer cells. *Infect. Immun.* **2004**, *72*, 5089–5096. [CrossRef] [PubMed]
124. Diaz-Zuniga, J.; Yanez, J.P.; Alvarez, C.; Melgar-Rodriguez, S.; Hernandez, M.; Sanz, M.; Vernal, R. Serotype-dependent response of human dendritic cells stimulated with *Aggregatibacter actinomycetemcomitans*. *J. Clin. Periodontol.* **2014**, *41*, 242–251. [CrossRef] [PubMed]
125. Aida, Y.; Kukita, T.; Takada, H.; Maeda, K.; Pabst, M.J. Lipopolysaccharides from periodontal pathogens prime neutrophils for enhanced respiratory burst: Differential effect of a synthetic lipid a precursor IVA (LA-14-PP). *J. Periodontal Res.* **1995**, *30*, 116–123. [CrossRef]
126. Yoshimura, A.; Hara, Y.; Kaneko, T.; Kato, I. Secretion of IL-1 beta, TNF-alpha, IL-8 and IL-1ra by human polymorphonuclear leukocytes in response to lipopolysaccharides from periodontopathic bacteria. *J. Periodontal Res.* **1997**, *32*, 279–286. [CrossRef]
127. Schytte Blix, I.J.; Helgeland, K.; Hvattum, E.; Lyberg, T. Lipopolysaccharide from Actinobacillus actinomycetemcomitans stimulates production of interleukin-1beta, tumor necrosis factor-alpha, interleukin-6 and interleukin-1 receptor antagonist in human whole blood. *J. Periodontal Res.* **1999**, *34*, 34–40. [CrossRef]
128. Blix, I.J.; Helgeland, K.; Kahler, H.; Lyberg, T. LPS from *Actinobacillus actinomycetemcomitans* and the expression of beta2 integrins and L-selectin in an ex vivo human whole blood system. *Eur. J. Oral Sci.* **1999**, *107*, 14–20. [CrossRef]
129. Grenier, D.; Leduc, A.; Mayrand, D. Interaction between *Actinobacillus actinomycetemcomitans* lipopolysaccharides and human hemoglobin. *FEMS Microbiol. Lett.* **1997**, *151*, 77–81. [CrossRef]
130. Ahlstrand, T.; Kovesjoki, L.; Maula, T.; Oscarsson, J.; Ihalin, R. *Aggregatibacter actinomycetemcomitans* LPS binds human interleukin-8. *J. Oral Microbiol.* **2019**, *11*, 1549931. [CrossRef]
131. Papapanou, P.N.; Sanz, M.; Buduneli, N.; Dietrich, T.; Feres, M.; Fine, D.H.; Flemmig, T.F.; Garcia, R.; Giannobile, W.V.; Graziani, F.; et al. Periodontitis: Consensus report of workgroup 2 of the 2017 World Workshop on the Classification of Periodontal and Peri-Implant Diseases and Conditions. *J. Clin. Periodontol.* **2018**, *45* (Suppl. 20), S162–S170. [CrossRef]
132. Barbour, S.E.; Ishihara, Y.; Fakher, M.; Al-Darmaki, S.; Caven, T.H.; Shelburne, C.P.; Best, A.M.; Schenkein, H.A.; Tew, J.G. Monocyte differentiation in localized juvenile periodontitis is skewed toward the dendritic cell phenotype. *Infect. Immun.* **2002**, *70*, 2780–2786. [CrossRef] [PubMed]
133. Diaz-Zuniga, J.; Melgar-Rodriguez, S.; Alvarez, C.; Monasterio, G.; Benitez, A.; Ciuchi, P.; Diaz, C.; Mardones, J.; Escobar, A.; Sanz, M.; et al. T-lymphocyte phenotype and function triggered by *Aggregatibacter actinomycetemcomitans* is serotype-dependent. *J. Periodontal Res.* **2015**, *50*, 824–835. [CrossRef] [PubMed]
134. Nicu, E.A.; Loos, B.G. Polymorphonuclear neutrophils in periodontitis and their possible modulation as a therapeutic approach. *Periodontology 2000* **2016**, *71*, 140–163. [CrossRef] [PubMed]
135. Tang, G.; Kawai, T.; Komatsuzawa, H.; Mintz, K.P. Lipopolysaccharides mediate leukotoxin secretion in *Aggregatibacter actinomycetemcomitans*. *Mol. Oral Microbiol.* **2012**, *27*, 70–82. [CrossRef]
136. Ahlstrand, T.; Torittu, A.; Elovaara, H.; Valimaa, H.; Pollanen, M.T.; Kasvandik, S.; Hogbom, M.; Ihalin, R. Interactions between the *Aggregatibacter actinomycetemcomitans* secretin HofQ and host cytokines indicate a link between natural competence and interleukin-8 uptake. *Virulence* **2018**, *9*, 1205–1223. [CrossRef]
137. Paino, A.; Tuominen, H.; Jaaskelainen, M.; Alanko, J.; Nuutila, J.; Asikainen, S.E.; Pelliniemi, L.J.; Pollanen, M.T.; Chen, C.; Ihalin, R. Trimeric form of intracellular ATP synthase subunit beta of *Aggregatibacter actinomycetemcomitans* binds human interleukin-1beta. *PLoS ONE* **2011**, *6*, e18929. [CrossRef]

138. Ahlstrand, T.; Tuominen, H.; Beklen, A.; Torittu, A.; Oscarsson, J.; Sormunen, R.; Pollanen, M.T.; Permi, P.; Ihalin, R. A novel intrinsically disordered outer membrane lipoprotein of *Aggregatibacter actinomycetemcomitans* binds various cytokines and plays a role in biofilm response to interleukin-1beta and interleukin-8. *Virulence* **2017**, *8*, 115–134. [CrossRef]

139. Paino, A.; Lohermaa, E.; Sormunen, R.; Tuominen, H.; Korhonen, J.; Pollanen, M.T.; Ihalin, R. Interleukin-1beta is internalised by viable *Aggregatibacter actinomycetemcomitans* biofilm and locates to the outer edges of nucleoids. *Cytokine* **2012**, *60*, 565–574. [CrossRef]

140. Paino, A.; Ahlstrand, T.; Nuutila, J.; Navickaite, I.; Lahti, M.; Tuominen, H.; Valimaa, H.; Lamminmaki, U.; Pollanen, M.T.; Ihalin, R. Identification of a novel bacterial outer membrane interleukin-1Beta-binding protein from *Aggregatibacter actinomycetemcomitans*. *PLoS ONE* **2013**, *8*, e70509. [CrossRef]

141. Kanangat, S.; Postlethwaite, A.; Cholera, S.; Williams, L.; Schaberg, D. Modulation of virulence gene expression in *Staphylococcus aureus* by interleukin-1beta: Novel implications in bacterial pathogenesis. *Microbes Infect.* **2007**, *9*, 408–415. [CrossRef] [PubMed]

142. Wu, M.; Guina, T.; Brittnacher, M.; Nguyen, H.; Eng, J.; Miller, S.I. The *Pseudomonas aeruginosa* proteome during anaerobic growth. *J. Bacteriol.* **2005**, *187*, 8185–8190. [CrossRef] [PubMed]

143. Mahdavi, J.; Royer, P.J.; Sjolinder, H.S.; Azimi, S.; Self, T.; Stoof, J.; Wheldon, L.M.; Brannstrom, K.; Wilson, R.; Moreton, J.; et al. Pro-inflammatory cytokines can act as intracellular modulators of commensal bacterial virulence. *Open Biol.* **2013**, *3*, 130048. [CrossRef] [PubMed]

144. Sperandio, V.; Torres, A.G.; Kaper, J.B. Quorum sensing *Escherichia coli* regulators B and C (QseBC): A novel two-component regulatory system involved in the regulation of flagella and motility by quorum sensing in E. coli. *Mol. Microbiol.* **2002**, *43*, 809–821. [CrossRef] [PubMed]

145. Moreira, C.G.; Sperandio, V. The Epinephrine/Norepinephrine/Autoinducer-3 Interkingdom Signaling System in *Escherichia coli* O157:H7. *Adv. Exp. Med. Biol.* **2016**, *874*, 247–261. [CrossRef] [PubMed]

146. Weigel, W.A.; Demuth, D.R.; Torres-Escobar, A.; Juarez-Rodriguez, M.D. *Aggregatibacter actinomycetemcomitans* QseBC is activated by catecholamines and iron and regulates genes encoding proteins associated with anaerobic respiration and metabolism. *Mol. Oral Microbiol.* **2015**, *30*, 384–398. [CrossRef]

147. Novak, E.A.; Shao, H.; Daep, C.A.; Demuth, D.R. Autoinducer-2 and QseC control biofilm formation and in vivo virulence of *Aggregatibacter actinomycetemcomitans*. *Infect. Immun.* **2010**, *78*, 2919–2926. [CrossRef]

148. Deatherage, B.L.; Cookson, B.T. Membrane vesicle release in bacteria, eukaryotes, and archaea: A conserved yet underappreciated aspect of microbial life. *Infect. Immun.* **2012**, *80*, 1948–1957. [CrossRef]

149. Uhlin, B.E.; Oscarsson, J.; Wai, S.N. Haemolysins. In *Pathogenic Escherichia Coli: Molecular and Cellular Microbiology*; Morabito, S., Ed.; Caister Academic Press: Norfolk, UK, 2014; pp. 161–180.

150. Rompikuntal, P.K.; Thay, B.; Khan, M.K.; Alanko, J.; Penttinen, A.M.; Asikainen, S.; Wai, S.N.; Oscarsson, J. Perinuclear localization of internalized outer membrane vesicles carrying active cytolethal distending toxin from *Aggregatibacter actinomycetemcomitans*. *Infect. Immun.* **2012**, *80*, 31–42. [CrossRef]

151. Demuth, D.R.; James, D.; Kowashi, Y.; Kato, S. Interaction of *Actinobacillus actinomycetemcomitans* outer membrane vesicles with HL60 cells does not require leukotoxin. *Cell. Microbiol.* **2003**, *5*, 111–121. [CrossRef]

152. Goulhen, F.; Hafezi, A.; Uitto, V.J.; Hinode, D.; Nakamura, R.; Grenier, D.; Mayrand, D. Subcellular localization and cytotoxic activity of the GroEL-like protein isolated from *Actinobacillus actinomycetemcomitans*. *Infect. Immun.* **1998**, *66*, 5307–5313. [PubMed]

153. Karched, M.; Ihalin, R.; Eneslätt, K.; Zhong, D.; Oscarsson, J.; Wai, S.N.; Chen, C.; Asikainen, S.E. Vesicle-independent extracellular release of a proinflammatory outer membrane lipoprotein in free-soluble form. *BMC Microbiol.* **2008**, *8*, 18. [CrossRef] [PubMed]

154. Kieselbach, T.; Zijnge, V.; Granström, E.; Oscarsson, J. Proteomics of *Aggregatibacter actinomycetemcomitans* Outer Membrane Vesicles. *PLoS ONE* **2015**, *10*, e0138591. [CrossRef] [PubMed]

155. Kieselbach, T.; Oscarsson, J. Dataset of the proteome of purified outer membrane vesicles from the human pathogen *Aggregatibacter actinomycetemcomitans*. *Data Brief* **2017**, *10*, 426–431. [CrossRef] [PubMed]

156. Rochester, D.F. Does respiratory muscle rest relieve fatigue or incipient fatigue? *Am. Rev. Respir. Dis.* **1988**, *138*, 516–517. [CrossRef]

157. Iino, Y.; Hopps, R.M. The bone-resorbing activities in tissue culture of lipopolysaccharides from the bacteria *Actinobacillus actinomycetemcomitans*, Bacteroides gingivalis and Capnocytophaga ochracea isolated from human mouths. *Arch. Oral Biol.* **1984**, *29*, 59–63. [CrossRef]

158. Reddi, K.; Meghji, S.; Wilson, M.; Henderson, B. Comparison of the osteolytic activity of surface-associated proteins of bacteria implicated in periodontal disease. *Oral Dis.* **1995**, *1*, 26–31. [CrossRef]
159. Choi, J.W.; Kim, S.C.; Hong, S.H.; Lee, H.J. Secretable Small RNAs via Outer Membrane Vesicles in Periodontal Pathogens. *J. Dent. Res.* **2017**, *96*, 458–466. [CrossRef]
160. O'Donoghue, E.J.; Krachler, A.M. Mechanisms of outer membrane vesicle entry into host cells. *Cell. Microbiol.* **2016**, *18*, 1508–1517. [CrossRef]
161. Kesty, N.C.; Mason, K.M.; Reedy, M.; Miller, S.E.; Kuehn, M.J. Enterotoxigenic *Escherichia coli* vesicles target toxin delivery into mammalian cells. *EMBO J.* **2004**, *23*, 4538–4549. [CrossRef]
162. Nice, J.B.; Balashova, N.V.; Kachlany, S.C.; Koufos, E.; Krueger, E.; Lally, E.T.; Brown, A.C. *Aggregatibacter actinomycetemcomitans* Leukotoxin Is Delivered to Host Cells in an LFA-1-Indepdendent Manner When Associated with Outer Membrane Vesicles. *Toxins* **2018**, *10*, 414. [CrossRef] [PubMed]
163. Ximenez-Fyvie, L.A.; Haffajee, A.D.; Socransky, S.S. Microbial composition of supra- and subgingival plaque in subjects with adult periodontitis. *J. Clin. Periodontol.* **2000**, *27*, 722–732. [CrossRef] [PubMed]
164. Noiri, Y.; Li, L.; Ebisu, S. The localization of periodontal-disease-associated bacteria in human periodontal pockets. *J. Dent. Res.* **2001**, *80*, 1930–1934. [CrossRef] [PubMed]
165. Christersson, L.A.; Albini, B.; Zambon, J.J.; Wikesjo, U.M.; Genco, R.J. Tissue localization *of Actinobacillus actinomycetemcomitans* in human periodontitis. I. Light, immunofluorescence and electron microscopic studies. *J. Periodontol.* **1987**, *58*, 529–539. [CrossRef] [PubMed]
166. Colombo, A.V.; da Silva, C.M.; Haffajee, A.; Colombo, A.P. Identification of intracellular oral species within human crevicular epithelial cells from subjects with chronic periodontitis by fluorescence in situ hybridization. *J. Periodontal Res.* **2007**, *42*, 236–243. [CrossRef]
167. Mendes, L.; Rocha, R.; Azevedo, A.S.; Ferreira, C.; Henriques, M.; Pinto, M.G.; Azevedo, N.F. Novel strategy to detect and locate periodontal pathogens: The PNA-FISH technique. *Microbiol. Res.* **2016**, *192*, 185–191. [CrossRef]
168. Willi, M.; Belibasakis, G.N.; Bostanci, N. Expression and regulation of triggering receptor expressed on myeloid cells 1 in periodontal diseases. *Clin. Exp. Immunol.* **2014**, *178*, 190–200. [CrossRef]
169. Thurnheer, T.; Belibasakis, G.N. Integration of non-oral bacteria into in vitro oral biofilms. *Virulence* **2015**, *6*, 258–264. [CrossRef]
170. Bao, K.; Bostanci, N.; Selevsek, N.; Thurnheer, T.; Belibasakis, G.N. Quantitative proteomics reveal distinct protein regulations caused by *Aggregatibacter actinomycetemcomitans* within subgingival biofilms. *PLoS ONE* **2015**, *10*, e0119222. [CrossRef]
171. Llama-Palacios, A.; Potupa, O.; Sanchez, M.C.; Figuero, E.; Herrera, D.; Sanz, M. *Aggregatibacter actinomycetemcomitans* Growth in Biofilm versus Planktonic State: Differential Expression of Proteins. *J. Proteome Res.* **2017**, *16*, 3158–3167. [CrossRef]
172. Costerton, J.W.; Stewart, P.S.; Greenberg, E.P. Bacterial biofilms: A common cause of persistent infections. *Science* **1999**, *284*, 1318–1322. [CrossRef] [PubMed]
173. Rathsam, C.; Eaton, R.E.; Simpson, C.L.; Browne, G.V.; Berg, T.; Harty, D.W.; Jacques, N.A. Up-regulation of competence- but not stress-responsive proteins accompanies an altered metabolic phenotype in *Streptococcus mutans* biofilms. *Microbiology* **2005**, *151*, 1823–1837. [CrossRef] [PubMed]
174. Takasaki, K.; Fujise, O.; Miura, M.; Hamachi, T.; Maeda, K. *Porphyromonas gingivalis* displays a competitive advantage over *Aggregatibacter actinomycetemcomitans* in co-cultured biofilm. *J. Periodontal Res.* **2013**, *48*, 286–292. [CrossRef] [PubMed]
175. Smith, K.P.; Voogt, R.D.; Ruiz, T.; Mintz, K.P. The conserved carboxyl domain of MorC, an inner membrane protein of *Aggregatibacter actinomycetemcomitans*, is essential for membrane function. *Mol. Oral Microbiol.* **2016**, *31*, 43–58. [CrossRef] [PubMed]
176. Smith, K.P.; Fields, J.G.; Voogt, R.D.; Deng, B.; Lam, Y.W.; Mintz, K.P. Alteration in abundance of specific membrane proteins of *Aggregatibacter actinomycetemcomitans* is attributed to deletion of the inner membrane protein MorC. *Proteomics* **2015**, *15*, 1859–1867. [CrossRef]
177. Zijnge, V.; Kieselbach, T.; Oscarsson, J. Proteomics of protein secretion by *Aggregatibacter actinomycetemcomitans*. *PLoS ONE* **2012**, *7*, e41662. [CrossRef]
178. Rylev, M.; Abduljabar, A.B.; Reinholdt, J.; Ennibi, O.K.; Haubek, D.; Birkelund, S.; Kilian, M. Proteomic and immunoproteomic analysis of *Aggregatibacter actinomycetemcomitans* JP2 clone strain HK1651. *J. Proteom.* **2011**, *74*, 2972–2985. [CrossRef]

179. Tendeng, C.; Bertin, P.N. H-NS in Gram-negative bacteria: A family of multifaceted proteins. *Trends Microbiol.* **2003**, *11*, 511–518. [CrossRef]
180. Juarez, A.; Nieto, J.M.; Prenafeta, A.; Miquelay, E.; Balsalobre, C.; Carrascal, M.; Madrid, C. Interaction of the nucleoid-associated proteins Hha and H-NS to modulate expression of the hemolysin operon in Escherichia coli. *Adv. Exp. Med. Biol.* **2000**, *485*, 127–131. [CrossRef]
181. Li, H.; Granat, A.; Stewart, V.; Gillespie, J.R. RpoS, H-NS, and DsrA influence EHEC hemolysin operon (ehxCABD) transcription in *Escherichia coli* O157:H7 strain EDL933. *FEMS Microbiol. Lett.* **2008**, *285*, 257–262. [CrossRef]
182. Wang, H.; Ayala, J.C.; Benitez, J.A.; Silva, A.J. RNA-seq analysis identifies new genes regulated by the histone-like nucleoid structuring protein (H-NS) affecting *Vibrio cholerae* virulence, stress response and chemotaxis. *PLoS ONE* **2015**, *10*, e0118295. [CrossRef] [PubMed]
183. Bao, K.; Belibasakis, G.N.; Selevsek, N.; Grossmann, J.; Bostanci, N. Proteomic profiling of host-biofilm interactions in an oral infection model resembling the periodontal pocket. *Sci. Rep.* **2015**, *5*, 15999. [CrossRef] [PubMed]
184. Maughan, H.S.S.; Wilson, L.; Redfield, R. Competence, DNA Uptake and Transformation in Pasteurellaceae. In *Pasteurellaceae Biology, Genomics and Molecular Aspects*; Kuhnert, P., Christensen, H., Eds.; Caister Academic Press: Norfolk, UK, 2008; pp. 79–88.
185. Fujise, O.; Lakio, L.; Wang, Y.; Asikainen, S.; Chen, C. Clonal distribution of natural competence in *Actinobacillus actinomycetemcomitans*. *Oral Microbiol. Immunol.* **2004**, *19*, 340–342. [CrossRef] [PubMed]
186. Jorth, P.; Whiteley, M. An evolutionary link between natural transformation and CRISPR adaptive immunity. *mBio* **2012**, *3*. [CrossRef]
187. Redfield, R.J.; Findlay, W.A.; Bosse, J.; Kroll, J.S.; Cameron, A.D.; Nash, J.H. Evolution of competence and DNA uptake specificity in the Pasteurellaceae. *BMC Evol. Biol.* **2006**, *6*, 82. [CrossRef]
188. Wang, Y.; Shi, W.; Chen, W.; Chen, C. Type IV pilus gene homologs pilABCD are required for natural transformation in *Actinobacillus actinomycetemcomitans*. *Gene* **2003**, *312*, 249–255. [CrossRef]
189. Tanaka, A.; Fujise, O.; Chen, C.; Miura, M.; Hamachi, T.; Maeda, K. A novel gene required for natural competence in *Aggregatibacter actinomycetemcomitans*. *J. Periodontal Res.* **2012**, *47*, 129–134. [CrossRef]
190. Hisano, K.; Fujise, O.; Miura, M.; Hamachi, T.; Matsuzaki, E.; Nishimura, F. The pga gene cluster in *Aggregatibacter actinomycetemcomitans* is necessary for the development of natural competence in Ca^{2+}-promoted biofilms. *Mol. Oral Microbiol.* **2014**, *29*, 79–89. [CrossRef]
191. Wang, Y.; Goodman, S.D.; Redfield, R.J.; Chen, C. Natural transformation and DNA uptake signal sequences in *Actinobacillus actinomycetemcomitans*. *J. Bacteriol.* **2002**, *184*, 3442–3449. [CrossRef]

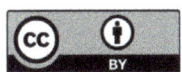

© 2019 by the authors. Licensee MDPI, Basel, Switzerland. This article is an open access article distributed under the terms and conditions of the Creative Commons Attribution (CC BY) license (http://creativecommons.org/licenses/by/4.0/).

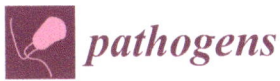

Case Report

JP2 Genotype of *Aggregatibacter actinomycetemcomitans* in Caucasian Patients: A Presentation of Two Cases

Alexandra Stähli *, Anton Sculean and Sigrun Eick

Department of Periodontology, School of Dental Medicine, University of Bern, Freiburgstrasse 7, 3010 Bern, Switzerland; anton.sculean@zmk.unibe.ch (A.S.); sigrun.eick@zmk.unibe.ch (S.E.)
* Correspondence: alexandra.staehli@zmk.unibe.ch

Received: 31 January 2020; Accepted: 25 February 2020; Published: 1 March 2020

Abstract: *Aggregatibacter actinomycetemcomitans* is a key pathogen that has been associated with periodontal disease. Its most important virulence factor is a leukotoxin capable of inactivating immune cells. The JP2 genotype of *Aggregatibacter actinomycetemcomitans* shows enhanced leukotoxic activity and is mostly present in individuals of North and West African origin with severe periodontitis. In this paper, two cases of Caucasians diagnosed with the JP2 genotype are presented. A 50-year-old female patient had three approximal sites with ≥ 6 mm clinical attachment loss (CAL) and eight sites with probing depth (PD) ≥ 5 mm. Microbiological diagnostics revealed *A. actinomycetemcomitans* JP2 genotype, but not *Porphyromonas gingivalis*. This JP2 genotype was highly leukotoxic to monocytic cells. The second case was a 55-year-old female patient with CAL of > 5 mm at all molars and PD of up to 12 mm. *A. actinomycetemcomitans* JP2 was identified, but not *P. gingivalis*. Her husband originated from North-Africa. In him, no *A. actinomycetemcomitans* was detected, but their 17-year-old daughter was diagnosed with periodontitis and was found to be positive for the JP2 genotype. Both patients were successfully treated with adjunctive antibiotics and the JP2 genotype was eliminated. In summary, here, the microbiological diagnosis was key for the treatment with adjunctive antibiotics.

Keywords: JP2 clone of *Aggregatibacter actinomycetemcomitans*; periodontitis; JP2 in Caucasian; microbiological diagnosis; adjunctive antibiotics

---

1. Introduction

Bacterial biofilm causes destruction of the periodontium in two ways: through direct action of bacteria and their products on the host-tissue and by activating the immune host response [1]. *Aggregatibacter actinomycetemcomitans* is one of the key pathogens in the course of periodontal disease. *A. actinomycetemcomitans* has been strongly associated with localized aggressive periodontitis [2], however, its mere presence could not be used to distinguish between chronic (CP) and aggressive forms of periodontitis (AP) [3]. In the Department of Periodontology, School of Dental Medicine, University of Bern, patients diagnosed with AP generally received antibiotics during nonsurgical periodontal therapy (i.e., hygienic phase). Retrospective analysis of our patients revealed that the prevalence of *A. actinomycetemcomitans* was higher in patients diagnosed with AP than in those diagnosed with CP [4]. Following periodontal therapy, especially surgical treatment, *A. actinomycetemcomitans* was less frequently detected in patients with AP than in those with CP [4]. *A. actinomycetemcomitans* possesses several virulence factors, that is, lipopolysaccharides that induce pro-inflammatory cytokines, a cytolethal distending toxin causing cell cycle arrest in T-cells, macrophages and epithelial cells, and a leukotoxin [5]. The leukotoxin produced by the bacterium is capable of killing or inactivating immune cells and of inducing the release of interleukin (IL)-1β [6].

Here, we focus on a subtype of *A. actinomycetemcomitans*, the highly leukotoxic JP2 genotype, which was first isolated from a child of African American origin with prepubertal periodontitis [7]. Later, it was found as a common isolate in individuals of North and West African descent with aggressive forms of periodontitis [8–12]. With respect to the JP2 genotype, a 530 base pair deletion in the promoter region of the leukotoxin gene is responsible for a 10- to 20-fold increased production of leukotoxin [13,14]. The JP2 clone is a subpopulation of the serotype b strains [15].

To date, seven serotypes of *A. actinomycetemcomitans*, designated from a to g, have been identified [16]. Among them, serotypes a, b, and c are globally dominant, whereby type c is the most prevalent [17]. Interestingly, they show different associations with disease depending on ethnicity, geographical localization, or periodontal status. For example, in the United States, serotype c was mostly associated with AP, but also other strains, and the JP2 genotype was found in patients suffering from periodontitis [18]. In Brazil, serotype c was found to be the most prevalent one and associated with both AP and CP. On the other hand, serotype b was also detected in periodontally healthy individuals [19]. Conversely, others found a connection between serotype b and aggressive periodontitis [20]. In Japan, serotype c was predominantly isolated from patients with AP, while the occurrence of serotype b was rare [21]. The specific JP2 genotype of *A. actinomycetemcomitans* was found to be strongly associated with severe periodontitis, particularly in Northern and Western Africa [22,23]. In Asia, the occurrence of the JP2 genotype has not been reported so far [23], and in Germany, it was detected in immigrants from North Africa living for more than 10 years in Germany, but not in Caucasians [24]. Dissemination of the JP2 genotype to non-African populations was only very rarely described [22]. Nevertheless, recent data obtained from nearly 3500 subgingival plaque samples of 1445 periodontitis patients in Sweden showed that the JP2 genotype was found in 1.2% of patients and most of them were of non-African descent [25]. Furthermore, serotype b was more often found in younger patients with periodontitis than in older cohorts [25].

In our department, microbiological diagnostics of subgingival biofilm samples is routinely performed. This includes subtyping of *A. actinomycetemcomitans* strains. After identifying the JP2 genotype in an immigrant from Morocco in 2013, such a clone was detected in two periodontitis patients of non-African origin. Here, the two cases starting with the diagnosis together with all steps of periodontal treatment are presented.

2. Results

2.1. Case 1

A 50-year-old female patient presented with localized CP according to the Classification System for Periodontal Diseases and Conditions set in 1999 [26]. At the initial examination, the patient was diagnosed with severe CP with three approximal sites with clinical attachment loss (CAL) $\geq$ 6 mm and eight sites with probing depth (PD) $\geq$ 5 mm (Table 1), as defined by the Centre for Disease Control and Prevention and the American Academy of Periodontology (CDC–AAP) [27,28]. No furcation involvement was detected. The patient reported to smoke occasionally. She was healthy and took no medications. Besides the third molars, teeth 16 and 27 were missing. The endodontically treated tooth 47 was scheduled for extraction because of an apical osteolysis. Besides this, the radiographs showed no further pathologies. No angular bony defects were visible and slight horizontal bone loss was noted. Microbiological diagnostics revealed high counts (more than 10^5) for *A. actinomycetemcomitans*, low counts (about 10^4) each for *Tannerella forsythia* and *Treponema denticola*, but no *Porphyromonas gingivalis*. Subtyping of *A. actinomycetemcomitans* showed a serotype b strain being positive for the deletion in the promotor region of in the leukotoxin operon (JP2 genotype). Another *A. actinomycetemcomitans* (without deletion in the promoter region of the leukotoxin operon) was not detected. At the next visit, she was asked for contact with people from North and Western Africa, but she had never been abroad before, nor had she closer contact to Africans. Further, additional biofilm was sampled to confirm the microbiological analysis and to culture the strain. Cultivation confirmed the high counts (10^5) and identification of *A. actinomycetemcomitans*. Determination of antibiotic resistance found a minimal inhibitory concentration (MIC) of ≤ 0.5 µg/mL for amoxicillin and 4 µg/mL for metronidazole. The MTT (3-(4,5-dimethylthiazol-2-yl)-2,5-diphenyltetrazolium bromide) tetrazolium assay confirmed a very high toxicity of that strain, being remarkably higher than those of the control JP2 genotype reference strain (HK1651) (Figure 1). Meanwhile, the patient improved her oral hygiene, and no *T. forsythia* and *T. denticola* were found anymore, but *A. actinomycetemcomitans* was still present in high counts. In order to eradicate *A. actinomycetemcomitans*, the further treatment plan entailed a hygienic phase with antibiotics (amoxicillin 375 mg and metronidazole 500 mg each tid for seven days). After the initial oral hygiene instruction and supragingival scaling, the patient showed good oral hygiene with a plaque index (O'Leary [29]) of < 20% of all tooth surfaces. Thereafter, subgingival scaling was performed in one session by hand curettes and an ultrasonic device with local anesthesia. Antibiotics as mentioned before and 0.02% chlorhexidine were given for 7 and 14 days, respectively. Tooth 47 was extracted. Three months after nonsurgical therapy, the patient was re-evaluated. The goals of periodontal therapy were achieved in all quadrants. There was no site with PD ≥ 5 mm and, therefore, no further surgical periodontal therapy was needed. Microbiological testing revealed an absence of *A. actinomycetemcomitans*, *P. gingivalis*, *T. forsythia*, and *T. denticola*. For supportive periodontal therapy, the patient was sent back to her dentist in private practice.

Table 1. Baseline data. PD, probing depth.

	Patient 1	Patient 2
Age (years)	50	55
Gender	f	f
Mean probing depth in mm	2.5	4.36
Number of sites ≥ 5 mm PD	8	43
Mean attachment loss in mm	2	5
Bleeding on probing in %	47	31
Plaque index in %	38	75
Number of teeth	26	29

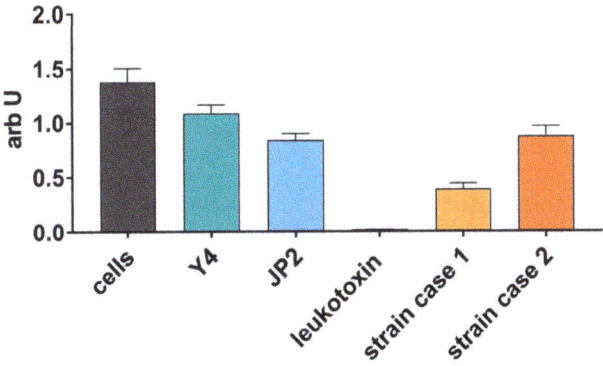

Figure 1. MTT ((3-(4,5-dimethylthiazol-2-yl)-2,5-diphenyltetrazolium bromide) tetrazolium) assay assessing the vitality of the MONO-MAC-6 cells after contact with the clinical *Aggregatibacter actinomycetemcomitans* JP2 genotype strains (case 1 and case 2) in comparison with *Aggregatibacter actinomycetemcomitans* leukotoxin, a reference JP2 genotype strain (HK1651) and Y4 strain.

2.2. Case 2

A 55-year-old female patient was referred to the clinic for periodontal treatment after having been diagnosed with chronic generalized periodontitis. The periodontal screening index [30] was 4 for each sextant and the periodontal chart showed CAL of > 5 mm at all molars. At teeth 11 and 22, PDs up to 12 mm were detected. In the maxilla, all molars showed a furcation involvement degree II at least at one side. Teeth numbers 18, 38, and 48 were missing. In the mandible, all molars showed degree I furcation involvement. The patient was systemically healthy and a non-smoker. On the radiographs, horizontal bone loss was detected at the distal aspects of teeth 16, 15, 25, and 26. Angular bony defects were observed mesially of all first molars as well as distally of tooth 11. Microbiological analysis revealed high counts (more than 10^5) for *A. actinomycetemcomitans*, low counts (about 10^4) each for *T. forsythia*, and moderate counts (about 10^5) for *T. denticola*, but no *P. gingivalis*. Subtyping of *A. actinomycetemcomitans* showed a serotype b strain being positive for the deletion in the promotor region of the leukotoxin operon (JP2 genotype). No other *A. actinomycetemcomitans* strain was identified. Her strain could be cultured (about 10^5 per sample) and showed low MIC values to amoxicillin (≤ 0.5 µg/mL) and a resistance to metronidazole (32 µg/mL). The toxicity of the strain to the MONO-MAC-6 cells was similar to that of the JP2 genotype reference strain (HK1651), but also higher than those of the Y4 strain (serotype b strain without deletion in the promotor region) (Figure 1).

At the next visit, she was asked for contacts with Africans and, indeed, she was married to a man from North Africa. Her husband agreed to a periodontal clinical diagnosis including a microbiological analysis. However, he was periodontally healthy and no *A. actinomycetemcomitans* was detected. In the following, her children also agreed to a periodontal clinical and microbiological diagnosis. The 17-year-old daughter was diagnosed with aggressive periodontitis together with a positive detection for *A. actinomycetemcomitans*, but no *P. gingivalis*. After this accidental diagnosis, the daughter also received periodontal therapy, including adjunctive antibiotics.

After a thorough oral hygiene instruction and supragingival scaling, the patient showed an excellent oral hygiene and a plaque index (O'Leary [29]) of less than 15%, and subgingival scaling was performed in two sessions within one week using hand curettes and local anesthesia. Upon the second session, antibiotics (amoxicillin 375 mg and metronidazole 500 mg each tid for seven days) were given because of the JP2 genotype detection and the severity of the tissue destruction. The reevaluation showed a conspicuous improvement with residual PD > 5 mm at teeth 11, 46, and 36. The latter further improved until the first recall so that surgical therapy was needed only for tooth 11 distally with PD of 9 mm and 46 mesially with PD of 7 mm. Now, the JP2 genotype of *A. actinomycetemcomitans* could not be detected anymore. For both teeth, a flap was raised using the simplified papilla preservation technique. After removal of granulation tissue, scaling and root planing was performed. Tooth 11 exhibited a three-wall defect with an intraosseous depth of 3.5 mm. Given the defect configuration, enamel matrix derivative and bone graft material were administered into the defect. Tooth 46 mesially exhibited a narrow angular bony defect of 3 mm depth, which was treated by means of an access flap surgery and application of an enamel matrix derivative. The patient was enrolled into a three-month recall at the Department of Periodontology. After one year, the recall interval was reduced to six months. A stable periodontal situation was noted with no PD > 4 mm. After another year, the patient was sent back to her dentist in private practice.

3. Discussion

In the present paper, we reported on two rare cases of *A. actinomycetemcomitans* JP2 genotype infection in Caucasians, highlighting the treatment sequences, the clinical outcomes, and the potential value of microbiological testing for the early detection of periodontal disease. Although, over the last 10 years, each *A. actinomycetemcomitans* positive sample has been screened for JP2 genotype presence, no further cases have been detected in our clinic up to now. This is in line with the findings of others who have only sporadically reported on the detection of JP2 genotype in non-African populations [31]. Conversely, the JP2 genotype is widespread and highly present in Northwest African populations.

The reason this genotype of *A. actinomycetemcomitans* has remained geographically restricted despite globalization is still an unanswered question. However, it cannot be excluded that a specific host tropism exists that favors the colonization among these populations.

The highly leukotoxic JP2 genotype is strongly associated with AP. In Northwest African countries, there is a higher prevalence of AP reported among the young population than in other parts of the world, where it is a rare disease with a prevalence of less than 1% [32,33]. In contrast, both patients presented here were, at the time of the baseline examination, between 50 and 55 years of age and diagnosed with CP. An association between young age and the presence of JP2 genotype has been observed, however, with the increasing age of the host, these strains seem to disappear [12]. A prospective longitudinal cohort study has demonstrated that, initially, periodontally healthy subjects harboring the JP2 clone are more likely to develop periodontal attachment loss; a much less pronounced disease risk was found for those not carrying the JP2 genotype [33]. In our cases, it is unclear at what age the patients were infected by the JP2 genotype and how fast the periodontal defects evolved. The 50-year-old patient had no association with North or West African countries. The 55-year-old patient was married to a North African man.

It is of interest to note that there was no detection of *P. gingivalis* in any of these two cases. The fact that *P. gingivalis* was not detected could be correlated with the ability of certain subgingival bacteria to modulate the leukotoxicity of *A. actinomycetemcomitans*. Antibodies raised against *A. actinomycetemcomitans* and its leukotoxin may be inactivated by proteases of other bacteria such as *P. gingivalis* [34]. Gingipains are the primary virulence factor of *P. gingivalis*, showing a proteolytic activity against a broad spectrum of proteins [35]. Further, it has been shown that leukotoxin is proteolytically degraded by the action of gingipains [34]. *P. gingivalis* was able to completely destroy the leukotoxin of *A. actinomycetemcomitans* within an hour [34].

A. actinomycetemcomitans leukotoxin affects immune cells to release IL-1β [6]. Here, we tested the toxicity of the JP2 genotype strains of the two cases on MONO-MAC-6 cells. The JP2 genotype reference strain (HK1651) was more toxic than the Y4 strain. The difference might be not very high, but can be related to the experimental conditions using a lower bacterial concentration and a different cell line than that reported before [36]. One JP2 genotype strain showed a similar cell toxicity to the JP2 genotype reference strain on MONO-MAC-6 cells. The patient with that strain showed periodontal defects at the molar region and at the maxillary incisors, reflecting the typical localization pattern of AP [37].

However, MTT cytotoxicity assay revealed strong cytotoxicity of the other strain, interestingly, the case with no contact to Africans. Here, we can only speculate if there is a difference in production of leukotoxin or in retaining it at the cell surface. Leukotoxin is enriched in outer-membrane-like vesicles [36]. The obviously very high toxicity may contribute to the infection of a person with no genetic predisposition. Here, it has to be pointed out that leukotoxicity may be different depending on the test method that was used [38]. Variation of leukotoxicity was not only observed among JP2- and non-JP2 genotype of *A. actinomycetemcomitans*, but also among the methods of Western blotting, ELISA, cell lysis assay, and mRNA expression assay [38].

After diagnosis, the patients received two sessions of oral hygiene instructions and supragingival scaling by means of ultrasonic and hand instruments. Thereafter, subgingival non-surgical instrumentation was performed with adjunctive antibiotic therapy (amoxicillin and metronidazole). Microbiological testing after the hygienic phase showed that *A. actinomycetemcomitans* was no longer detected. In these cases, the microbiological characterization of *A. actinomycetemcomitans* strains influenced the therapeutic approach, namely to administer or not adjunctive systemic antibiotics. Otherwise, in view of the increasing bacterial resistance, patients diagnosed with CP are not treated with adjunctive amoxicillin and metronidazole during non-surgical mechanical therapy. The in vitro resistance of the strains to amoxicillin and metronidazole was determined. These data cannot be transferred directly to the clinic. A synergism between metronidazole and amoxicillin is well known, as amoxicillin increases the uptake of metronidazole in the bacterial cells [39]. First, this combination was successfully used to treat patients with *A. actinomycetemcomitans* associated periodontitis [40].

Nonetheless, it is well documented that, in patients diagnosed with CP or AP, better clinical outcomes can be obtained if systemic antibiotics are administered in conjunction with subgingival mechanical debridement, irrespective of their microbiological profile [41]. Therefore, in general, microbiological testing was found to be clinically irrelevant for the treatment strategy. It was demonstrated that the presence of putative periodontal pathogens quantified before the treatment was not key for the outcome of scaling and root planing (SRP) with or without amoxicillin and metronidazole [42].

A study evaluating the treatment response of patients infected with JP2 or non-JP2 genotype of *A. actinomycetemcomitans* has shown that patients infected with JP2 genotype had higher PD, CAL, and gingival inflammation than those infected with non-JP2 genotype at baseline. Patients with persisting JP2 genotype after full-mouth SRP and adjunctive administration of amoxicillin and metronidazole had increased gingival inflammation compared with patients where the JP2 strain was eliminated [43]. In the non-JP2 genotype-infected group, the clinical improvements in terms of PD reduction and CAL gain were statistically significantly higher compared with patients infected with the JP2 genotype. These data appear to suggest that the persistence of JP2 genotype in periodontal pocket diminishes the treatment response, which in turn may favor the progression of periodontitis.

In our material, we presented two cases of Caucasians infected with JP2 genotype who were successfully treated with full-mouth SRP and amoxicillin and metronidazole. The microbiological diagnosis was the key decision making factor for selecting the treatment strategy, including the use of amoxicillin and metronidazole. Additionally, it is important to point out that the microbiological diagnosis has finally led to a screening of the patients' family members and the diagnosis of an AP in the teenage daughter of one patient.

4. Materials and Methods

The two patients of non-African origin with detection of the JP2 genotype underwent active periodontal therapy at the Department of Periodontology during the years 2014 and 2015. Both patients were diagnosed with CP according to the classification set in 1999 [26]. The severity and extent of periodontal destruction varied considerably. For each patient, pooled samples of the deepest pockets of each quadrant were analyzed for the major bacteria associated with periodontal diseases using nucleic acid-based strip technology (micro-IDent®plus11, Hain Lifescience, Nehren, Germany) [4]. Identification of the serotype b strains and JP2 genotype strains was performed using the PCR technique [24].

Then, after asking for an additional biofilm sample, cultivation and isolation of the *A. actinomycetemcomitans* strain were performed. After confirming the identification (JP2 genotype), determination of antibiotic resistance to amoxicillin and metronidazole was done using the microbroth-dilution technique. Further, the toxicity to monocytic cells of human origin (MONO-MAC-6; DSMZ no. ACC 124) was assessed. Those were maintained in RPMI 1640 medium containing 10% fetale bovine serum (FBS) and, after washing, adjusted to 10^6/mL in RPMI 1640. Forty hour cultures of *A. actinomycetemcomitans* strains on agar plates were adjusted to 2×10^7/mL in RPMI 1640. Both suspension were mixed 1:1 and the vitality of MONO-MAC-6 cells was determined after 6 h of incubation at 37 °C with 5% of CO_2 using the MTT assay, according to Mosmann [44]. As controls, *A. actinomycetemcomitans* HK1651 (JP2 genotype) and *A. actinomycetemcomitans* Y4 (both strains obtained from ATCC, #ATCC 700685, and ATCC 43718), as well as leukotoxin (2.5 µg/mL; purified as described by Kachlany et al. [45] from culture supernatant of a control *A. actinomycetemcomitans* HK1651 strain added by a final centrifugation using a 10 kDa centrifugal filter to remove proteins of lower weights), were used.

5. Conclusions

Colonization of Caucasians by the JP2 genotype of *A. actinomycetemcomitans* is rare. In the present study, the microbiological diagnosis played the key role for selecting the use of adjunctive systemic antibiotics, as well as for the ensuring an accurate periodontal diagnosis and adequate treatment for the patient's teenage daughter.

Author Contributions: Conceptualization, S.E. and A.S. (Alexandra Stähli); methodology, S.E.; treatment, A.S. (Alexandra Stähli); writing—original draft preparation, A.S. (Alexandra Stähli) and S.E.; writing—review and editing, A.S. (Anton Sculean). All authors have read and agreed to the published version of the manuscript.

Funding: This research received no external funding.

Acknowledgments: Anna Magdoń (Laboratory of Oral Microbiology, Department of Periodontology, School of Dental Medicine, University of Bern) is acknowledged for identification and characterization of *A. actinomycetemcomitans* strains.

Conflicts of Interest: The authors declare no conflict of interest.

References

1. Tonetti, M. Etiology and pathogenesis. In Proceedings of the 1st European Workshop on Periodontology, Thurgau, Switzerland, 1–4 February 1993; Lang, N.P., Karring, T., Eds.; Quintessenz Verlags-GmbH: Berlin, Germany, 1993; pp. 54–89.
2. Faveri, M.; Figueiredo, L.C.; Duarte, P.M.; Mestnik, M.J.; Mayer, M.P.; Feres, M. Microbiological profile of untreated subjects with localized aggressive periodontitis. *J. Clin. Periodontol.* **2009**, *36*, 739–749. [CrossRef] [PubMed]
3. Mombelli, A.; Casagni, F.; Madianos, P.N. Can presence or absence of periodontal pathogens distinguish between subjects with chronic and aggressive periodontitis? A systematic review. *J. Clin. Periodontol.* **2002**, *29* (Suppl. 3), 10–21. [CrossRef]
4. Eick, S.; Nydegger, J.; Burgin, W.; Salvi, G.E.; Sculean, A.; Ramseier, C. Microbiological analysis and the outcomes of periodontal treatment with or without adjunctive systemic antibiotics-a retrospective study. *Clin. Oral Investig.* **2018**, *22*, 3031–3041. [CrossRef] [PubMed]
5. Gholizadeh, P.; Pormohammad, A.; Eslami, H.; Shokouhi, B.; Fakhrzadeh, V.; Kafil, H.S. Oral pathogenesis of Aggregatibacter actinomycetemcomitans. *Microb. Pathog.* **2017**, *113*, 303–311. [CrossRef] [PubMed]
6. Johansson, A. Aggregatibacter actinomycetemcomitans leukotoxin: A powerful tool with capacity to cause imbalance in the host inflammatory response. *Toxins* **2011**, *3*, 242–259. [CrossRef] [PubMed]
7. Tsai, C.C.; Shenker, B.J.; DiRienzo, J.M.; Malamud, D.; Taichman, N.S. Extraction and isolation of a leukotoxin from Actinobacillus actinomycetemcomitans with polymyxin B. *Infect. Immun.* **1984**, *43*, 700–705. [CrossRef] [PubMed]
8. Poulsen, K.; Theilade, E.; Lally, E.T.; Demuth, D.R.; Kilian, M. Population structure of Actinobacillus actinomycetemcomitans: A framework for studies of disease-associated properties. *Microbiology* **1994**, *140 Pt 8*, 2049–2060. [CrossRef]
9. Haubek, D.; Poulsen, K.; Westergaard, J.; Dahlen, G.; Kilian, M. Highly toxic clone of Actinobacillus actinomycetemcomitans in geographically widespread cases of juvenile periodontitis in adolescents of African origin. *J. Clin. Microbiol.* **1996**, *34*, 1576–1578. [CrossRef]
10. Haubek, D.; Dirienzo, J.M.; Tinoco, E.M.; Westergaard, J.; Lopez, N.J.; Chung, C.P.; Poulsen, K.; Kilian, M. Racial tropism of a highly toxic clone of Actinobacillus actinomycetemcomitans associated with juvenile periodontitis. *J. Clin. Microbiol.* **1997**, *35*, 3037–3042. [CrossRef]
11. Haubek, D.; Ennibi, O.K.; Poulsen, K.; Poulsen, S.; Benzarti, N.; Kilian, M. Early-onset periodontitis in Morocco is associated with the highly leukotoxic clone of Actinobacillus actinomycetemcomitans. *J. Dent. Res.* **2001**, *80*, 1580–1583. [CrossRef]
12. Haraszthy, V.I.; Hariharan, G.; Tinoco, E.M.; Cortelli, J.R.; Lally, E.T.; Davis, E.; Zambon, J.J. Evidence for the role of highly leukotoxic Actinobacillus actinomycetemcomitans in the pathogenesis of localized juvenile and other forms of early-onset periodontitis. *J. Periodontol.* **2000**, *71*, 912–922. [CrossRef]
13. Brogan, J.M.; Lally, E.T.; Poulsen, K.; Kilian, M.; Demuth, D.R. Regulation of Actinobacillus actinomycetemcomitans leukotoxin expression: Analysis of the promoter regions of leukotoxic and minimally leukotoxic strains. *Infect. Immun.* **1994**, *62*, 501–508. [CrossRef] [PubMed]
14. Hritz, M.; Fisher, E.; Demuth, D.R. Differential regulation of the leukotoxin operon in highly leukotoxic and minimally leukotoxic strains of Actinobacillus actinomycetemcomitans. *Infect. Immun.* **1996**, *64*, 2724–2729. [CrossRef] [PubMed]
15. Haubek, D. The highly leukotoxic JP2 clone of Aggregatibacter actinomycetemcomitans: Evolutionary aspects, epidemiology and etiological role in aggressive periodontitis. *APMIS Suppl.* **2010**, *130*, 1–53. [CrossRef]
16. Takada, K.; Saito, M.; Tsuzukibashi, O.; Kawashima, Y.; Ishida, S.; Hirasawa, M. Characterization of a new serotype g isolate of Aggregatibacter actinomycetemcomitans. *Mol. Oral Microbiol.* **2010**, *25*, 200–206. [CrossRef]

17. Brigido, J.A.; da Silveira, V.R.; Rego, R.O.; Nogueira, N.A. Serotypes of Aggregatibacter actinomycetemcomitans in relation to periodontal status and geographic origin of individuals-a review of the literature. *Med. Oral Patol. Oral Cir. Bucal* **2014**, *19*, e184. [CrossRef] [PubMed]
18. Chen, C.; Wang, T.; Chen, W. Occurrence of Aggregatibacter actinomycetemcomitans serotypes in subgingival plaque from United States subjects. *Mol. Oral Microbiol.* **2010**, *25*, 207–214. [CrossRef] [PubMed]
19. Teixeira, R.E.; Mendes, E.N.; Roque de Carvalho, M.A.; Nicoli, J.R.; Farias Lde, M.; Magalhaes, P.P. Actinobacillus actinomycetemcomitans serotype-specific genotypes and periodontal status in Brazilian subjects. *Can. J. Microbiol.* **2006**, *52*, 182–188. [CrossRef]
20. Cortelli, J.R.; Aquino, D.R.; Cortelli, S.C.; Roman-Torres, C.V.; Franco, G.C.; Gomez, R.S.; Batista, L.H.; Costa, F.O. Aggregatibacter actinomycetemcomitans serotypes infections and periodontal conditions: A two-way assessment. *Eur. J. Clin. Microbiol. Infect. Dis.* **2012**, *31*, 1311–1318. [CrossRef]
21. Thiha, K.; Takeuchi, Y.; Umeda, M.; Huang, Y.; Ohnishi, M.; Ishikawa, I. Identification of periodontopathic bacteria in gingival tissue of Japanese periodontitis patients. *Oral Microbiol. Immunol.* **2007**, *22*, 201–207. [CrossRef]
22. Haubek, D.; Johansson, A. Pathogenicity of the highly leukotoxic JP2 clone of Aggregatibacter actinomycetemcomitans and its geographic dissemination and role in aggressive periodontitis. *J. Oral Microbiol.* **2014**, *6*. [CrossRef] [PubMed]
23. Kim, T.S.; Frank, P.; Eickholz, P.; Eick, S.; Kim, C.K. Serotypes of Aggregatibacter actinomycetemcomitans in patients with different ethnic backgrounds. *J. Periodontol.* **2009**, *80*, 2020–2027. [CrossRef] [PubMed]
24. Jentsch, H.; Cachovan, G.; Guentsch, A.; Eickholz, P.; Pfister, W.; Eick, S. Characterization of Aggregatibacter actinomycetemcomitans strains in periodontitis patients in Germany. *Clin. Oral Investig.* **2012**, *16*, 1589–1597. [CrossRef] [PubMed]
25. Claesson, R.; Hoglund-Aberg, C.; Haubek, D.; Johansson, A. Age-related prevalence and characteristics of Aggregatibacter actinomycetemcomitans in periodontitis patients living in Sweden. *J. Oral Microbiol.* **2017**, *9*, 1334504. [CrossRef]
26. Armitage, G.C. Development of a classification system for periodontal diseases and conditions. *Ann. Periodontol.* **1999**, *4*, 1–6. [CrossRef]
27. Eke, P.I.; Page, R.C.; Wei, L.; Thornton-Evans, G.; Genco, R.J. Update of the case definitions for population-based surveillance of periodontitis. *J. Periodontol.* **2012**, *83*, 1449–1454. [CrossRef]
28. Page, R.C.; Eke, P.I. Case definitions for use in population-based surveillance of periodontitis. *J. Periodontol.* **2007**, *78*, 1387–1399. [CrossRef]
29. O'Leary, T.J.; Drake, R.B.; Naylor, J.E. The plaque control record. *J. Periodontol.* **1972**, *43*, 38. [CrossRef]
30. Diamanti-Kipioti, A.; Papapanou, P.N.; Moraitaki-Tsami, A.; Lindhe, J.; Mitsis, F. Comparative estimation of periodontal conditions by means of different index systems. *J. Clin. Periodontol.* **1993**, *20*, 656–661. [CrossRef]
31. Claesson, R.; Lagervall, M.; Hoglund-Aberg, C.; Johansson, A.; Haubek, D. Detection of the highly leukotoxic JP2 clone of Aggregatibacter actinomycetemcomitans in members of a Caucasian family living in Sweden. *J. Clin. Periodontol.* **2011**, *38*, 115–121. [CrossRef]
32. Albandar, J.M.; Buischi, Y.A.; Barbosa, M.F. Destructive forms of periodontal disease in adolescents. A 3-year longitudinal study. *J. Periodontol.* **1991**, *62*, 370–376. [CrossRef] [PubMed]
33. Haubek, D.; Ennibi, O.K.; Poulsen, K.; Vaeth, M.; Poulsen, S.; Kilian, M. Risk of aggressive periodontitis in adolescent carriers of the JP2 clone of Aggregatibacter (Actinobacillus) actinomycetemcomitans in Morocco: A prospective longitudinal cohort study. *Lancet* **2008**, *371*, 237–242. [CrossRef]
34. Johansson, A.; Hanstrom, L.; Kalfas, S. Inhibition of Actinobacillus actinomycetemcomitans leukotoxicity by bacteria from the subgingival flora. *Oral Microbiol. Immunol.* **2000**, *15*, 218–225. [CrossRef] [PubMed]
35. Guo, Y.; Nguyen, K.A.; Potempa, J. Dichotomy of gingipains action as virulence factors: From cleaving substrates with the precision of a surgeon's knife to a meat chopper-like brutal degradation of proteins. *Periodontol 2000* **2010**, *54*, 15–44. [CrossRef]
36. Kato, S.; Kowashi, Y.; Demuth, D.R. Outer membrane-like vesicles secreted by Actinobacillus actinomycetemcomitans are enriched in leukotoxin. *Microb. Pathog.* **2002**, *32*, 1–13. [CrossRef]
37. Baer, P.N. The case for periodontosis as a clinical entity. *J. Periodontol.* **1971**, *42*, 516–520. [CrossRef]
38. Jensen, A.B.; Lund, M.; Norskov-Lauritsen, N.; Johansson, A.; Claesson, R.; Reinholdt, J.; Haubek, D. Differential cell lysis among periodontal strains of JP2 and Non-JP2 genotype of aggregatibacter actinomycetemcomitans serotype B is not reflected in dissimilar expression and production of leukotoxin. *Pathogens* **2019**, *8*, 211. [CrossRef]

39. Pavicic, M.J.; van Winkelhoff, A.J.; Pavicic-Temming, Y.A.; de Graaff, J. Amoxycillin causes an enhanced uptake of metronidazole in Actinobacillus actinomycetemcomitans: A mechanism of synergy. *J. Antimicrob. Chemother.* **1994**, *34*, 1047–1050. [CrossRef]
40. van Winkelhoff, A.J.; Rodenburg, J.P.; Goene, R.J.; Abbas, F.; Winkel, E.G.; de Graaff, J. Metronidazole plus amoxycillin in the treatment of Actinobacillus actinomycetemcomitans associated periodontitis. *J. Clin. Periodontol.* **1989**, *16*, 128–131. [CrossRef]
41. Mombelli, A.; Cionca, N.; Almaghlouth, A.; Decaillet, F.; Courvoisier, D.S.; Giannopoulou, C. Are there specific benefits of amoxicillin plus metronidazole in Aggregatibacter actinomycetemcomitans-associated periodontitis? Double-masked, randomized clinical trial of efficacy and safety. *J. Periodontol.* **2013**, *84*, 715–724. [CrossRef]
42. Cionca, N.; Giannopoulou, C.; Ugolotti, G.; Mombelli, A. Microbiologic testing and outcomes of full-mouth scaling and root planing with or without amoxicillin/metronidazole in chronic periodontitis. *J. Periodontol.* **2010**, *81*, 15–23. [CrossRef] [PubMed]
43. Cortelli, S.C.; Costa, F.O.; Kawai, T.; Aquino, D.R.; Franco, G.C.; Ohara, K.; Roman-Torres, C.V.; Cortelli, J.R. Diminished treatment response of periodontally diseased patients infected with the JP2 clone of Aggregatibacter (Actinobacillus) actinomycetemcomitans. *J. Clin. Microbiol.* **2009**, *47*, 2018–2025. [CrossRef] [PubMed]
44. Mosmann, T. Rapid colorimetric assay for cellular growth and survival: Application to proliferation and cytotoxicity assays. *J. Immunol. Methods* **1983**, *65*, 55–63. [CrossRef]
45. Kachlany, S.C.; Fine, D.H.; Figurski, D.H. Purification of secreted leukotoxin (LtxA) from Actinobacillus actinomycetemcomitans. *Protein. Expr. Purif.* **2002**, *25*, 465–471. [CrossRef]

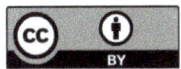

© 2020 by the authors. Licensee MDPI, Basel, Switzerland. This article is an open access article distributed under the terms and conditions of the Creative Commons Attribution (CC BY) license (http://creativecommons.org/licenses/by/4.0/).

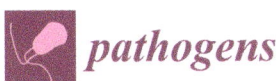

Article

Distinct Signaling Pathways Between Human Macrophages and Primary Gingival Epithelial Cells by *Aggregatibacter actinomycetemcomitans*

Ellen S. Ando-Suguimoto [1],*, Manjunatha R. Benakanakere [2],*, Marcia P.A. Mayer [1] and Denis F. Kinane [3]

1. Department of Microbiology, Institute of Biomedical Sciences, University of São Paulo, São Paulo 05508-020, Brazil; mpamayer@icb.usp.br
2. Department of Periodontics, School of Dental Medicine, University of Pennsylvania, Philadelphia, PA 19104, USA
3. Department of Periodontology, School of Dental Medicine, University of Geneva Faculty of Medicine, 12114 Geneva, Switzerland; dfkinane@outlook.com
* Correspondence: ellensuguimoto@gmail.com (E.S.A.S.); bmanju@upenn.edu (M.R.B.); Tel.: +55-11-3091-7348 (E.S.A.S.); +1-215-746-4189 (M.R.B.)

Received: 28 November 2019; Accepted: 23 March 2020; Published: 27 March 2020

Abstract: In aggressive periodontitis, the dysbiotic microbial community in the subgingival crevice, which is abundant in Aggregatibacter actinomycetemcomitans, interacts with extra- and intracellular receptors of host cells, leading to exacerbated inflammation and subsequent tissue destruction. Our goal was to understand the innate immune interactions of A. actinomycetemcomitans with macrophages and human gingival epithelial cells (HGECs) on the signaling cascade involved in inflammasome and inflammatory responses. U937 macrophages and HGECs were co-cultured with A. actinomycetemcomitans strain Y4 and key signaling pathways were analyzed using real-time PCR, Western blotting and cytokine production by ELISA. A. actinomycetemcomitans infection upregulated the transcription of TLR2, TLR4, NOD2 and NLRP3 in U937 macrophages, but not in HGECs. Transcription of IL-1β and IL-18 was upregulated in macrophages and HGECs after 1 h interaction with A. actinomycetemcomitans, but positive regulation persisted only in macrophages, resulting in the presence of IL-1β in macrophage supernatant. Immunoblot data revealed that A. actinomycetemcomitans induced the phosphorylation of AKT and ERK1/2, possibly leading to activation of the NF-κB pathway in macrophages. On the other hand, HGEC signaling induced by A. actinomycetemcomitans was distinct, since AKT and 4EBP1 were phosphorylated after stimulation with A. actinomycetemcomitans, whereas ERK1/2 was not. Furthermore, A. actinomycetemcomitans was able to induce the cleavage of caspase-1 in U937 macrophages in an NRLP3-dependent pathway. Differences in host cell responses, such as those seen between HGECs and macrophages, suggested that survival of A. actinomycetemcomitans in periodontal tissues may be favored by its ability to differentially activate host cells.

Keywords: *A. actinomycetemcomitans*; inflammasome; immune response; periodontal disease

---

1. Introduction

Periodontitis is an infectious inflammatory disease that leads to the destruction of tooth-supporting tissues by an imbalanced immune response [1–5]. The inflammatory process is induced by a dysbiotic microbial community, with the Gram-negative facultative species *Aggregatibacter actinomycetemcomitans* associated the rapid progression rate of periodontitis, which was previously denominated localized aggressive periodontitis and is now classified as molar/incisor pattern periodontitis [6,7]. *A. actinomycetemcomitans* is also associated with endocarditis [8] and may play a role in cardiovascular disease and arthritis [9,10]. The dysbiosis induced by *A. actinomycetemcomitans* may be the result of an immunological palsy induced by its virulence factors, such as leukotoxin (Ltx) and cytolethal distending toxin (Cdt) [11,12], which are associated with its ability to invade non-phagocytic cells [13].

During infection, the immune response is induced by microbial-associated molecular patterns (MAMPS), which are recognized by pattern-recognition receptors (PRRs) in eukaryotic cells. PRRs are found extracellularly as Toll-Like Receptors (TLRs) and are expressed on the cell surface, with their stimulation by MAMPS resulting from the activation of NF-κB, MAPK and IRF signaling pathways, culminating in the production of a number of cytokines, chemokines and immunomodulatory factors [14]. PRRs are also present in the cytoplasm and are here called Nod-Like Receptors (NLRs), with nucleotide binding domain/leucine rich repeats, including NLRP1, NLRP3, NLRC4, NOD1, NOD2, and AIM2 receptors; these detect intracellular microorganisms and their products [15–17]. Although both pathogenic and commensal microbes are recognized by PPRs, pathogens often induce the production of endogenous danger signals (danger-associated molecular patterns (DAMPs)) [18]. The cytosol senses DAMPS via NLRs, leading to the formation of multiprotein cytoplasmic complexes called inflammasomes [19]. These complexes activate caspase-1, which results in the release of mature interleukin-1β (IL-1β) and interleukin-18 (IL-18), thereby inducing pyroptosis and apoptosis [20].

A. actinomycetemcomitans is recognized by Toll-Like Receptor 4 (TLR4) and TLR2 [21]. Gingival epithelial cells (GECs) are the first defense barrier against pathogens in periodontal tissues; *A. actinomycetemcomitans* adheres to and invades epithelial cells [22]. The interaction of *A. actinomycetemcomitans* with GECs induces the expression of ICAM-1, TNF, GM-CSF, IL-6 and IL-8 and causes apoptosis in monocytes mediated by interaction with TLR2 [22–24]. Furthermore, macrophages infected with *A. actinomycetemcomitans* secrete IL-1β [25,26] and IL-18, a response which is associated with the purinergic receptor $P2X_7$, an endogenous danger signal receptor [27].

Inflammasome activation may play a key role in periodontitis. The expression of NLRP3, which is involved in inflammasomes, is higher in chronic and aggressive periodontitis gingival tissues than in healthy tissues, especially at the periodontal epithelium layer [28]. In periodontal disease, NLRP3 salivary levels are higher in aggressive periodontitis cases compared to periodontally healthy subjects [29].

A. actinomycetemcomitans cytolethal distending toxin (AaCdt) was shown to be involved in NLRP3 activation in THP-1 monocytes and release of mature IL-1β [30], but other bacterial factors may be also associated with this response to *A. actinomycetemcomitans,* since infection of human monocytes with leukotoxin- and Cdt-deficient strains still resulted in upregulation of NLRP3, IL-1β and IL-18 expression [31]. *A. actinomycetemcomitans* was also shown to activate the inflammasome pathway in nonimmune cells. NRLP3 upregulation and secretion of mature IL-1β and IL-18 were observed in human osteoblastic MG63 cells upon exposure to *A. actinomycetemcomitans*, leading to apoptosis [32]. Furthermore, NOD1 and NOD2 were activated in human embryonic kidney cells in the presence of *A. actinomycetemcomitans* [33].

The response to a pathogen depends not only on the stimulus, but also on the cell type; however, there are no data regarding whether *A. actinomycetemcomitans* is able to activate inflammasomes in epithelial cells, as reviewed previously [34]. Given the significance of gingival epithelial cells and macrophages in aggressive periodontitis, the present study evaluated the signaling network initiated by *A. actinomycetemcomitans* in gingival epithelial cells and macrophages and, consequently, the induction of immune and inflammasome responses.

2. Results

A. actinomycetemcomitans is associated with localized aggressive periodontitis, however, the molecular mechanisms of the innate immune response in distinct myeloid and nonmyeloid cells of the oral cavity are unknown. We set out to understand the differential activation immune vs. nonimmune cells by *A. actinomycetemcomitans*. We stimulated the U937 cell line to differentiate into macrophages and primary human gingival epithelial cells (HGECs) via *A. actinomycetemcomitans* Y4 at different time points to determine the innate immune responses. The innate immune genes, in particular *TLR2*, *TLR4* and *NLRP3*, were upregulated in U937 macrophages co-cultured with *A. actinomycetemcomitans* after two and three hours of incubation, where *NLRP3* doubled its expression compared to the control after two hours of co-culture and was downregulated after four and eight hours, whereas *NOD2* mRNA reached maximum levels after 8 h of stimulation, increasing expression by two times. On the other hand, infection of HGECs with *A. actinomycetemcomitans* did not result in altered transcription profile of genes encoding these receptors (Tables 1 and 2).

Table 1. Effect of co-culture of *A. actinomycetemcomitans* strain Y4 (Aa- MOI 1:100) with human gingival epithelial cells (HGECs) for 1, 2, 3, 4 and 8 h on the relative transcription of *TLR4*, *TLR2*, *NLRP3*, *NOD1*, *NOD2*, *IL-1β*, *IL-18* and *TNF-α* detected by real-time PCR and expressed in terms of fold-change in comparison with control. Control consisted of infected cells at 0 h. Transcription of the target gene was normalized according to mRNA levels of GAPDH; = data are shown as fold-change ± standard deviation (SD) representative of three independent experiments.

Gene Expression (HGECs)	Control (0 h)	Aa 1 h	Aa 2 h	Aa 3 h	Aa 4 h	Aa 8 h
				Fold-Change (±SD)		
tlr-4	1.00	0.79 (±0.14)	0.74 (±0.10)	0.68 (±0.08)	0.39 (±0.04)	0.32 (±0.01)
tlr-2	1.00	0.78 (±0.01)	0.66 (±0.09)	0.47 (±0.04)	0.41 (±0.03)	0.46 (±0.04)
nlrp3	1.00	1.15 (±0.23)	0.76 (±0.11)	0.64 (±0.09)	0.50 (±0.03)	1.07 (0.05)
nod1	1.00	1.15 (±0.24)	1.38 (±0.20)	0.80 (±0.00)	0.58 (±0.02)	0.42 (0 05)
nod2	1.00	0.77 (0.09)	0.77 (±0.09)	0.72 (±0.08)	0.77 (±0.01)	0.76 (0.03)
il-1β	1.00	1.22 (±0.06) *	0.72 (±0.01)	0.33 (±0.01)	0.51 (±0.02)	0.13 (±0.01)
Il-18	1.00	1.27 (±0.12) *	0.93 (±0.09)	0.70 (±0.05)	0.64 (±0.09)	0.43 (±0.02)
tnf	1.00	0.88 (±0.05)	0.98 (±0.06)	2.00 (±0.21) *	3.72 (±0.13) *	0.94 (±0.09)

* Statistically significant difference in comparison with control (ANOVA–Tukey's, p < 0.05).

Table 2. Effect of co-culture of *A. actinomycetemcomitans* strain Y4 (Aa- MOI 1:100) with U937 macrophages for 1, 2, 3, 4 and 8 h on the relative transcription of *TLR4*, *TLR2*, *NLRP3*, *NOD1*, *NOD2 IL-1β*, *IL-18* and *TNF-α* detected by real-time PCR and expressed in fold-change in comparison with control. Control consisted of infected cells at 0 h. Transcription of target gene was normalized according to mRNA levels of GAPDH; data are shown as fold-change ± SD representative of three independent experiments.

Gene Expression (U937 cells)	Control (0 h)	Aa 1 h	Aa 2 h	Aa 3 h	Aa 4 h	Aa 8 h
				Fold-change (±SD)		
tlr-4	1.00	1.27 (±0.03) *	1.30 (±0.10) *	1.15 (±0.01) *	0.44 (±0.00)	0.25 (±0.00)
tlr-2	1.00	1.18 (±0.10)	1.51 (±0.18) *	1.47 (±0.14) *	0.75 (±0.04)	0.68 (±0.01)
nlrp3	1.00	0.92 (±0.01)	2.03 (±0.17) *	1.85 (0.18) *	0.70 (±0.02)	0.83 (0.04)
nod1	1.00	1.24 (±0.03)	1.07 (±0.05)	1.13 (±0.40)	1.90 (±0.17)	0.76 (0.09)
nod2	1.00	1.25 (0.07) *	1.24 (±0.02) *	1.29 (±0.07) *	1.67 (±0.13) *	2.34 (0.06) *
il-1b	1.00	10.75 (±0.43) *	31.79 (±0.30) *	43.19 (±1.01) *	26.75 (±2.88) *	54.56 (±7.20) *
Il-18	1.00	1.62 (±0.05) *	1.34 (±0.16) *	1.42 (±0.17) *	1.23 (±0.13)	0.83 (±0.01)
tnf	1.00	7.18 (±0.41)	85.13 (±6.84) *	134.96 (±26.93) *	85.53 (±1.44) *	68.86 (±2.54) *

* Statistically significant difference in comparison with control (ANOVA–Tukey's, p < 0.05).

Cytokine gene expression, *IL-1β*, *IL-18* and *TNF* mRNA levels, increased after co-culture of macrophages with *A. actinomycetemcomitans* (Table 2). On the other hand, the interaction of *A. actinomycetemcomitans* with HGECs resulted in a small increase in *IL-1β* and *IL-18* mRNA levels after one hour of co-culture, and decreased at later time points (Table 1). *TNF* mRNA levels increased after two hours of co-culture of *A. actinomycetemcomitans*, with U937 macrophages reaching the peak after three hours of co-culture (134 times increase), and after three and four hours with HGECs (2 and 3.72 times increase, respectively). Production of IL-1β increased after *A. actinomycetemcomitans* challenge in U937 macrophages but not in HGECs. The *A. actinomycetemcomitans* challenge induced production of TNF in U937 macrophages after two hours, whereas in HGECs, TNF was induced after a prolonged period (Figure 1).

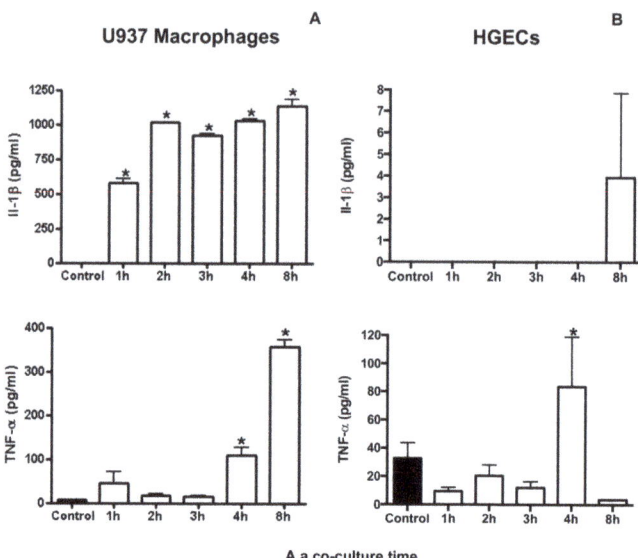

Figure 1. Effect of co-culture of *A. actinomycetemcomitans* strain Y4 (Multiplicity of infection (MOI) 1:100) with U937 macrophages (**A**) or HGECs (**B**) for 1, 2, 3, 4 and 8 h on the levels of IL-1β and TNF-α levels in cell supernatants. Control consisted of infected cells at 0 h. Data (pg cytokine/mL) are presented as mean ± SD representative of three independent experiments. * Statistically significant difference in comparison with control (ANOVA–Tukey's, $p < 0.05$).

Since transcription of *TLR2, TLR4 and NLRP3* was upregulated in U937 macrophages, we determined the activation of signaling molecules downstream of TLRs. Signaling pathway analysis indicated that NF-κB was activated (phosphorylation of serine 32 in IκB-α) and pro caspase-1 was induced and cleaved in *A. actinomycetemcomitans* infected-macrophages (Figure 2A). Infection with *A. actinomycetemcomitans* induced activation of ERK1/2 (phosphorylation of T 202/Y204 residues in ERK1) after 15 min of co-culture and AKT (phosphorylation serine 473 in AKT) after 120 min of co-culture. However, p4EBP1 and pcFos levels did not increase in *A. actinomycetemcomitans*-infected macrophages.

Interestingly, signaling induced by *A. actinomycetemcomitans* was distinct in HGECs. In these epithelial cells, AKT and 4EBP1were phosphorylated after stimulation with *A. actinomycetemcomitans*, whereas ERK1/2 was not phosphorylated (Figure 2B). On the other hand, the phosphorylation of Serine 473 (Ser 473), indicative of AKT activation, was not observed until 60 min of stimulation with *A. actinomycetemcomitans*; these data indicated that AKT activation was under the levels observed in noninfected cells at the early stages of co-culture.

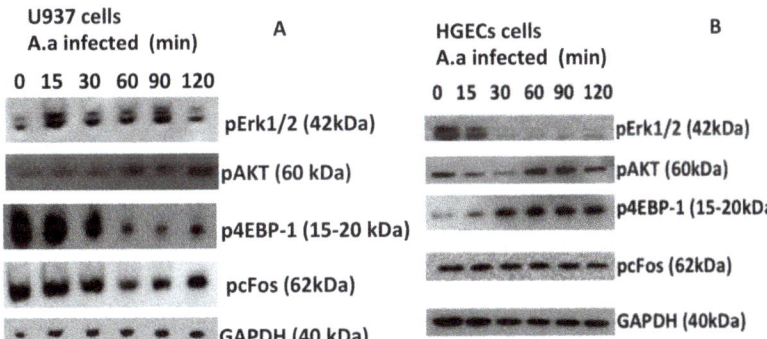

Figure 2. Different pathways are activated by *A. actinomycetemcomitans* in macrophages and HGECs. Western blot was used to evaluate the phosphorylation of ERK1/2, 4EBP-1, cFos and AKT in U937 macrophages (**A**) and in HGECs (**B**) after infection with *A. actinomycetemcomitans* strain Y4 (MOI 1:100) at different time points. GAPDH was used as the control. The data shown are representative of three independent experiments.

IL-1β and TNF-α transcription and protein levels (Table 2 and Figure 1) were increased in *A. actinomycetemcomitans*-infected macrophages within a few hours of incubation, mainly because of the activation of NF-κB in these cells (Figure 3). These results suggested that, in macrophages, NF-κB activation by *A. actinomycetemcomitans* is dependent on AKT–ERK1/2 activation, although more profound studies should still be performed. NF-κB activation induced the release of pro-IL-1β and pro-IL-18, which, in the context of the inflammasome, are processed to their mature forms by caspase-1 in macrophages, as shown by the increased production of active caspase-1 in cells co-cultured with *A. actinomycetemcomitans* (Figure 3). The data indicated that infected macrophages exhibited *NLRP3* upregulation and release of IL-1.

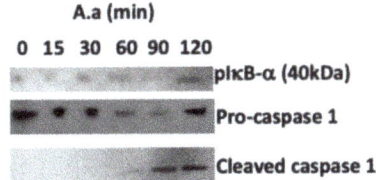

Figure 3. Western blot image showing increased levels of phosphorylated IκB (pIkB-α), (indicative of NF-κB activation), decreased levels of procaspase-1 and increased levels of cleaved caspase-1 (indicative of inflammasome activation in U937 macrophages) after co-culture of *A. actinomycetemcomitans* strain Y4 (MOI 1:100) at different time points. GAPDH was used as the control. The data shown are representative of three independent experiments.

The inflammasome response was analyzed in cells by silencing NLRP3. siNLRP3 macrophages infected with *A. actinomycetemcomitans* exhibited decreased *IL-1β* and *IL-18* mRNA levels, but not *TNF-α* (Figure 4). Taken together, *A. actinomycetemcomitans* distinctly activated innate immune and inflammasomes in myeloid cells (Figure 5) and nonmyeloid cells.

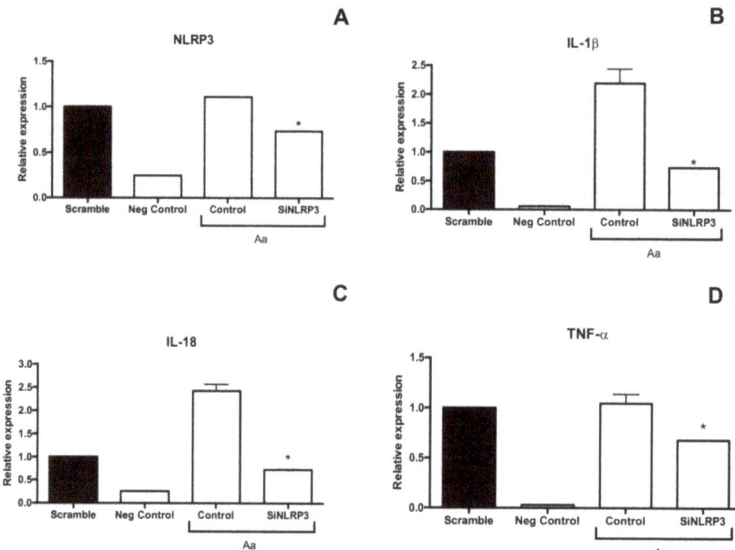

Figure 4. Effect of siNLRP3 silencing in *A. actinomycetemcomitans* Y4-infected U937 macrophages (MOI 1:100, 24 h of co-culture) on the relative expression of *NLRP3* (**A**), *IL-1β* (**B**), *IL-18* (**C**) and *TNF-α* (**D**) detected by real time PCR. Scramble: Scramble control without *A. actinomycetemcomitans* (pool of nontargeting Sirna); negative control: Cells without *A. actinomycetemcomitans*; control: Positive control: Cells with *A. actinomycetemcomitans* without *NLRP3* silencing; siNLRP3: Cells with silencing of *NLRP3* and co-culture with *A. actinomycetemcomitans*. * Statistically significant difference in comparison with electroporated cells with *A. actinomycetemcomitans* and scramble control (ANOVA–Tukey's, $p < 0.05$). Data shown in fold-change relative to the scramble are presented as mean ± SD representative of three independent experiments.

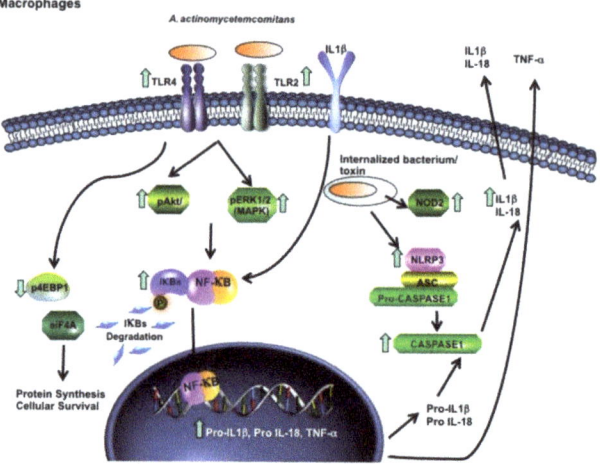

Figure 5. U937 macrophage response after co-culture with *A. actinomycetemcomitans* Y4. Arrows mean up- or downregulation of gene transcription for *TLR4, TLR2, NOD2, NLRP3, Pro-IL-1β, Pro-IL-18* and *TNF-α*, and for phosphorylation of 4EBP1, AKT, pERK1/2, IκB-α and caspase-1. *A. actinomycetemcomitans* was able to induce an inflammatory response and inflammasome activation in macrophages. Adapted from Qiagen's website (https://www.qiagen.com/br/shop/genes-and-pathways/pathway-central/?q=).

3. Discussion

The immune response elicited by the dysbiotic community in aggressive periodontitis induced inflammation, resulting in tissue destruction and bone resorption [35]. In this study, we analyzed two important host cell defenses, namely, a first barrier of epithelial cells and a second specialized cell, the macrophages of myeloid origin.

Human gingival epithelial cells and macrophages displayed distinct responses after challenge with *A. actinomycetemcomitans*. The expression of innate immune receptors was not altered by *A. actinomycetemcomitans* infection in HGECs, suggesting that the epithelial barrier was a weak response, resulting in a discrete increase in IL-1β and IL-18 production after one hour of co-culture and decreased expression thereafter. These data were in accordance with others demonstrating that *A. actinomycetemcomitans* did not induce IL-1β production by gingival epithelial cells [36,37]. Moreover, the increase in mRNA expression of TNF after three hours indicated that the primary HGECs respond to the bacteria stimuli, as demonstrated in immortalized OBA-09 cells [22].

On the other hand, transcription of genes encoding TLR2, TLR4, NLRP3 and NOD2 was upregulated in *A. actinomycetemcomitans*-infected macrophages, suggesting a rapid innate immune response against the pathogen. Previous studies in macrophages [38,39] and dendritic cells [40] corroborated our observation that *A. actinomycetemcomitans* leads to increased expression of TLR2 and TLR4 between two and three hours and one and three hours, respectively. After this period of co-culture, there was a decrease in TLR2 and TLR4 expression, concomitant to an increase in the expression of internal receptors such as NLRP3 and NOD2, suggesting phagocytosis of *A. actinomycetemcomitans* and/or its products.

The engagement of microbial components with TLR2 and TLR4 mediates transcriptional responses through activation of NF-κB, leading to the production of pro-inflammatory cytokines, including TNF-α and inactive pro-IL-1β [39]. Furthermore, the response of macrophages to *A. actinomycetemcomitans* infection was obvious, with immediate and continuous upregulation of *TNF-α*, *IL-1β* and, to a lesser extent, *IL-18*.

A. actinomycetemcomitans phagocytosis by macrophages was impaired due to cytolethal distending toxin production, but the ability to produce nitric oxide (NO) and TNF-α was still functional in the intoxicated macrophages [41]. The upregulation of extra- and intracellular receptors for PAMPS and DAMPS in macrophages reinforced these observations. Binding of PAMPS to TLRs and NOD2 activates the NF-kB pathway, inducing the expression of inflammatory cytokines [42]. When the signaling transduction pathways were analyzed, as shown in Figure 4, the mitogen activated pathway (MAPK) ERK1/2 was activated in *A. actinomycetemcomitans*-infected macrophages, which was suggestive of NF-κB activation after 120 min of incubation, as indicated increased levels of pIkB-α at this time point (Figure 5). The increased level of phosphorylated serine–threonine kinase (pAKT), also observed after 120 min of macrophage interaction with *A. actinomycetemcomitans*, indicated activation of the PI3K/AKT kinase pathway, which indirectly activates NF-κB via proteasome degradation of IκB. The phosphorylation of 4EBP1 at Thr37/46 decreases its association with eIF4E and consequently inhibits the mRNA translation of growth, thereby promoting protein synthesis [43]. Our results demonstrated that in the late co-culture period, there were decreased levels of phosphorylated 4EBP1, suggesting that *A. actinomycetemcomitans* was not able to affect the viability of the macrophages.

Interestingly, the signaling pathway responses in HGECs were different from those of macrophages, with decreased levels of phosphorylated ERK1/2 and increased levels of 4EBP1 in the phosphorylated form. Additionally, AKT phosphorylation was not observed up to 30 min after interaction of *A. actinomycetemcomitans* with HGECs, which was in accordance with the pro-apoptotic phenotype of epithelial cells reported after 60 min of bacteria–HGEC interaction (Handfield et al., 2005). AKT is key in cellular survival [44] and was only activated when the infected cells were incubated for a prolonged period. Inhibition of the AKT/mTOR pathway in infected macrophages and at early stages of infection in HGECs may exert bacterial clearance effects. AKT inhibition promoted by *Streptococcus pneumoniae* was associated with infection progression and inhibition of autophagy [45,46]. In contrast, attenuation of the AKT/mTor pathway enhanced autophagy and *Salmonella ssp.* clearance [47], indicating that subversion of this pathway may result in different outcomes according to the infecting agent.

Another studied protein was pc-FOS, which is one of the downstream factors induced by ERK1/2 pathway [48]. c-FOS phosphorylation is involved in osteoclastogenesis, leading to differentiation of precursor cells into osteoclasts due to the production of colony-stimulating factor 1 (CSF-1) and receptor activator of the NF-kB ligand (RANKL) [49]. Although previous data indicated that *A. actinomycetemcomitans* lipopolysaccharide (LPS) induced c-FOS phosphorylation in human gingival fibroblasts [50], our data indicated no increase in pc-FOS after co-culture with live *A. actinomycetemcomitans*, suggesting that ERK1/2 pathway activation did not induce c-FOS phosphorylation in the HGECs or U937 macrophages.

After *A. actinomycetemcomitans* infection, increased levels of IL-1β, TNF-α and IL-18 transcripts were observed in macrophages (Figure 1). Activation of NF-κB leads to pro-IL1 production, whereas pro-IL-18 is constitutively expressed but its expression increases after cellular activation [51,52]. The increase in IL-1β levels after one to three hours and in TNF-α levels after prolonged incubation with *A. actinomycetemcomitans*-infected macrophages possibly indicated that the binding of IL-1β to its receptor IL-1R1 led to a cascade of downstream events, eventually resulting in the expression of TNF-α. Silencing of NRLP3 indicated that activation of this intracellular receptor mediates pro-IL-1β and pro-IL-18 production in infected macrophages (Figure 5). However, the release of the mature and bioactive IL-1 family of cytokines, including IL-1β and IL-18 [51,52], is mediated by caspase-1 in inflammasomes [53]. Our data also indicated that *A. actinomycetemcomitans* Y4 infection in macrophages led to cleavage of procaspase-1 to caspase-1(Figures 4 and 5), resulting in the release of active IL-1β. This observation contradicted a previous study which reported that *A. actinomycetemcomitans* Y4 was not able to induce caspase-1 expression in monocytes, despite the increased expression of IL-1β [31].

On the other hand, the response of HGECs to *A. actinomycetemcomitans* resulted in a slight increase in transcript levels of *IL-1β* and *IL-18* after one hour of incubation, which returned to levels below those achieved in control cells thereafter (Table 1). Furthermore, the levels of TNF-α and IL-1β in cell supernatants were high in infected macrophages, but not in HGECS, shortly after incubation with *A. actinomycetemcomitans* (Figure 1). These data were in accordance with others reporting that HGEC interaction with *A. actinomycetemcomitans* extracts for eight hours did not result in IL-1β production, and increased levels of this cytokine were observed only after 12 h of incubation [54]. Other data indicated that *A. actinomycetemcomitans* infection leads to upregulation of *IL-1β* in HGECs after 60 min of incubation [55]. However, we showed that this upregulation was not maintained after longer interaction periods and did not result in the production of significant amounts of pro-IL-1β. When we analyzed the TNF levels, we observed a small increase of this cytokine in the presence of *A. actinomycetemcomitans*, however, in the presence of *Porphyromonas gingivalis*, the increase was higher after 24 h of co-culture with HGECs, showing that the cells were responsive to another periodontal pathogen [56]. Despite a limited number of samples of HGCEs from different donors, this study was in accordance with the low inflammatory response in the presence of *A. actinomycetemcomitans* when co-cultured with immortalized gingival cells OBA-9 (unpublished data). Furthermore, differences between this work and other studies regarding the tested *A. actinomycetemcomitans* strain, as well as differences in the origins of the monocytic cells and distinct macrophage phenotypes, may have contributed to conflicting data [31]. Overall, our results were in accordance with those that previously verified that *A. actinomycetemcomitans* and its product, Cdt, were able to induce inflammasome activation in macrophages [30,57].

Thus, our data indicated that, although macrophages responded to *A. actinomycetemcomitans* infection by upregulating the expression of intra- and extracellular receptors and production of cytokines (Figure 4), HGEC response to *A. actinomycetemcomitans* was mild, differing from that of other periodontopathogens, such as *P. gingivalis* [36].

Induction of inflammasomes in response to the microbial community was shown to control the microbiota in the gut, whereas its depletion induced dysbiosis [58]. Macrophages promptly recognize *A. actinomycetemcomitans* and its products, activating inflammasomes, which may be important in control of oral dysbiosis, but may also result in tissue destruction and perpetuation of inflammation. However, epithelial cells are the first barrier against pathogens and their response is important for the subsequent immune response. Epithelial cells internalize *A. actinomycetemcomitans* and a pro-apoptotic phenotype is induced by this species [55]. Thus, the low response to the pathogen by epithelial cells may be an additional factor of evasion of host defense mechanisms, facilitating colonization and dissemination to the underlying tissues in oral mucosa. This study demonstrated the differences between the responses of macrophages and gingival epithelial cells in the presence of *A. actinomycetemcomitans*.

4. Material and Methods

4.1. Eukaryotic Cells and Bacteria Culture Conditions

Gingival tissue was obtained from young healthy adult patients after third molar extractions (HGECs) by approval of the Institutional Review Board [5,56]. HGECs at the 3rd passage were harvested, seeded at a density of 0.5×10^5 cells/well on 6-well plates in KSFM (Keratinocyte Serum Free Medium) medium (Life Technologies, Carlsbad, CA, USA) supplemented with 10 mg/mL insulin, 5 µg/mL transferrin (Sigma-Aldrich, St Louis, MO, USA), 50 µg/mL bovine pituitary extract (BPE) (Life Technologies), 3-factor supplement (10 µM of 2-mercaptoethanol, 10 µM ethanolamine and 10 nM NA-Selenite- Sigma-Aldrich), 1% penicillin–streptomycin solution (Sigma-Aldrich) and 25 µg/L of fungizone (Life Technologies).

The human monocytic cell line U937 [59] was maintained in suspension culture in RPMI-1640 (Life Technologies, Carlsbad, CA, USA) supplemented with 10% (v/v) heat-inactivated fetal bovine serum (FBS) (Hyclone, Logan, UT, USA), 1% penicillin–streptomycin solution (Sigma-Aldrich) and 25 µg/L of fungizone and amphotericin B solution (Gibco, Scotland, UK), at 37 °C in a humidified atmosphere of 5% CO_2. U937 cells were differentiated into adherent macrophage-like cells by exposure of 4×10^6 cells to 20 nM phorbol 12-myristate 13-acetate (PMA) (Sigma-Aldrich) for 24 h and left to differentiate for an additional 48 h in 5% CO_2 at 37 °C [60].

A. actinomycetemcomitans strain Y4 serotype b was grown under microaerophilic conditions at 37 °C in tryptic soy broth (Sigma-Aldrich) supplemented with 0.6% weight/volume yeast extract.

4.2. Co-culture Assay

HGECs or differentiated U937 macrophages cultivated in media (5% fetal bovine serum) without antibiotics were infected with *A. actinomycetemcomitans* Y4 cells culture at mid log-phase at an multiplicity of infection (MOI) of 1:100 (eukaryotic cell:bacteria). After incubation for 1, 2, 3, 4 and 8 h for U937 macrophages and HGECs, the supernatants were collected and cells were washed twice with 1x phosphate saline buffer (PBS) prior to total RNA extraction. In order to verify the activation of signaling pathways in *A. actinomycetemcomitans*-infected cells, the co-cultures were obtained as described at time points 0, 15, 30, 60, 90 and 120 min, and the cell lysates were used in a Western blot assay. Noninfected HGECs and U937 macrophages were used as negative controls. The study was performed in three independent experiments and the HGECs were obtained from three different donors.

4.3. Gene Expression

Expression of inflammasome-related genes in infected HGECs and U973 macrophages was assessed by reverse transcription followed by real-time PCR (RT-qPCR). Total RNA was extracted from cultured U937 cells and HGECs using the RNeasy mini kit (Qiagen, Hilden, Germany), according to the manufacturer's instruction. Ten micrograms of RNA was used to obtain first strand cDNA synthesis using the High-Capacity cDNA Archive kit (Applied Biosystems, Foster City, CA, USA) in a total volume of 100 µL. Real-time PCR was performed using an ABI 7500 system (Applied Biosystem). The transcription of genes encoding the receptors NLRP3 (Hs00918082_m1), NOD1 (Hs01036720_m1), NOD2 (Hs01550753_m1), TLR2 (Hs02621280_s1) and TLR4 (Hs00152939_m1) and cytokines IL-1β

(Hs01555410_m1), IL-18 (Hs01038788_m1) and TNF-α (Hs00174128_m1) were evaluated using Taqman probes for human and theTaqMan Gene Expression Master Mix (Applied Biosystem). Transcription of human GAPDH (Hs02786624_g1) was used as an endogenous control. Results were analyzed using $2^{-\Delta\Delta Ct}$, where the results were normalized using the housekeeping gene or gene of interest from the reference sample in the case of cells at 0 h and compared with genes of the other samples using the threshold cycle (Ct) values from the real-time reaction [61].

4.4. Activation of Inflammasome-Related Signaling Pathways

The amount of phosphorylated proteins indicative of activation of different pathways and other proteins involved in inflammasomes were determined in HGECs and U937 macrophages co-cultured with *A. actinomycetemcomitans* by Western blotting. The cells were washed twice with 1x PBS, suspended in 1x SDS-PAGE loading dye (BioRad, Hercules, CA, USA) and boiled. SDS-PAGE was carried out according to the Laemmli method [62]. The gel was transferred to the nitrocellulose membrane (Life Technologies) at 4 °C in a Mini-Trans-Blot cell (Life Technologies) apparatus for 2 h at 370 mA. The primary antibodies were for phosphorylated ERK1/2 (pERK1/2) at T202/Y204, pAKT (Ser 473), p4EBP-1 (Trr 37/46) and pc-Fos (Ser 32). In U937 cells, pIκB-α (Ser32) (Cell Signaling, Danvers, MA, USA), caspase-1 p10 (C20) and cleaved caspase p10 were also evaluated. As a control, the antibody anti-GAPDH (Santa Cruz Biotechnology, Dallas, TX, USA) was used at 1:1000 dilution. The secondary antibody was anti-rabbit IgG, HPR-linked and diluted at 1:2000. Protein detection was performed using Amershan ECL Prime Western Blotting Detection reagent (GE Healthcare, Uppsala, Sweden). After detecting one protein, the primary and secondary antibody detected previously was removed using Restore™ Western Blot Stripping Buffer (Thermo-Scientific) and the same gel was used to detect other proteins. The results are representative of three independent experiments and cells at 0 h were used as the control.

4.5. Cytokines Quantification

Levels of secreted IL-1β and TNF-α were determined in the supernatants of U937 and HGEC that were co-cultured with *A. actinomycetemcomitans* by ELISA using an R&D systems kit (Minneapolis, MN, USA). The plates were read in a microplate reader at an optical density (OD) of 450 nm. The amounts of each cytokine were determined after comparison with the respective standard curve.

4.6. Silencing of NLRP3

In order to confirm inflammasome activation by *A. actinomycetemcomitans* in macrophages, silencing of NLRP3 was performed. U937 cells (2×10^6 cells) were transfected with siNLRP3 (Dharmacon-Thermo Scientific, Waltham, MA, USA) using the Amaxanucleofactor kit V (Lonza, Allendale, NJ, USA). Cell suspensions were centrifuged at 90× g for 10 min, the medium was removed and 1 μM of siNLRP3 in 100 μL of nucleofactor V buffer were added. As a negative control, scramble siRNA (siControl non-targeting siRNA Pool, Horizon Discovery, UK) was used. The samples were electroporated in nucleofactor program V-001 (Lonza), RPMI medium was added and the cells were transferred into 6-well plates with 2.5 mL of phorbol 12-myristate 13-acetate (PMA) in RPMI medium and incubated for 24 h. Co-cultures of transfected U937 macrophages with *A. actinomycetemcomitans* were performed as described. Transcription of genes encoding NRLP3, IL-1β, IL-18 and TNF-α was determined by RT-qPCR and the production of cytokines in the cell supernatants was measured by ELISA.

4.7. Statistical Analysis

Comparisons between samples were performed by one-way ANOVA followed by post-Tukey's test (Graphpad Prism version 4.0, La Jolla, CA, USA). Results were considered significant when $p < 0.05$.

5. Conclusions

Taken together, our data indicated that *A. actinomycetemcomitans* enhanced the expression of NLRP3, TLR4, TLR2 and NOD2 in macrophages but not in HGECs, consequently inducing distinct signaling pathways and cytokine production and demonstrating varied innate immune responses depending on the cell type.

Author Contributions: Conceptualization, E.A.S., M.R.B., M.P.A.M; methodology, E.A.S., M.R.B; software, E.A.S.; validation, E.A.S., M.R.B..; formal analysis, E.A.S.; investigation, E.A.S, M.R.B.; resources, M.R.B.; data curation, E.A.S.; writing—original draft preparation, E.A.S.; writing—review and editing, E.A.S, M.R.B., M.P.A.M., D.F.K..; visualization, E.A.S.; supervision, M.R.B., M.P.A.M.; project administration, M.R.B.; funding acquisition, E.A.S., M.R.B., D.F.K. All authors have read and agreed to the published version of the manuscript.

Funding: This research was funded by FAPESP grants 2012/05887-0, 2015/18273-9 and the School of Dental Medicine, University of Pennsylvania.

Acknowledgments: We thank Joseph DiRienzo for providing *A. actinomycetemcomitans* strain Y4. E.A.S was supported by FAPESP grant 2012/05887-0 and 2015/18273-9. M.R.B was supported by internal funding by the School of Dental Medicine, University of Pennsylvania, Philadelphia.

Conflicts of Interest: The authors declare no conflict of interest.

References

1. Graves, D. Cytokines that promote periodontal tissue destruction. *J. Periodontol.* **2008**, *79*, 1585–1591. [CrossRef]
2. Kinane, D.F.; Bartold, P.M. Clinical relevance of the host responses of periodontitis. *Periodontology 2000* **2007**, *43*, 278–293. [CrossRef] [PubMed]
3. Benakanakere, M.; Kinane, D.F. Innate cellular responses to the periodontal biofilm. *Front. Oral Biol.* **2012**, *15*, 41–55. [PubMed]
4. Hajishengallis, G. Periodontitis: From microbial immune subversion to systemic inflammation. *Nat. Rev. Immunol.* **2015**, *15*, 30–44. [CrossRef] [PubMed]
5. Benakanakere, M.; Abdolhosseini, M.; Hosur, K.; Finoti, L.S.; Kinane, D.F. TLR2 promoter hypermethylation creates innate immune dysbiosis. *J. Dent. Res.* **2015**, *94*, 183–191. [CrossRef] [PubMed]
6. Fine, D.H.; Markowitz, K.; Furgang, D.; Fairlie, K.; Ferrandiz, J.; Nasri, C.; McKiernan, M.; Gunsolley, J. Aggregatibacter actinomycetemcomitans and its relationship to initiation of localized aggressive periodontitis: Longitudinal cohort study of initially healthy adolescents. *J. Clin. Microbiol.* **2007**, *45*, 3859–3869. [CrossRef] [PubMed]
7. Norskov-Lauritsen, N.; Claesson, R.; Birkeholm Jensen, A.; Aberg, C.H.; Haubek, D. Aggregatibacter Actinomycetemcomitans: Clinical Significance of a Pathobiont Subjected to Ample Changes in Classification and Nomenclature. *Pathogens* **2019**, *8*, 243. [CrossRef]
8. Paturel, L.; Casalta, J.P.; Habib, G.; Nezri, M.; Raoult, D. Actinobacillus actinomycetemcomitans endocarditis. *Clin. Microbiol. Infect.* **2004**, *10*, 98–118. [CrossRef]
9. Calandrini, C.A.; Ribeiro, A.C.; Gonnelli, A.C.; Ota-Tsuzuki, C.; Rangel, L.P.; Saba-Chujfi, E.; Mayer, M.P. Microbial composition of atherosclerotic plaques. *Oral Dis.* **2014**, *20*, e128–e134. [CrossRef]
10. Konig, M.F.; Abusleme, L.; Reinholdt, J.; Palmer, R.J.; Teles, R.P.; Sampson, K.; Rosen, A.; Nigrovic, P.A.; Sokolove, J.; Giles, J.T.; et al. Aggregatibacter actinomycetemcomitans-induced hypercitrullination links periodontal infection to autoimmunity in rheumatoid arthritis. *Sci. Transl. Med.* **2016**, *8*. [CrossRef]
11. Fine, D.H.; Markowitz, K.; Fairlie, K.; Tischio-Bereski, D.; Ferrendiz, J.; Furgang, D.; Paster, B.J.; Dewhirst, F.E. A consortium of Aggregatibacter actinomycetemcomitans, Streptococcus parasanguinis, and Filifactor alocis is present in sites prior to bone loss in a longitudinal study of localized aggressive periodontitis. *J. Clin. Microbiol.* **2013**, *51*, 2850–2861. [CrossRef] [PubMed]
12. Shenker, B.J.; Boesze-Battaglia, K.; Scuron, M.D.; Walker, L.P.; Zekavat, A.; Dlakic, M. The toxicity of the Aggregatibacter actinomycetemcomitans cytolethal distending toxin correlates with its phosphatidylinositol-3,4,5-triphosphate phosphatase activity. *Cell. Microbiol.* **2016**, *18*, 223–243. [CrossRef] [PubMed]

13. Kajiya, M.; Komatsuzawa, H.; Papantonakis, A.; Seki, M.; Makihira, S.; Ouhara, K.; Kusumoto, Y.; Murakami, S.; Taubman, M.A.; Kawai, T. Aggregatibacter actinomycetemcomitans Omp29 is associated with bacterial entry to gingival epithelial cells by F-actin rearrangement. *PLoS ONE* **2011**, *6*, e18287. [CrossRef] [PubMed]
14. Chattopadhyay, S.; Sen, G.C. Tyrosine phosphorylation in Toll-like receptor signaling. *Cytokine Growth Factor Rev.* **2014**, *25*, 533–541. [CrossRef]
15. Martinon, F.; Tschopp, J. NLRs join TLRs as innate sensors of pathogens. *Trends Immunol.* **2005**, *26*, 447–454. [CrossRef]
16. Ferrand, J.; Ferrero, R.L. Recognition of Extracellular Bacteria by NLRs and Its Role in the Development of Adaptive Immunity. *Front. Immunol.* **2013**, *4*, 344. [CrossRef]
17. Brewer, S.M.; Brubaker, S.W.; Monack, D.M. Host inflammasome defense mechanisms and bacterial pathogen evasion strategies. *Curr. Opin. Immunol.* **2019**, *60*, 63–70. [CrossRef]
18. Abderrazak, A.; Syrovets, T.; Couchie, D.; El Hadri, K.; Friguet, B.; Simmet, T.; Rouis, M. NLRP3 inflammasome: From a danger signal sensor to a regulatory node of oxidative stress and inflammatory diseases. *Redox Biol.* **2015**, *4*, 296–307. [CrossRef]
19. Franchi, L.; Muñoz-Planillo, R.; Núñez, G. Sensing and reacting to microbes through the inflammasomes. *Nat. Immunol.* **2012**, *13*, 325–332. [CrossRef]
20. Tsuchiya, K. Inflammasome-associated cell death: Pyroptosis, apoptosis, and physiological implications. *Microbiol. Immunol.* **2020**. [CrossRef]
21. Kikkert, R.; Laine, M.L.; Aarden, L.A.; van Winkelhoff, A.J. Activation of toll-like receptors 2 and 4 by gram-negative periodontal bacteria. *Oral Microbiol. Immunol.* **2007**, *22*, 145–151. [CrossRef] [PubMed]
22. Umeda, J.E.; Demuth, D.R.; Ando, E.S.; Faveri, M.; Mayer, M.P. Signaling transduction analysis in gingival epithelial cells after infection with Aggregatibacter actinomycetemcomitans. *Mol. Oral Microbiol.* **2012**, *27*, 23–33. [CrossRef] [PubMed]
23. Dickinson, B.C.; Moffatt, C.E.; Hagerty, D.; Whitmore, S.E.; Brown, T.A.; Graves, D.T.; Lamont, R.J. Interaction of oral bacteria with gingival epithelial cell multilayers. *Mol. Oral Microbiol.* **2011**, *26*, 210–220. [CrossRef] [PubMed]
24. Kato, S.; Nakashima, K.; Nagasawa, T.; Abiko, Y.; Furuichi, Y. Involvement of Toll-like receptor 2 in apoptosis of Aggregatibacter actinomycetemcomitans-infected THP-1 cells. *J. Microbiol. Immunol. Infect.* **2013**, *46*, 164–170. [CrossRef]
25. Kelk, P.; Claesson, R.; Chen, C.; Sjöstedt, A.; Johansson, A. IL-1beta secretion induced by Aggregatibacter (Actinobacillus) actinomycetemcomitans is mainly caused by the leukotoxin. *Int. J. Med Microbiol.* **2008**, *298*, 529–541. [CrossRef]
26. Kelk, P.; Claesson, R.; Hänström, L.; Lerner, U.H.; Kalfas, S.; Johansson, A. Abundant secretion of bioactive interleukin-1beta by human macrophages induced by Actinobacillus actinomycetemcomitans leukotoxin. *Infect. Immun.* **2005**, *73*, 453–458. [CrossRef]
27. Kelk, P.; Abd, H.; Claesson, R.; Sandstrom, G.; Sjostedt, A.; Johansson, A. Cellular and molecular response of human macrophages exposed to Aggregatibacter actinomycetemcomitans leukotoxin. *Cell Death Dis.* **2011**, *2*, e126. [CrossRef]
28. Xue, F.; Shu, R.; Xie, Y. The expression of NLRP3, NLRP1 and AIM2 in the gingival tissue of periodontitis patients: RT-PCR study and immunohistochemistry. *Arch. Oral Biol.* **2015**, *60*, 948–958. [CrossRef]
29. Isaza-Guzman, D.M.; Medina-Piedrahita, V.M.; Gutierrez-Henao, C.; Tobon-Arroyave, S.I. Salivary Levels of NLRP3 Inflammasome-Related Proteins as Potential Biomarkers of Periodontal Clinical Status. *J. Periodontol.* **2017**, *88*, 1329–1338. [CrossRef]
30. Shenker, B.J.; Ojcius, D.M.; Walker, L.P.; Zekavat, A.; Scuron, M.D.; Boesze-Battaglia, K. Aggregatibacter actinomycetemcomitans cytolethal distending toxin activates the NLRP3 inflammasome in human macrophages, leading to the release of proinflammatory cytokines. *Infect. Immun.* **2015**, *83*, 1487–1496. [CrossRef]
31. Belibasakis, G.N.; Johansson, A. Aggregatibacter actinomycetemcomitans targets NLRP3 and NLRP6 inflammasome expression in human mononuclear leukocytes. *Cytokine* **2012**, *59*, 124–130. [CrossRef] [PubMed]

32. Zhao, P.; Liu, J.; Pan, C.; Pan, Y. NLRP3 inflammasome is required for apoptosis of Aggregatibacter actinomycetemcomitans-infected human osteoblastic MG63 cells. *Acta Histochem.* **2014**, *116*, 1119–1124. [CrossRef] [PubMed]
33. Thay, B.; Damm, A.; Kufer, T.A.; Wai, S.N.; Oscarsson, J. Aggregatibacter actinomycetemcomitans outer membrane vesicles are internalized in human host cells and trigger NOD1- and NOD2-dependent NF-kappaB activation. *Infect. Immun.* **2014**, *82*, 4034–4046. [CrossRef] [PubMed]
34. Yilmaz, O.; Lee, K.L. The inflammasome and danger molecule signaling: At the crossroads of inflammation and pathogen persistence in the oral cavity. *Periodontology 2000* **2015**, *69*, 83–95. [CrossRef]
35. Fukushima, H.; Jimi, E.; Okamoto, F.; Motokawa, W.; Okabe, K. IL-1-induced receptor activator of NF-kappa B ligand in human periodontal ligament cells involves ERK-dependent PGE2 production. *Bone* **2005**, *36*, 267–275. [CrossRef]
36. Stathopoulou, P.G.; Benakanakere, M.R.; Galicia, J.C.; Kinane, D.F. Epithelial cell pro-inflammatory cytokine response differs across dental plaque bacterial species. *J. Clin. Periodontol.* **2010**, *37*, 24–29. [CrossRef]
37. Uchida, Y.; Shiba, H.; Komatsuzawa, H.; Takemoto, T.; Sakata, M.; Fujita, T.; Kawaguchi, H.; Sugai, M.; Kurihara, H. Expression of IL-1 beta and IL-8 by human gingival epithelial cells in response to Actinobacillus actinomycetemcomitans. *Cytokine* **2001**, *14*, 152–161. [CrossRef]
38. Gelani, V.; Fernandes, A.P.; Gasparoto, T.H.; Garlet, T.P.; Cestari, T.M.; Lima, H.R.; Ramos, E.S.; de Souza Malaspina, T.S.; Santos, C.F.; Garlet, G.P.; et al. The role of toll-like receptor 2 in the recognition of Aggregatibacter actinomycetemcomitans. *J. Periodontol.* **2009**, *80*, 2010–2019. [CrossRef]
39. Park, S.R.; Kim, D.J.; Han, S.H.; Kang, M.J.; Lee, J.Y.; Jeong, Y.J.; Lee, S.J.; Kim, T.H.; Ahn, S.G.; Yoon, J.H.; et al. Diverse Toll-like receptors mediate cytokine production by Fusobacterium nucleatum and Aggregatibacter actinomycetemcomitans in macrophages. *Infect. Immun.* **2014**, *82*, 1914–1920. [CrossRef]
40. Diaz-Zuniga, J.; Monasterio, G.; Alvarez, C.; Melgar-Rodriguez, S.; Benitez, A.; Ciuchi, P.; Garcia, M.; Arias, J.; Sanz, M.; Vernal, R. Variability of the dendritic cell response triggered by different serotypes of Aggregatibacter actinomycetemcomitans or Porphyromonas gingivalis is toll-like receptor 2 (TLR2) or TLR4 dependent. *J. Periodontol.* **2015**, *86*, 108–119. [CrossRef]
41. Ando-Suguimoto, E.S.; da Silva, M.P.; Kawamoto, D.; Chen, C.; DiRienzo, J.M.; Mayer, M.P. The cytolethal distending toxin of Aggregatibacter actinomycetemcomitans inhibits macrophage phagocytosis and subverts cytokine production. *Cytokine* **2014**, *66*, 46–53. [CrossRef]
42. Tsai, W.H.; Huang, D.Y.; Yu, Y.H.; Chen, C.Y.; Lin, W.W. Dual roles of NOD2 in TLR4-mediated signal transduction and -induced inflammatory gene expression in macrophages. *Cell. Microbiol.* **2011**, *13*, 717–730. [CrossRef] [PubMed]
43. Qin, X.; Jiang, B.; Zhang, Y. 4E-BP1, a multifactor regulated multifunctional protein. *Cell Cycle* **2016**, *15*, 781–786. [CrossRef] [PubMed]
44. Vanhaesebroeck, B.; Alessi, D.R. The PI3K-PDK1 connection: More than just a road to PKB. *Biochem. J.* **2000**, *346*, 561–576. [PubMed]
45. Kim, J.Y.; Paton, J.C.; Briles, D.E.; Rhee, D.K.; Pyo, S. Streptococcus pneumoniae induces pyroptosis through the regulation of autophagy in murine microglia. *Oncotarget* **2015**, *6*, 44161–44178. [CrossRef] [PubMed]
46. Li, P.; Shi, J.; He, Q.; Hu, Q.; Wang, Y.Y.; Zhang, L.J.; Chan, W.T.; Chen, W.X. Streptococcus pneumoniae induces autophagy through the inhibition of the PI3K-I/Akt/mTOR pathway and ROS hypergeneration in A549 cells. *PLoS ONE* **2015**, *10*, e0122753. [CrossRef] [PubMed]
47. Owen, K.A.; Meyer, C.B.; Bouton, A.H.; Casanova, J.E. Activation of focal adhesion kinase by Salmonella suppresses autophagy via an Akt/mTOR signaling pathway and promotes bacterial survival in macrophages. *PLoS Pathog.* **2014**, *10*, e1004159. [CrossRef] [PubMed]
48. Monje, P.; Hernandez-Losa, J.; Lyons, R.J.; Castellone, M.D.; Gutkind, J.S. Regulation of the transcriptional activity of c-Fos by ERK. A novel role for the prolyl isomerase PIN1. *J. Biol. Chem.* **2005**, *280*, 35081–35084. [CrossRef]
49. Arai, A.; Mizoguchi, T.; Harada, S.; Kobayashi, Y.; Nakamichi, Y.; Yasuda, H.; Penninger, J.M.; Yamada, K.; Udagawa, N.; Takahashi, N. Fos plays an essential role in the upregulation of RANK expression in osteoclast precursors within the bone microenvironment. *J. Cell Sci.* **2012**, *125*, 2910–2917. [CrossRef]
50. Gutierrez-Venegas, G.; Castillo-Aleman, R. Characterization of the transduction pathway involved in c-fos and c-jun expression induced by Aggregatibacter actinomycetemcomitans lipopolysaccharides in human gingival fibroblasts. *Int. Immunopharmacol.* **2008**, *8*, 1513–1523. [CrossRef]

51. Latz, E.; Xiao, T.S.; Stutz, A. Activation and regulation of the inflammasomes. *Nat. Rev. Immunol.* **2013**, *13*, 397–411. [CrossRef] [PubMed]
52. Hajishengallis, G.; Wang, M.; Liang, S. Induction of distinct TLR2-mediated proinflammatory and proadhesive signaling pathways in response to Porphyromonas gingivalis fimbriae. *J. Immunol.* **2009**, *182*, 6690–6696. [CrossRef] [PubMed]
53. Sahoo, M.; Ceballos-Olvera, I.; del Barrio, L.; Re, F. Role of the inflammasome, IL-1beta, and IL-18 in bacterial infections. *Sci. World J.* **2011**, *11*, 2037–2050. [CrossRef] [PubMed]
54. Sfakianakis, A.; Barr, C.E.; Kreutzer, D.L. Actinobacillus actinomycetemcomitans-induced expression of IL-1alpha and IL-1beta in human gingival epithelial cells: Role in IL-8 expression. *Eur. J. Oral Sci.* **2001**, *109*, 393–401. [CrossRef]
55. Handfield, M.; Mans, J.J.; Zheng, G.; Lopez, M.C.; Mao, S.; Progulske-Fox, A.; Narasimhan, G.; Baker, H.V.; Lamont, R.J. Distinct transcriptional profiles characterize oral epithelium-microbiota interactions. *Cell. Microbiol.* **2005**, *7*, 811–823. [CrossRef]
56. Stathopoulou, P.G.; Galicia, J.C.; Benakanakere, M.R.; Garcia, C.A.; Potempa, J.; Kinane, D.F. Porphyromonas gingivalis induce apoptosis in human gingival epithelial cells through a gingipain-dependent mechanism. *BMC Microbiol.* **2009**, *9*, 107. [CrossRef]
57. Kim, S.; Park, M.H.; Song, Y.R.; Na, H.S.; Chung, J. Aggregatibacter actinomycetemcomitans-Induced AIM2 Inflammasome Activation Is Suppressed by Xylitol in Differentiated THP-1 Macrophages. *J. Periodontol.* **2016**, *87*, e116–126. [CrossRef]
58. Palm, N.W.; de Zoete, M.R.; Flavell, R.A. Immune-microbiota interactions in health and disease. *Clin. Immunol.* **2015**. [CrossRef]
59. Sundstrom, C.; Nilsson, K. Establishment and characterization of a human histiocytic lymphoma cell line (U-937). *Int. J. Cancer* **1976**, *17*, 565–577. [CrossRef]
60. Minta, J.O.; Pambrun, L. In vitro induction of cytologic and functional differentiation of the immature human monocytelike cell line U-937 with phorbol myristate acetate. *Am. J. Pathol.* **1985**, *119*, 111–126.
61. Pfaffl, M.W. A new mathematical model for relative quantification in real-time RT-PCR. *Nucleic Acids Res.* **2001**, *29*, e45. [CrossRef] [PubMed]
62. Laemmli, U.K. Cleavage of structural proteins during the assembly of the head of bacteriophage T4. *Nature* **1970**, *227*, 680–685. [CrossRef] [PubMed]

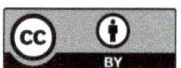

© 2020 by the authors. Licensee MDPI, Basel, Switzerland. This article is an open access article distributed under the terms and conditions of the Creative Commons Attribution (CC BY) license (http://creativecommons.org/licenses/by/4.0/).

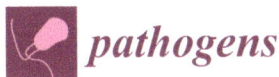

Article

Chemical Composition, Antimicrobial activity, In Vitro Cytotoxicity and Leukotoxin Neutralization of Essential Oil from *Origanum vulgare* against *Aggregatibacter actinomycetemcomitans*

Sanae Akkaoui [1], Anders Johansson [2], Maâmar Yagoubi [3], Dorte Haubek [4], Adnane El hamidi [5], Sana Rida [6], Rolf Claesson [7] and OumKeltoum Ennibi [8],*

1. Research laboratory in oral biology and biotechnology, Faculty of dental medicine, Mohammed V University in Rabat, Rabat 10 000, Morocco; sanae.akkaoui@um5s.net.ma
2. Division of Molecular Periodontology, Department of Odontology, Umeå University, 901 87 Umeå, Sweden; anders.p.johansson@umu.se
3. Microbiology Laboratory, faculty of medicine and pharmacy, Mohammed V University in Rabat, Rabat 10 000, Morocco; m.yagoubi@um5s.net.ma
4. Section for Pediatric Dentistry, Department of Dentistry and Oral Health, AarhusUniversity, 8000 Aarhus, Denmark; dorte.haubek@dent.au.dk
5. Materials, Nanotechnologies and Environment laboratory, Faculty of Sciences, Mohammed V University in Rabat, Rabat 10 000, Morocco; adnane_el@hotmail.com
6. Department of endodontics, Research laboratory in oral biology and biotechnology, Faculty of Dental Medicine, Mohammed V University in Rabat, Rabat 10 000, Morocco; s.rida@um5s.net.ma
7. Division of Oral Microbiology, Department of Odontology, Umeå University, 901 87 Umeå, Sweden; rolf.claesson@umu.se
8. Department of Periodontology, Research laboratory in oral biology and biotechnology, Faculty of Dental Medicine, Mohammed V University in Rabat, Rabat 10 000, Morocco
* Correspondence: o.ennibi@um5s.net.ma

Received: 27 January 2020; Accepted: 3 March 2020; Published: 5 March 2020

Abstract: In this study, the essential oil of *Origanum vulgare* was evaluated for putative antibacterial activity against six clinical strains and five reference strains of *Aggregatibacter actinomycetemcomitans*, in comparison with some antimicrobials. The chemical composition of the essential oil was analyzed, using chromatography (CG) and gas chromatography–mass spectrometry coupled (CG–MS). The major compounds in the oil were Carvacrol (32.36%), α-terpineol (16.70%), *p*-cymene (16.24%), and Thymol (12.05%). The antimicrobial activity was determined by an agar well diffusion test. A broth microdilution method was used to study the minimal inhibitory concentration (MIC). The minimal bactericidal concentration (MBC) was also determined. The cytotoxicity of the essential oil (IC50) was <125 µg/mL for THP-1 cells, which was high in comparison with different MIC values for the *A. actinomycetemcomitans* strains. *O. vulgare* essential oil did not interfere with the neutralizing capacity of *Psidium guajava* against the *A. actinomycetemcomitans* leukotoxin. In addition, it was shown that the *O. vulgare* EO had an antibacterial effect against *A. actinomycetemcomitans* on a similar level as some tested antimicrobials. In view of these findings, we suggest that *O.vulgare* EO may be used as an adjuvant for prevention and treatment of periodontal diseases associated to *A. actinomycetemcomitans*. In addition, it can be used together with the previously tested leukotoxin neutralizing *Psidium guajava*.

Keywords: *Aggregatibacter actinomycetemcomitans*; periodontitis; *Origanum vulgare*; essential oil; antimicrobial activity; minimum inhibitory concentration; minimal bactericidal concentration; cytotoxicity; leukotoxin neutralization

1. Introduction

Aggregatibacter actinomycetemcomitans is a capnophilic Gram-negative coccobacillus, widely known as one of the putative pathogens associated with periodontitis, mainly in adolescents and young adults [1]. Pathogenesis of periodontitis is very complex, including immunogenetic factors, life style, proportion, and composition of specific periodontitis associated bacterial species, including *A. actinomycetemcomitans* in the oral biofilm [2]. The contribution of *A. actinomycetemcomitans* in initiation and progression of the disease is due to various virulent factors released in periodontal tissues [3]. A total of seven serotypes (a,b,c,d,e,f, and g) [2,4] of *A. actinomycetemcomitans* have been isolated from periodontal lesions worldwide. Patients seem to be colonized by a single serotype for life [2]. Among virulence factors of the bacterium, the leukotoxin (LtxA) is the most studied [3,5]. It activates or kills immune cells, helping the bacterium to survive in a site of infection. A specific variant of *A. actinomycetemcomitans* produces more LtxA than other variants [6]. This highly leukotoxic clone, JP2, has been associated with aggressive forms of periodontitis in Morocco [7,8]. According to the 2017 World Workshop of Periodontology, aggressive periodontitis is included in the category of "periodontitis", which is characterized based on stages and grades. Extension and distribution of periodontal lesions allow distinguishing localized, generalized, and molar-incisor distribution forms [9].

Aggressive periodontitis treatment of is based on mechanical debridement with antimicrobials as adjuvants. This aims to allow the elimination of *A. actinomycetemcomitans* and other bacterial species which penetrate the periodontal epithelial tissue [10]. However, given the increasing resistance of oral bacteria to antimicrobials and the side effects caused by antiseptic agents often used in dentistry (i.e., dental staining and taste alteration) [11], the search for new natural agents as alternative therapeutic products with fewer side effects (e.g., gastric problems) and less bacterial-resistance development has become a necessity.

Morocco has, by its geographical diversity, great natural resources for cultivation of medicinal and aromatic plants. Surveys performed in Morocco among the population in different regions have shown a frequent therapeutic use of this natural heritage in traditional medicine [12,13].

Many studies through the world have been carried out to screen medicinal and pharmacological properties of different plants and essential oils, to integrate them into the therapeutic arsenal, according to standards of quality and effectiveness [14,15].

However, the use of medicinal plants and essential oils is limited in dentistry, and their antimicrobial activities on oral bacteria are not widely studied. We have previously reported that, in Moroccan population, *O.vulgare* is used as a mouthwash in traditional medicine [13].

O. vulgare is a widespread aromatic plant naturally growing in different parts of the world, including Northern Africa, the Mediterranean area, the Arabian Peninsula, Central Asia, and Europe [16,17]. It belongs to Lamiaceae family, and it is known for being a rich source of EOs, which have proven to possess a large variety of biological activities because of their chemical compounds [18]. The abundance of different compounds of EOs of Origanum species may show some variations because of ecological and environmental effects, geographical location, and time of collection [19–21].

We have additionally evaluated the possibility to neutralize the LtxA by administrating a mouth rinse with LtxA neutralizing agents released from leaves of *Psidium guajava* [22].

The aim of the present work was to study the antibacterial activity of *O. vulgare* EO of Moroccan origin on *A. actinomycetemcomitans*. In addition, we explored its cytotoxicity and checked how it cooperates with the leukotoxin neutralizing properties.

2. Results

2.1. Chemical Composition of the Essential Oil

The chemical analysis of *O. vulgare* EO was performed by using gas chromatography/mass spectrometry (GC/MS) technique. The 25 identified components and their relative percentage are summarized in Table 1. The major constituents were as follows: Carvacrol (32.36%), α-terpineol (16.70), p-cymene (16.25%), and Thymol (12.06%) (Figure 1). Thus, the EO of O. vulgare is dominated by oxygenated monoterpenes.

Table 1. Chemical composition of O. vulgare EO.

No	Compound	Formula	RT (min)	RI	Conc. (%)
1	α-Thujene	$C_{10}H_{16}$	13.768	927	0.20
2	α-pinene	$C_{10}H_{16}$	14.179	936	0.44
3	1-octen-3-ol	$C_8H_{16}O$	16.403	942	1.69
4	3-Octanone	$C_8H_{16}O$	16.877	989	0.53
5	Dehydrocineole	$C_{10}H_{16}O$	17.291	995	0.39
6	3-Octanol	$C_8H_{18}O$	17.351	997	0.42
7	p-cymene	$C_{10}H_{14}$	19.335	1028	16.25
8	Limonene	$C_{10}H_{16}$	19.575	1031	0.28
9	Eucalyptol	$C_{10}H_{18}O$	19.782	1035	0.82
10	γ-terpinene	$C_{10}H_{16}$	21.457	1061	1.03
11	Cis-Sabinene hydrate	$C_{10}H_{18}O$	22.01	1068	0.43
12	1-hepten-3-ol	$C_7H_{14}O$	22.641	1084	0.21
13	Linalool	$C_{10}H_{18}O$	24.005	1101	2.16
14	Borneol	$C_{10}H_{18}O$	28.615	1167	0.37
15	Terpinen-4-ol	$C_{10}H_{18}O$	29.372	1179	0.77
16	p-Cimen-8-ol	$C_{10}H_{14}O$	29.822	1185	0.82
17	α-terpineol	$C_{10}H_{18}O$	30.296	1189	16.70
18	Pulegone	$C_{10}H_{16}O$	33.591	1251	0.49
19	Thymol methyl ether	$C_{11}H_{16}O$	33.721	1235	6.60
20	p-Cymen-3-ol	$C_{10}H_{14}O$	36.33	1287	0.88
21	Thymol	$C_{10}H_{14}O$	36.787	1290	12.06
22	p-Thymol	$C_{10}H_{14}O$	37.024	1291	0.74
23	Carvacrol	$C_{10}H_{14}O$	37.524	1300	32.36
24	Caryophyllene	$C_{15}H_{24}$	45.356	1418	0.93
25	Caryophyllene oxide	$C_{15}H_{24}O$	55.195	1582	2.42

RT: retention time; RI: retention index; Conc.: Concentration

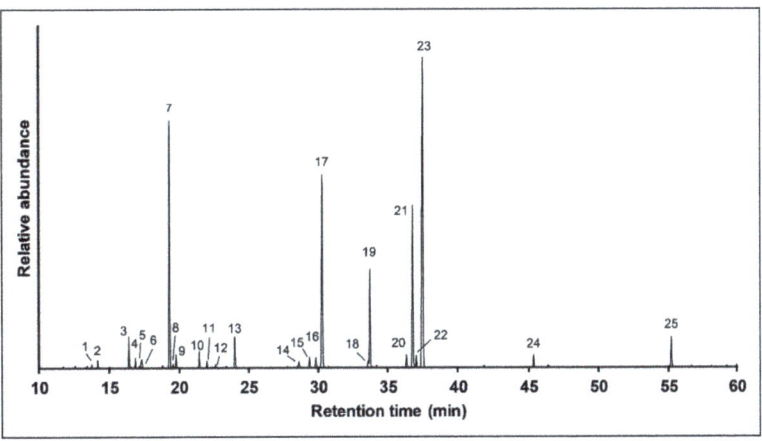

Figure 1. Chromatography/mass spectrometry (GC/MS) chromatogram of O.vulgare EO.

2.2. Antimicrobial Activity

The inhibition zones obtained respectively when the O. vulgare EO, Amoxicillin (AM), Amoxicillin and clavulanic acid (AMC), and Doxycycline (DO) were tested against six clinical strains and five reference strains of A. actinomycetemcomitans are shown in Table 2. All tested strains showed inhibition zones in the presence of the EO (27.6 µg) (37–69 mm). The susceptibility to the antimicrobials varied among the strains (Table 2).

Table 2. Mean diameter of inhibition zones (mm) obtained by the agar diffusion method and the interpretation according to the European Committee on Antimicrobial Susceptibility Testing Breakpoint tables for interpretation of MICs and zone diameters Version 9.0, valid from 2019-01-01.

A. a. strains	Inhibition Zone Diameter (mm) [1] *									p-value
	EO	Antimicrobials								
	O. vulgare 27.6 µg	AMC [2] 25 µg	AML [3] 25 µg	DO [4] 30 µg	SP [5] 100 µg	CIP [6] 5 µg	MH [7] 30 µg	VA [8] 30 µg	MTZ [9] 5 µg	
		Breakpoints								
		S ≥ 15 R < 15	note[10]	note[11]	no info	S ≥ 30 R < 30	S ≥ 24 R < 21	no info	no info	
clinical strain 1	37.33 ± 2.08 S	31.66 ± 1.15 S	30.33 ± 0.57 S	25.00 ± 0.00 ** S	29.66 ± 0.57 –	28.33 ± 0.57 R	36.00 ± 1.73 S	0.00 –	0.00 R	<0.001
clinical strain 2	51.33 ± 0.57 ** S	32.66 ± 0.57 ** S	29.33 ± 1.15 ** S	23.33 ± 0.57 S	22.66 ± 0.57 –	26.66 ± 0.57 ** R	36.33 ± 0.57 ** S	14.33 ± 0.57 ** –	0.00 R	<0.001
clinical strain 3	65.66 ± 0.57 ** S	30.66 ± 0.57 S	30.66 ± 1.15 S	25.66 ± 0.57 S	28.66 ± 1.15 –	29.33 ± 1.15 R	38.33 ± 2.08 ** S	15.66 ± 0.57 ** –	0.00 R	<0.001
clinical strain 4	63.66 ± 0.57 ** S	32.00 ± 1.00 S	28.66 ± 1.15 S	27.66 ± 0.57 S	27.66 ± 1.15 –	33.00 ± 1.00 S	39.33 ± 0.57 ** S	15.00 ± 0.00 ** –	0.00 R	<0.001
clinical strain 5	65.33 ± 0.57 ** S	31.00 ± 1.73 S	27.33 ± 0.57 ** S	23.33 ± 0.57 ** S	28.33 ± 0.57 –	31.66 ± 0.57 S	38.00 ± 1.73 ** S	14.66 ± 0.57 ** –	0.00 R	<0.001
clinical strain 6	56.33 ± 1.52 ** S	31.00 ± 0.00 S	27.66 ± 0.57 S	22.66 ± 0.57 ** S	27.00 ± 1.00 –	31.66 ± 0.57 S	34.66 ± 0.57 ** S	15.33 ± 0.57 ** –	0.00 R	<0.001
ATCC 43717 (Suny aB75)	69.66 ± 0.57 ** S	40.33 ± 0.57 ** S	25.66 ± 0.57 S	28.33 ± 0.57 S	29.33 ± 0.57 –	30.66 ± 0.57 S	33.66 ± 0.57 ** S	24.66 ± 0.57 –	0.00 R	<0.001
ATTC 43718 Y4	65.33 ± 0.57 ** S	25.33 ± 0.57 S	34.33 ± 0.57 S	28.66 ± 0.57 S	28.66 ± 1.15 ** –	31.00 ± 1.00 ** S	33.33 ± 0.57 S	24.33 ± 0.57 –	0.00 R	<0.001
HK1651 (JP2)	67.66 ± 1.52 ** S	28.33 ± 0.57 S	27.66 ± 0.57 S	28.33 ± 0.57 S	27.33 ± 0.57 –	34.33 ± 0.57 S	32.00 ± 1.73 S	23.66 ± 0.57 ** –	0.00 R	<0.001
HK 921 (JP2)	37.00 ± 1.73 S	29.66 ± 0.57 S	27.66 ± 0.57 S	29.00 ± 0.00 S	25.66 ± 0.57 –	34.66 ± 0.57 S	29.33 ± 1.15 S	20.33 ± 0.57 ** –	0.00 R	<0.001
HK1605 (non JP2)	46.00 ± 1.00 ** S	29.33 ± 0.57 S	22.66 ± 0.57 ** S	26.66 ± 1.15 ** S	29.33 ± 1.15 –	29.33 ± 1.15 ** R	32.00 ± 1.00 ** S	19.66 ± 0.57 ** –	0.00 R	<0.001

Calculation of Inhibition Zone Diameter includes the diameter of the well (6mm). * Mean ± Standard deviation; R: resistant;S: susceptible; EO: essential oil. ** $p < 0.01$: the inhibition zone diameter of a group (EO or antimicrobials) vs. the inhibition diameters of all other groups for each strain. [1] Diameter of inhibition zones, including diameter of well 6 mm. [2] Amoxicillin + Clavulanic Ac; [3] Amoxicillin; [4] Doxycycline; [5] Spiramycine; [6] Ciprofloxacine; [7] Minocycline; [8] Vancomycin; [9] Metronidazol. [10] Breakpoint is missing for Amoxicillin; however, susceptibility can be inferred from ampicillin, for which the breakpoint is: S ≥ 16 and R < 16 mm. [11] breakpoint is missing for Doxycycline; however, isolates susceptible to tetracycline are also susceptible to Doxycycline. Breakpoint for tetracycline is: S ≥ 25 and R < 22.

The serial diffusion test in 96-well microplates showed MIC values in the ranges of 0.05 to 1.51 µg/mL and 0.09 to 2.01 µg/mL for MBCs (Table 3). For MBC/MIC ratio, all the values found were lower than 4, considering EO as bactericidal agents.

Table 3. Minimum inhibitory concentrations (MIC) and minimum bactericidal concentrations (MBC) of *O. vulgare* EO for the selected *A. actinomycetemcomitans* strains.

A. *Actinomycetemcomitans* Strains	*O. vulgare* EO		
	MIC(µg/mL) *	MBC (µg/mL) *	MIC/MBC *
clinical strain 1	1.00 ± 0.43	1.51 ± 0.00	0.99 ± 0.87
clinical strain 2	0.49 ± 0.21	0.62 ± 0.21	1.34 ± 0.58
clinical strain 3	0.15 ± 0.51	0.18 ± 0.00	1.00 ± 0.00
clinical strain 4	0.12 ± 0.05	0.15 ± 0.51	0.49 ± 0.05
clinical strain 5	0.12 ± 0.05	0.15 ± 0.05	1.00 ± 0.86
clinical strain 6	0.49 ± 0.21	0.75 ± 0.00	0.66 ± 0.29
ATTC 43717 (Suny aB75)	0.09 ± 0.00	0.09 ± 0.00	1.00 ± 0.00
Y4 ATTC 43718	0.18 ± 0.00	0.18 ± 0.00	1.00 ± 0.00
HK1651 (JP2)	0.09 ± 0.00	0.09 ± 0.00	1.00 ± 0.00
HK 921(JP2)	1.51 ± 0.00	2.01 ± 0.87	0.83 ± 0.28
HK1605 (non JP2)	0.62 ± 0.21	0.75 ± 0.00	0.83 ± 0.29

* Mean± standard deviation.

2.3. Cytotoxicity

The *O. vulgare* EO showed a dose-dependent cytotoxic effect in cultures of PMA-differentiated THP-1 cells (Figure 2). Concentrations of oil above 125 µg/mL caused substantial decreased cell viability after 24 h of exposure.

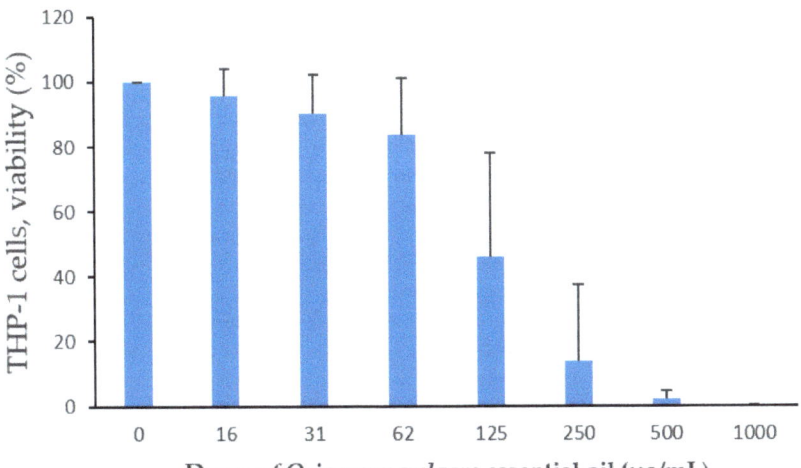

Figure 2. Cytotoxicity of *O.vulgare* essential oil.

PMA-differentiated THP-1 cells were exposed to different concentrations of oil for 24 h and cell viability determined with neutral red uptake staining. Mean ± standard deviation of three independent experiments are shown.

2.4. A. actinomycetemcomitans Leukotoxin Neutralization

The *O. vulgare* EO showed no neutralizing effect on *A. actinomycetemcomitans* leukotoxicity estimated in cultures of PMA-differentiated THP-1 cells (Table 4). The presence of oil from *O. vulgare* did not affect the inhibitory effect on leukotoxicity exhibited by the extract from the *Psidium guajava* leaves.

Table 4. Leukotoxicity (200 ng/mL) in presence of *Psidium guajava* or *O. vulgare* EO alone or in combination after 2 h incubation in cultures of PMA-differentiated THP-cells. Result is expressed as percent viable cells in relation to control cells (100%) based on quantitative neutral red uptake analyses. Mean ± SD of triplicate analyses.

Concentration (µL/mL)	Oil (%)	Guava (%)	Association oil and Guava (%)	p
0	99.99 ± 0.93 *	100 ± 0.93	100 ± 0.93	<0.001
4	93.82 ± 3.13 *	93.55 ± 0.98	96.27 ± 0.98	<0.001
8	95.73 ± 0.31 *	91.92 ± 2.72	106.33 ± 1.65	<0.001
16	98.99 ± 0.41 *	106.60 ± 6.14	90.01 ± 8.17	<0.001
31	102.52 ± 1.22 *	108.51 ± 10.02	105.79 ± 20.35	<0.001
62	78.86 ± 3.86 *	85.39 ± 7.24	93.55 ± 2.52	<0.001
125	59.28 ± 1.72 *	98.72 ± 6.81	84.30 ± 2.61	<0.001
250	−4.07 ± 0.31 *	93.01 ± 4.31	98.99 ± 9.99	<0.001

* Significant difference ($p < 0.001$).

3. Discussion

The use of natural products, such as Eos, as antibacterial agents is expanding in oral hygiene and dentistry. In Morocco, a major herbal-producing nation, many studies have been carried out on the antimicrobial activity of Moroccan plant extracts and EOs [23,24].

However, there are few reports on the effects of Moroccan EOs on periodontal pathogens. The EO of *O. vulgare* was selected for this study on the basis of its traditional use for the treatment of oral diseases [13].

The results of the present study showed that the essential oil of *O. vulgare* exhibited a strong antimicrobial activity against all tested clinical and reference strains of *A. actinomycetemcomitans*.

The antimicrobial activity of an EO is well-known, and it is linked to its main constituents. The *O. vulgare* EOs is characterized by the dominance of various antibacterial compounds. Chemical analyses of this oil revealed that the main constituents of the oil were carvacrol 32.36%, α-terpineol 16.70%, p-cymene 16.24%, and thymol 12.05% (Figure 1 and Table 1). All these compounds have strong antibacterial activity, as shown in previous studies [25–27]. Linalool (an alcohol) is one of the components of the essential oil of *O. vulgare* present in lower concentration (Table 1). However, this compound was found to have antimicrobial activity against various oral and non-oral microbes [28–30].

In this study, we used the agar diffusion test to study the antibacterial activity of *O. vulgare* EO against clinical and reference strains of *A. actinomycetemcomitans*. Substantial antibacterial activity against both JP2 and non-JP2 strains was observed. The diameters of the inhibition zones obtained were greater than 20 mm, (going from 37.00 ± 1.73 mm for strain HK 921(JP2), to 69.66 ± 0.57 mm for strain ATCC 43717 Sunny aB75) (Table 3). The studied strains showed a high sensitivity to the studied essential oil when 27.6 µg of it was used.

For analyzing the susceptibility of the *A. actinomycetemcomitans* strains to the tested antimicrobials, and according to the EUCAST (European Committee on Antimicrobial Susceptibility Testing), breakpoints for *Haemophilus influenzae* was used, as there is not one associated to *A. actinomycetemcomitans* [31].

Based on the EUCAST interpretation values, all 11 tested *A. actinomycetemcomitans* strains were susceptible to AMC and MH. All isolates were also susceptible to AML if ampicillin-derived breakpoints were used. Furthermore, eight strains were susceptible to DO if tetracycline-derived breakpoints were used. Susceptibility to SP, VA and MTZ could not be validated, since no breakpoints for *H. influenzae* are available in the EUCAST database. Inhibition zones are usually absent when susceptibility of *A. actinomycetemcomitans* to MTZ is tested under aerobic conditions.

For studying the antibacterial effect of the essential oil to the selected *A. actinomycetemcomitans* strains, compared with corresponding effect of the antimicrobials, the inhibition zones were used. Since all inhibition zones induced by the essential oil (27.6 µg) were significantly larger, it indicates that the oil has a substantial antibacterial effect on *A. actinomycetemcomitans*.

A range of different antimicrobials have been used as adjuvant for treatment of periodontitis during the last decades. This has raised questions about risk for resistance development among the antimicrobials and also doubts about the beneficial value of this treatment strategy. However, a range of clinical studies have shown that use of a combination of MTZ and AML in conjunction with standard periodontal treatment of aggressive forms of periodontitis achieves better clinical and microbiological results than treatment without these antimicrobials [32–34].

Regarding resistance development among these antimicrobials, different results are reported. However, the breakpoint for MTZ is not available. Thus, susceptibility testing of this antimicrobial is not relevant. Based on usage of breakpoint value for *Haemophilus influenzae*, most reports of susceptibility of *A. actinomycetemcomitans* to AML show that the prevalence of resistant isolates of the bacterium is low [35]. In addition, when isolates earlier found to be resistant to this antimicrobial were retested, the opposite result was achieved [36].

For the microdilution test, the results obtained for MIC are mainly in accordance with the diameters of the inhibition zones observed in the well diffusion test. On the other hand, the *O. vulgare* EO showed bactericidal activity with promising MBC results and an MBC/MIC ratio below 4. The MBC values were similar or almost identical to those of MIC. *O. vulgare* EO had the highest inhibitory activity against ATTC 43717 (Suny aB75) (CMI = 0.09 µg/mL) and the highest bactericidal effect against the reference strains ATTC 43717 (Suny aB75) and HK1651 (JP2) (CMB= 0.09 µg/mL) (Table 3). These results are consistent with those obtained in previous work on other tested non-oral Gram-negative bacteria [37–39] reflecting a higher antibacterial activity on this oral bacterium.

The cytotoxicity of the essential oil of *O. vulgare* EO *in* concentrations was below 125 µg/mL when analyzed in cultures of human macrophages (THP-1 cells). The IC50-value for the oil was much lower than the MIC-values for antibacterial effect, suggesting an advantage for its use as a clinical chemical agent. EO seems to be toxic for cells. Previously, it has been shown that carvacrol and other oregano constituents can be cytotoxic at high doses [40,41]. Thus, further investigations are needed to achieve maximum positive antimicrobial effect of *O.vulgare* EO without cytotoxic effects. In addition, this oil did not interfere with the LtxA neutralizing capacity of extract from *Psidium guajava* leaves. It has been shown that components extracted from *Psidium guajava* bind to LtxA and completely abolish its activity [42].

A mouth rinse containing water extract from *Psidium guava* leaves has been tested on adolescents in Morocco with the presence of *A. actinomycetemcomitans* from the JP2 genotype in their subgingival plaque [22]. Results from this pilot study are limited, but they indicate that LtxA neutralization alone was not sufficient for eradication of *A. actinomycetemcomitans* and its pro-inflammatory effect.

A. actinomycetemcomitans is a germ that is mostly associated with aggressive forms of periodontitis. One of its virulence factors is LtxA, which plays an important role in pathogenicity. Periodontal infections due to strains that produce high levels of LtxA are strongly associated with a serious disease. LtxA selectively kills human leukocytes and can affect the body's functioning local defensive mechanisms [5]. Previous studies on the role of LtxA in host–parasite interactions have focused mainly on polymorphonuclear leukocytes (PMN) [43,44]. In periodontal inflammation, macrophages have an important role in regulating inflammatory reactions and tissue degradation and remodeling [45]. LtxA causes a rapid inflammatory cell death in macrophages, which might cause an imbalance in the pro-inflammatory response [46].

We can conclude that the *O. vulgare* EO has the potential to be used as a preventive or therapeutic agent against periodontitis in individuals colonized with *A. actinomycetemcomitans*. Its cytotoxic properties can be overcome by the possibility to cooperate with the LtxA neutralizing compounds of *Psidium guajava*.

4. Materials and Methods

The present study was carried out after obtaining approval from the Biomedical Ethics Committee (Ref. 400/2010); the individual patient's written informed consent was obtained before the collection of the plaque samples for the study.

4.1. Plant Material and Extraction of Essential Oil

The aerial part of *O. vulgare* was purchased at a local market in Rabat, Morocco. A portion (100 g) of the aerial parts of the plants was hydrodistilled during 3 hours, using a Clevenger system. The obtained essential oil was dried over anhydrous sodium sulphate and, after filtration, stored at +4 °C, until it was tested and analyzed.

4.2. Gas Chromatography Coupled with Mass Spectrometry (GC/MS)

The chemical composition of the EO was analyzed by using a gas chromatograph (Perkin Elmer Clarus™ GC-680) fitted to a mass spectrometer (Q-8 MS Ion Trap), operating in electron-impact EI (70 eV) mode. Non-polar column HP-5MS (Methylpolysiloxane 5% phenyl, 60 m × 0.25 mm × 0.25 µm thickness) was used (the GC/MS was done at the Platform of physicalchemistry analysis and characterization, Faculty of Sciences, Mohammed V University in Rabat, Morocco). The chromatographic conditions were as follows: injector temperatures at 280 °C; carrier gas, helium at flow rate of 1 mL/min; temperature program ramp from 60 to 200 °C, at gradient of 2 °C/min. After holding 1 min at 200 °C, another ramp was operated from 200 until 300 °C, at 20 °C/min, and final hold for 5 min. The GC/MS system was controlled by Turbomass™ software; a library search was carried out, using the combination of NIST MS Search and literature. The NIST version was 2.0 g, built May 19, 2011. The relative number of individual components of the total oil was expressed as a percentage of each peak area relative to total peak areas. The retention indices (RI) were obtained by injecting in HP-5MS a mixture of continuous series of straight chain hydrocarbons (C8-C31), under the same conditions as described above.

4.3. A. actinomycetemcomitans Strains

The antimicrobial capacity of *O.vulgare* EO and of following selected antimicrobials, Amoxicillin (AM), Amoxicillin and clavulanic acid (AMC), Doxycycline (DO), Ciprofloxacin (CIP), Minocycline (MN), Vancomycin (VA), and Metronidazole(MTZ) was tested against six clinical isolates and the following reference strains: ATTC 43717 (Suny aB75), Y4 (ATCC 43718), HK1651(JP2), HK 921 (JP2), and HK1605 (non JP2). HK 1651 was obtained from Department of Odontology, Umeå University, Sweden. HK 921 (JP2) and HK1605 (non JP2) were obtained from Department of Dentistry and Oral Health Aarhus University, Denmark.

The bacterial strains and essential oil were stored at the laboratory of oral biology and biotechnology, Faculty of Dental Medicine, Mohammed V University in Rabat. The tests were performed at the same laboratory.

4.4. Subgingival Plaque Sampling

The clinical *A. actinomycetemcomitans* strains were obtained from subgingival plaque samples collected from patients with periodontitis. The patients were recruited at the Clinical Department of Periodontology in the Center of Consultations and Dental Treatments (CCTD) in Rabat-Morocco.

The sampled patients were diagnosed with aggressive periodontitis and had pockets of 5 mm or greater confirmed by clinical and radiological examination. Subgingival sampling of periodontal biofilm was performed, using absorbent paper point (medium size, Maillefer, Ballaigues, Switzerland). Then, the papers were pooled and placed in a tube containing 1.5 mL of phosphate buffer saline (PBS). All plaque samples were collected by the same examiner.

4.5. Culture and Isolation

Once in the laboratory, the sample was vortexed before being seeded into the culture medium Dentaid-1 [47] and used for selective isolation and growth of *A actinomycetemcomitans*. Plates were incubated at 37 °C, in air, with 5% CO_2; and after 3–5 days, they were carefully examined for the presence of *A. actinomycetemcomitans*. Identification of the bacterium was based on colony morphology, positive catalase reaction, and negative oxidase reaction. Putative *A. actinomycetemcomitans* colonies were further elucidated by microscopy, Gram stain, and enzymatic activity, including indole and fermentation of glucose, xylose, maltose, and mannitol [48]. The isolates were then stored at −80 °C in glycerol broth.

4.6. In Vitro Antimicrobial Susceptibility Assay

The antimicrobial effect of *O. vulgare* was tested in two ways. The agar well diffusion method was used to determine the antibacterial activity in comparison with corresponding activity of selected antimicrobials. A microdilution assay was used for the calculation of MIC (minimum inhibitory concentration). MBC (minimal bactericidal concentration) of the oil was also determined.

4.6.1. Agar Well Diffusion Method

Agar well diffusion method [49–51] was used to evaluate the antimicrobial activity of essential oil from *O. vulgare*.

Initially, the bacterial strains were cultivated on slant cultures for 24 hours. Subsequently, bacterial suspensions were prepared in 0.85% NaCl, and the turbidity was adjusted to McFarland 0.5 (approximately 1×10^8 CFU/mL). The turbidity was confirmed by a Sensititre®Nephelometer. At first, the agar plates were seeded by swabbing with a cotton swab. Then, 30 µL of the essential oil (27.6 µg) was added to wells (diameter 6 mm) made in the center of each agar plate after 15 minutes [52,53]. Doxycycline (disc: 30 µg) was used as positive control [54]. The plates were incubated at 37 °C, in an aerobic atmosphere containing 5% CO_2, for 48 hours. All tests were carried out in triplicate, in separate experiments. Diameters of the inhibition zones were measured as (mm), including the diameter of the well. The antibacterial activity was considered if an inhibition halo of growth larger than 6 mm (size of the well) was produced.

4.6.2. Minimum Inhibitory Concentration (MIC) Determination

The MIC of *O. vulgare* EO was determined by using a broth assay in 96-well microplates (Sigma-Aldrich, USA), as recommended by NCCLS, for the determination of the MIC (NCCLS, 1999). All tests were performed in Mueller Hinton broth (MHB) supplemented with Tween 80, (final concentration of 0.5% v/v), aimed to improve the solubility. The bacterial strains were cultured overnight, at 37°C, in Dentaid-1. The turbidity of the inoculums was adjusted to McFarland 0.5. The turbidity of the suspensions was confirmed with the Sensititre®Nephelometer. Serial dilutions ranging from 48.42 to 0.09 mg/mL of the EO were prepared in a 96-well microplate, including one growth control with "MHB + Tween 80", one sterile control containing "MHB and Tween 80", and another sterile control made of "MHB +Tween 80 +EO". Amoxicillin (10 mg/mL) was used as positive control. The plates were incubated under normal atmospheric conditions, at 37 °C, for 24 hours. After incubation time, 40 µL of 2 mg/mL Triphenyl Tetrazolium Chloride (TTC) indicator solution (indicator of microorganism growth) was added to all wells of the microplate. Subsequently, the plates were re-incubated for 2 hours, at 37 °C [55]. Bacterial growth was monitored when the TTC indicator was red.

4.6.3. Minimum Bactericidal Concentration (MCB) Determination

To measure the minimum bactericidal concentration (MBC), 10 µL of cultures was taken from wells of the microplate of MIC, with no visible turbidity, inoculated on blood agar plates, and incubated for 48 hours, at 37 °C, under 5% CO_2 [56]. MBC was defined to be the lowest concentration of essential oil that killed 99.9% of the microorganisms in culture on the agar plate after the incubation time.

The MBC/MIC ratio was calculated to show the nature of the antibacterial effect of essential oils. In a ratio less than 4, the essential oil was classified as a bactericidal essential oil, and in a ratio more than 4, it was classified as a bacteriostatic essential oil [57].

Each MIC and MBC value was obtained from three independent experiments.

4.7. Cell Culture

Cells of the human acute monocytic leukemia cell line THP-1 (ATCC 16) were cultured in RPMI-1640 (Sigma-Aldrich, St. Louis, MI, USA) with 10% fetal bovine serum (FBS) (Sigma-Aldrich), at 37 °C, in 5% CO_2. Before determination of leukotoxic activity, the THP-1 cells were seeded in 96-well cell-culture plates, at a cell density of 10^5 cells/mL in 100 µL culture medium supplemented with 50 nMphorbol 12-myristate 13-acetate (PMA, Sigma-Aldrich), and incubated for 24 hours. The PMA-activated THP-1 cells exhibited adherent properties and enhanced sensitivity to the LtxA.

After differentiation with phorbol 12-myristate 13-acetate (PMA), THP-1 cells acquire a macrophage phenotype, which is similar to primary human macrophages in many aspects [58,59]. This is the common way to use THP-1 cells in cell assays. The adherent phenotype is macrophage-like and easier to study in cytotoxicity assays.

Twenty-four hours prior to LtxA exposure, the culture medium was discarded, and 100 µL fresh medium without PMA was added to each well of the THP-1 monolayer.

4.8. Cytotoxicity Assay

The cell monolayers of PMA-differentiated THP-1 cells were exposed to different concentrations of the oil for 24 h, at conditions described above. The proportion of viable cells in each well was determined by the neutral red uptake method and expressed in relation to that of the control cells cultured in plane medium [60]. Cytotoxicity (LD_{50}) was expressed as the lowest concentration (ppm) that kills ≥ 50% of the cells.

4.9. LtxA Purification

LtxA was purified from *A. actinomycetemcomitans* strain HK 1519, described in detail previously [61]. The purified LtxA was basically free from lipopolysaccharides (LPS) (<0.001% of total protein) and visualized by SDS-polyacrylamide gel separation.

4.10. Preparation of Psidium Guajava Leave Extract

Guava leaves were collected in Ghana by Dr. F.Kwamin and transported with a courier to Umeå University, Umeå, Sweden. Guava leaves at a concentration of 250 g/liter of water, were boiled for 10 minutes before the leaves were removed by filtration, and cleared from debris by centrifugation. The supernatant was aliquoted and stored in a refrigerator until use. The amount of dry substance was determined by evaporation of the extract, which contained 10.0 mg/mL H_2O.

4.11. LxtA Neutralization Assay

The cell monolayers of PMA-differentiated THP-1 cells were exposed to different concentrations of the oil or guava for 15 min, before the LtxA (200 ng/mL) was added. The different mixtures were incubated for 2 h, at conditions described above. The proportion of viable cells in each well was determined by the neutral red uptake method, as described above.

4.12. Statistical Analyses

Statistical analysis was carried out by using SPSS for Windows (SPSS, Inc., Chicago, IL, USA). Inhibition zone diameter, MIC, MBC, MBC/MIC, and cell viability values, as continuous variables with a normal distribution, were expressed as mean ± standard deviation. For statistical differences between the inhibition diameter of the nine antimicrobial agents (EO, AMC, AMX, DO, SP, CIP, MH, VA, and MTZ), and the cell viability in presence of EO, Guava, and the association "EO +Guava", the One-Way Analysis of Variance (ANOVA) with Bonferroni correction was performed. A p-value < 0.05 was considered as statistically significant. Statistical analyses were carried out, using SPSS for Windows (SPSS, Inc., Chicago, IL, USA).

5. Conclusions

The present study indicates that *O. vulgare* EO may find application as an antibacterial agent on periodontitis associated with *A. actinomycetemcomitans* and shows the possibility of *Psidium guajava* to overcome its cytotoxic properties. However, further investigations on mechanisms of action and toxicity need to be continued.

Author Contributions: S.A., extraction of essential oil, culture and isolation of *A. actinomycetemcomitans*, in vitro antimicrobial susceptibility assay, statistical analyses, and drafting the manuscript; A.J., cell culture, LtxA purification, cytotoxicity assay, LtxA neutralization assay, and the drafting of the manuscript; M.Y., culture and isolation of *A. actinomycetemcomitans*. D.H., culture and isolation of *A. actinomycetemcomitans*. A.E.h., gas chromatography coupled with mass spectrometry (GC/MS) assay; R.C., in vitro antimicrobial susceptibility assay. O.E., recruitment of patients, subgingival plaque sampling, culture and isolation of *A. actinomycetemcomitans*, drafting the manuscript, and work supervision; S.R., helped with funds. All authors have read and agreed to the published version of the manuscript.

Funding: This research received funding from CNRST (National Center for scientific and Technological Research (PPR116/2016), Morocco.

Acknowledgments: The authors are thankful to Francis Kwamin at Ghana University for the collection of Guava leaves.

Conflicts of Interest: The authors declare no conflict of interest.

References

1. Henderson, B.; Ward, J.M.; Ready, D. Aggregatibacter (Actinobacillus) actinomycetemcomitans: A triple A*periodontopathogen? *Periodontology 2000* **2010**, *54*, 78–105. [CrossRef] [PubMed]
2. Asikainen, S.; Chen, C. Oral ecology and person-to-person transmission of Actinobacillus actinomycetemcomitans and Porphyromonas gingivalis. *Periodontology 2000* **1999**, *20*, 65–81. [CrossRef] [PubMed]
3. Zambon, J.J.; Haraszthy, V.I. The laboratory diagnosis of periodontal infections. *Periodontology 2000* **1995**, *7*, 69–82. [CrossRef] [PubMed]
4. Könönen, E.; Müller, H.P. Microbiology of aggressive periodontitis. *Periodontology 2000* **2014**, *65*, 46–78. [CrossRef] [PubMed]
5. Johansson, A. Aggregatibacter actinomycetemcomitans leukotoxin: A powerful tool with capacity to cause imbalance in the host inflammatory response. *Toxins* **2011**, *3*, 242–259. [CrossRef]
6. Brogan, J.M.; Lally, E.T.; Poulsen, K.; Kilian, M.; Demuth, D.R. Regulation of Actinobacillus actinomycetemcomitans leukotoxin expression: Analysis of the promoter regions of leukotoxic and minimally leukotoxic strains. *Infect. Immun.* **1994**, *62*, 501–508. [CrossRef]
7. Haubek, D.; Ennibi, O.K.; Poulsen, K.; Væth, M.; Poulsen, S.; Kilian, M. Risk of aggressive periodontitis in adolescent carriers of the JP2 clone of Aggregatibacter (Actinobacillus) actinomycetemcomitans in Morocco: A prospective longitudinal cohort study. *Lancet* **2008**, *371*, 237–242. [CrossRef]
8. Ennibi, O.K.; Benrachadi, L.; Bouziane, A.; Haubek, D.; Poulsen, K. The highly leukotoxic JP2 clone of Aggregatibacter actinomycetemcomitans in localized and generalized forms of aggressive periodontitis. *Acta Odontol. Scand.* **2012**, *70*, 318–322. [CrossRef]

9. Caton, J.G.; Armitage, G.; Berglundh, T.; Chapple, I.L.; Jepsen, S.; Kornman, K.S.; Mealey, B.L.; Papapanou, P.N.; Sanz, M.; Tonetti, M.S. A new classification scheme for periodontal and peri-implant diseases and conditions–Introduction and key changes from the 1999 classification. *J. Periodontol.* **2018**, *89*, S1–S8. [CrossRef]
10. Wang, C.-Y.; Wang, H.-C.; Li, J.-M.; Wang, J.-Y.; Yang, K.-C.; Ho, Y.-K.; Lin, P.-Y.; Lee, L.-N.; Yu, C.-J.; Yang, P.-C. Invasive infections of Aggregatibacter (Actinobacillus) actinomycetemcomitans. *J. Microbiol. Immunol. Infect.* **2010**, *43*, 491–497. [CrossRef]
11. Walker, C.B. The acquisition of antibiotic resistance in the periodontal microflora. *Periodontology 2000* **1996**, *10*, 79–88. [CrossRef] [PubMed]
12. Jouad, H.; Haloui, M.; Rhiouani, H.; ElHilaly, J.; Eddouks, M. Ethnobotanical survey of medicinal plants used for the treatment of diabetes, cardiac and renal diseases in the North centre region of Morocco (Fez–Boulemane). *J. Ethnopharmacol.* **2001**, *77*, 175–182. [CrossRef]
13. Akkaoui, S.; Ennibi, O.k. Use of traditional plants in management of halitosis in a Moroccan population. *J. Intercult. Ethnopharmacol.* **2017**, *6*, 267. [CrossRef] [PubMed]
14. Kharbach, M.; Marmouzi, I.; ElJemli, M.; Bouklouze, A.; VanderHeyden, Y. Recent advances in untargeted and targeted approaches applied in herbal-extracts and essential-oils finger printing-Areview. *J. Pharm. Biomed. Anal.* **2020**, *177*, 112849. [CrossRef]
15. Barnes, J. Quality, efficacy and safety of complementary medicines: Fashions, facts and the future. Part I. *Regul. Qual. Br. J. Clin. Pharmacol.* **2003**, *55*, 226–233. [CrossRef] [PubMed]
16. DeMartino, L.; DeFeo, V.; Nazzaro, F. Chemical composition and in vitro antimicrobial and mutagenic activities of seven Lamiacea eessential oils. *Molecules* **2009**, *14*, 4213–4230. [CrossRef]
17. Fikry, S.; Khalil, N.; Salama, O. Chemical profiling, biostatic and biocidal dynamics of Origanum vulgare L. essentialoil. *AMB Express* **2019**, *9*, 41. [CrossRef]
18. Raut, J.S.; Karuppayil, S.M. A status review on the medicinal properties of essential oils. *Ind. Crop. Prod.* **2014**, *62*, 250–264. [CrossRef]
19. Johnson, C.B.; Kazantzis, A.; Skoula, M.; Mitteregger, U.; Novak, J. Seasonal, populational and ontogenic variation in the volatile oil content and composition of individuals of Origanum vulgare subsp.Hirtum, assessed by GC headspacean alysis and by SPME sampling of individual oil glands. *Phytochem. Anal. Int. J. Plant Chem. Biochem. Technol.* **2004**, *15*, 286–292.
20. Lotti, C.; Ricciardi, L.; Rainaldi, G.; Ruta, C.; Tarraf, W.; DeMastro, G. Morphological, Biochemical, and Molecular Analysis of Origanum vulgare L. *Open Agric. J.* **2019**, *13*, 116–124. [CrossRef]
21. Khan, M.; Khan, S.T.; Khan, M.; Mousa, A.A.; Mahmood, A.; Alkhathlan, H.Z. Chemical diversity in leaf and stem essential oils of Origanum vulgare L. and their effects on microbicidal activities. *AMB Express* **2019**, *9*, 176. [CrossRef] [PubMed]
22. Ennibi, O.K.; Claesson, R.; Akkaoui, S.; Reddahi, S.; Kwamin, F.; Haubek, D.; Johansson, A. High salivary levels of JP2 genotype of Aggregatibacter actinomycetemcomitans is associated with clinical attachment lossin Moroccan adolescents. *Clin. Exp. Dent. Res.* **2019**, *5*, 44–51. [CrossRef] [PubMed]
23. Chaouki, W.; Leger, D.Y.; Eljastimi, J.; Beneytout, J.-L.; Hmamouchi, M. Antiproliferative effect of extracts from Aristolochia baetica and Origanum compactum on human breast cancer cell lineMCF-7. *Pharm. Biol.* **2010**, *48*, 269–274. [CrossRef] [PubMed]
24. Hmamouchi, M.; Hamamouchi, J.; Zouhdi, M.; Bessiere, J. Chemical and antimicrobial properties of essential oils of five Moroccan Pinaceae. *J. Essent. Oil Res.* **2001**, *13*, 298–302. [CrossRef]
25. CanBaser, K. Biological and pharmacological activities of carvacrol and carvacrol bearing essentialoils. *Curr. Pharm. Des.* **2008**, *14*, 3106–3119. [CrossRef]
26. Park, S.-N.; Lim, Y.K.; Freire, M.O.; Cho, E.; Jin, D.; Kook, J.-K. Antimicrobial effect of linalool and α-terpineol against periodontopathic and cariogenic bacteria. *Anaerobe* **2012**, *18*, 369–372. [CrossRef]
27. Bagamboula, C.; Uyttendaele, M.; Debevere, J. Inhibitory effect of thyme and basil essential oils, carvacrol, thymol, estragol, linalool and p-cymene towards Shigella sonnei and S.flexneri. *Food Microbiol.* **2004**, *21*, 33–42. [CrossRef]
28. Lin, Z.-K.; Hua, Y.; Gu, Y. The chemical constituents of the essential oil from the flowers, leaves and peels of Citrus aurantium. *Act. Bot. Sin.* **1986**, *28*, 641–645.
29. Alipour, G.; Dashti, S.; Hosseinzadeh, H. Review of pharmacological effects of Myrtus communis L. *and ist active constituents. Phytother. Res.* **2014**, *28*, 1125–1136. [CrossRef]

30. Cha, J.-D.; Jung, E.-K.; Kil, B.-S.; Lee, K.-Y. Chemical composition and antibacterial activity of essential oil from Artemisia feddei. *J. Microbiol. Biotechnol.* **2007**, *17*, 2061–2065.
31. European Committee on Antimicrobial Susceptibility Testing. Breakpoint Tables for Interpretation of MICs and Zone Diameters; Version 9.0. 2019. Available online: http://www.eucast.org/fileadmin/src/media/PDFs/EUCAST_files/Breakpoint_tables/Dosages_EUCAST_Breakpoint_Tables_v_9.0.pdf (accessed on 2 March 2020).
32. Winkel, E.; VanWinkelhoff, A.; Timmerman, M.; VanderVelden, U.; VanderWeijden, G. Amoxicillin plus metronidazole in the treatment of adult periodontitis patients: A double-blind placebo-controlled study. *J. Clin. Periodontol.* **2001**, *28*, 296–305. [CrossRef] [PubMed]
33. Zandbergen, D.; Slot, D.E.; Niederman, R.; VanderWeijden, F.A. The concomitant administration of systemic amoxicillin and metronidazole compared to scaling and root planing alone in treating periodontitis:=a systematic review=. *BMC Oral Health* **2016**, *16*, 27. [CrossRef] [PubMed]
34. Keestra, J.; Grosjean, I.; Coucke, W.; Quirynen, M.; Teughels, W. Non-surgical periodontal therapy with systemic antibiotics in patients with untreated chronic periodontitis: A systematic review and meta-analysis. *J. Periodontal Res.* **2015**, *50*, 294–314. [CrossRef] [PubMed]
35. Mínguez, M.; Ennibi, O.; Perdiguero, P.; Lakhdar, L.; Abdellaoui, L.; Sánchez, M.; Sanz, M.; Herrera, D. Antimicrobial susceptibilities of Aggregatibacter actinomycetemcomitans and Porphyromonas gingivalis strains from periodontitis patients in Morocco. *Clin. Oral Investig.* **2019**, *23*, 1161–1170. [CrossRef]
36. Jensen, A.B.; Haubek, D.; Claesson, R.; Johansson, A.; Nørskov-Lauritsen, N. Comprehensive antimicrobial susceptibility testing of a large collection of clinical strains of Aggregatibacter actinomycetemcomitans does not identify resistance to amoxicillin. *J. Clin. Periodontol.* **2019**, *46*, 846–854. [CrossRef] [PubMed]
37. Chao, S.C.; Young, D.G.; Oberg, C.J. Screening for inhibitory activity of essential oils on selected bacteria, fungi and viruses. *J. Essent. Oil Res.* **2000**, *12*, 639–649. [CrossRef]
38. Oussalah, M.; Caillet, S.; Saucier, L.; Lacroix, M. Antimicrobial effects of selected plant essential oils on the growth of a Pseudomonas putida strain isolated from meat. *Meat Sci.* **2006**, *73*, 236–244. [CrossRef]
39. Bouhdid, S.; Skali, S.; Idaomar, M.; Zhiri, A.; Baudoux, D.; Amensour, M.; Abrini, J. Antibacterial and antioxidant activities of Origanum compactum essential oil. *Afr. J. Biotechnol.* **2008**, *7*, 1563–1570.
40. Llana-Ruiz-Cabello, M.; Gutiérrez-Praena, D.; Pichardo, S.; Moreno, F.J.; Bermúdez, J.M.; Aucejo, S.; Cameán, A.M. Cytotoxicity and morphological effects induced by carvacrol and thymol on the human cell line Caco-2. *Food Chem. Toxicol.* **2014**, *64*, 281–290. [CrossRef]
41. Bauer, B.W.; Radovanovic, A.; Willson, N.-L.; Bajagai, Y.S.; Van, T.T.H.; Moore, R.J.; Stanley, D. Oregano: A potential prophylactic treatment for the intestinal microbiota. *Heliyon* **2019**, *5*, e02625. [CrossRef]
42. Kwamin, F.; Gref, R.; Haubek, D.; Johansson, A. Interactions of extracts from selected chewing stick sources with Aggregatibacter actinomycetemcomitans. *Bmc Res. Notes* **2012**, *5*, 203. [CrossRef] [PubMed]
43. Johansson, A.; Claesson, R.; Hänström, L.; Sandström, G.; Kalfas, S. Polymorphonuclear leukocyte degranulation induced by leukotoxin from Actinobacillus actinomycetemcomitans. *J. Periodontal Res.* **2000**, *35*, 85–92. [CrossRef] [PubMed]
44. Claesson, R.; Johansson, A.; Hanstrom, L.; Kalfas, S. Release and activation of matrix metalloproteinase 8 from human neutrophils triggered by the leukotoxin of Actinobacillus actinomycetemcomitans. *J.Periodontal. Res.* **2002**, *37*, 353–359. [CrossRef] [PubMed]
45. Kelk, P.; Abd, H.; Claesson, R.; Sandström, G.; Sjöstedt, A.; Johansson, A. Cellular and molecular response of human macrophages exposed to Aggregatibacter actinomycetemcomitans leukotoxin. *Cell. Death Dis.* **2009**, *2*, e126. [CrossRef] [PubMed]
46. Åberg, C.H.; Kelk, P.; Johansson, A. Aggregatibacter actinomycetemcomitans: Virulence of its leukotoxin and association with aggressive periodontitis. *Virulence* **2015**, *6*, 188–195. [CrossRef]
47. Alsina, M.; Olle, E.; Frias, J. Improved, Low-Cost Selective Culture Medium for Actinobacillusactinomycetemcomitans. *J. Clin. Microbiol.* **2001**, *39*, 509–513. [CrossRef] [PubMed]
48. Zbinden, R. Aggregatibacter, Capnocytophaga, Eikenella, Kingella, Pasteurella, and other fastidious or rarely encountered gram-negative rods. In *Manual of Clinical Microbiology*, 11th ed.; American Society of Microbiology: Washington, DC, USA, 2015; pp. 652–666.
49. Balouiri, M.; Sadiki, M.; Ibnsouda, S.K. Methods for in vitro evaluating antimicrobial activity: A review. *J. Pharm. Anal.* **2016**, *6*, 71–79. [CrossRef]

50. Magaldi, S.; Mata-Essayag, S.; DeCapriles, C.H.; Perez, C.; Colella, M.; Olaizola, C.; Ontiveros, Y. Well diffusion for antifungal susceptibility testing. *Int. J. Infect. Dis.* **2004**, *8*, 39–45. [CrossRef]
51. Valgas, C.; Souza, S.M.d.; Smânia, E.F.; SmâniaJr, A. Screening methods to determinean tibacterial activity of natural products. *Braz. J. Microbiol.* **2007**, *38*, 369–380. [CrossRef]
52. Adwan, G.; Abu-shanab, B.; Adwan, K. In vitro activity of certain drugs in combination with plant extracts against Staphylococcus aureus in fections. *Afr. J. Biotechnol.* **2009**, *8*, 4239–4241.
53. Boyanova, L.; Gergova, G.; Nikolov, R.; Derejian, S.; Lazarova, E.; Katsarov, N.; Mitov, I. Activity of Bulgarian propolis against 94 Helicobacter pylori strains invitro by agar-well diffusion, agar dilution and disc diffusion methods. *J. Med Microbiol.* **2005**, *54*, 481–483. [CrossRef] [PubMed]
54. Oettinger-Barak, O.; Dashper, S.G.; Catmull, D.V.; Adams, G.G.; Sela, M.N.; Machtei, E.E.; Reynolds, E.C. Antibiotic susceptibility of Aggregatibacter actinomycetemcomitans JP2 in a biofilm. *J. Oral Microbiol.* **2013**, *5*, 20320. [CrossRef] [PubMed]
55. Hammer, K.; Dry, L.; Johnson, M.; Michalak, E.; Carson, C.; Riley, T. Susceptibility of oral bacteria to Melaleuca alternifolia(teatree) oil in vitro. *Oral Microbiol. Immunol.* **2003**, *18*, 389–392. [CrossRef] [PubMed]
56. Hammer, K.A.; Carson, C.F.; Riley, T.V. Antimicrobial activity of essential oils and other plant extracts. *J. Appl. Microbiol.* **1999**, *86*, 985–990. [CrossRef]
57. Levison, M.E. Pharmacodynamics of antimicrobial drugs. *Infect. Dis. Clin.* **2004**, *18*, 451–465. [CrossRef]
58. Maeß, M.B.; Wittig, B.; Cignarella, A.; Lorkowski, S. Reduced PMA enhances the responsiveness of transfected THP-1 macrophages to polarizing stimuli. *J. Immunol. Methods* **2014**, *402*, 76–81. [CrossRef]
59. Lund, M.E.; To, J.; O'Brien, B.A.; Donnelly, S. The choice of phorbol12-myristate13-acetate differentiation protocol in fluences the response of THP-1 macrophages to apro-inflammatory stimulus. *J. Immunol. Methods* **2016**, *430*, 64–70. [CrossRef]
60. Repetto, G.; DelPeso, A.; Zurita, J.L. Neutral red uptake assay for thee stimation of cell viability/cytotoxicity. *Nat. Protoc.* **2008**, *3*, 1125. [CrossRef]
61. Johansson, A.; Hänström, L.; Kalfas, S. Inhibition of Actinobacillus actinomycetemcomitans leukotoxicity by bacteria from the subgingival flora. *Oral Microbiol. Immunol.* **2000**, *15*, 218–225. [CrossRef]

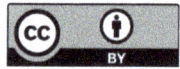

© 2020 by the authors. Licensee MDPI, Basel, Switzerland. This article is an open access article distributed under the terms and conditions of the Creative Commons Attribution (CC BY) license (http://creativecommons.org/licenses/by/4.0/).

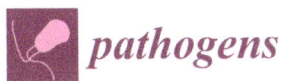

Article

Aggregatibacter actinomycetemcomitans LtxA Hijacks Endocytic Trafficking Pathways in Human Lymphocytes

Edward T Lally [1], Kathleen Boesze-Battaglia [1], Anuradha Dhingra [1], Nestor M Gomez [1], Jinery Lora [1], Claire H Mitchell [1], Alexander Giannakakis [1], Syed A Fahim [1], Roland Benz [2] and Nataliya Balashova [1,*]

[1] Department of Basic and Translational Sciences, School of Dental Medicine, University of Pennsylvania, Philadelphia, PA 19104, USA; kslpt@verizon.net (E.T.L.); battagli@upenn.edu (K.B.-B.); dhingra@upenn.edu (A.D.); tuk53759@temple.edu (N.M.G.); jlora@upenn.edu (J.L.); chm@upenn.edu (C.H.M.); alek@sas.upenn.edu (A.G.); razafahim1991@gmail.com (S.A.F.)
[2] Department of Life Science and Chemistry, Jacobs University Bremen, 28759 Bremen, Germany; r.benz@jacobs-university.de
* Correspondence: natbal@upenn.edu; Tel.: +215-898-5073; Fax: +215-898-2050

Received: 17 December 2019; Accepted: 16 January 2020; Published: 21 January 2020

Abstract: Leukotoxin (LtxA), from oral pathogen *Aggregatibacter actinomycetemcomitans*, is a secreted membrane-damaging protein. LtxA is internalized by β2 integrin LFA-1 (CD11a/CD18)-expressing leukocytes and ultimately causes cell death; however, toxin localization in the host cell is poorly understood and these studies fill this void. We investigated LtxA trafficking using multi-fluor confocal imaging, flow cytometry and Rab5a knockdown in human T lymphocyte Jurkat cells. Planar lipid bilayers were used to characterize LtxA pore-forming activity at different pHs. Our results demonstrate that the LtxA/LFA-1 complex gains access to the cytosol of Jurkat cells without evidence of plasma membrane damage, utilizing dynamin-dependent and presumably clathrin-independent mechanisms. Upon internalization, LtxA follows the LFA-1 endocytic trafficking pathways, as identified by co-localization experiments with endosomal and lysosomal markers (Rab5, Rab11A, Rab7, and Lamp1) and CD11a. Knockdown of Rab5a resulted in the loss of susceptibility of Jurkat cells to LtxA cytotoxicity, suggesting that late events of LtxA endocytic trafficking are required for toxicity. Toxin trafficking via the degradative endocytic pathway may culminate in the delivery of the protein to lysosomes or its accumulation in Rab11A-dependent recycling endosomes. The ability of LtxA to form pores at acidic pH may result in permeabilization of the endosomal and lysosomal membranes.

Keywords: *Aggregatibacter actinomycetemcomitans*; RTX toxin; localized aggressive periodontitis; LFA-1; leukotoxin (LtxA); endocytosis

1. Introduction

The RTX (Repeats in ToXin) toxins are membrane-damaging proteins secreted by some Gram-negative bacteria [1]. The organisms producing these proteins are important human and animal pathogens, implicating the toxins' role in the bacterial virulence. RTX toxins' common features are using the type I secretion system as a mode of export across the bacterial envelope, employing an uncleaved C-terminal recognition signal [2–4], and the characteristic nonapeptide glycine- and aspartate-rich repeat binding of Ca^{2+} ions [5,6]. The toxins are modified with fatty acid moieties attached to internal lysine residues, which is an unusual characteristic for bacterial proteins [7–10]. RTX toxins can be divided into three groups: (i) broadly cytolytic RTX hemolysins, (ii) species-specific RTX leukotoxins, and (iii) large, multifunctional, autoprocessing RTX toxins (MARTX) [1]. RTX leukotoxins exhibit a narrow cell type and species specificity due to cell-specific binding through protein receptors of the β_2 integrin family [1]. The β_2 integrins are expressed on the surface of leukocytes and share a common β_2 subunit, CD18, which is combined with either one of the unique α chains, α_L (CD11a), α_M (CD11b), α_X (CD11c), or α_D (CD11d) [11].

Aggregatibacter actinomycetemcomitans (*Aa*), a facultative anaerobe and common inhabitant of the human aerodigestive tract, causes localized aggressive periodontitis (LAP) [12]. LAP is a rapidly progressing periodontal disease that results in loss of tooth attachment and alveolar bone destruction in adolescents. If left untreated in teenagers, the infection will lead to the loss of the permanent first molars and central incisors [13]. Recent data indicate that *Aa* plays a role in the early stages of the disease. Specific *Aa* virulence factors can trigger the disease by suppressing the host response, which will allow for the overgrowth of *Aa* and other "toxic" bacteria in the local environment [12]. The pivotal virulence factor of *Aa* is an RTX leukotoxin, LtxA, that kills both human innate and adaptive immune cells [14]. *Aa* isolated from LAP patients predominantly belongs to a single clone, JP2 [15], which is characterized by increased LtxA production, implicating a role for LtxA in disease development [16]. Analysis of a primary LtxA sequence consisting of 1055 amino acids predicts four LtxA domains [17]. The hydrophobic domain encompasses residues 1–420 and incorporates cholesterol recognition amino acid consensus (CRAC) [18]. CRAC motif mediates LtxA binding to cholesterol and is essential for LtxA association with the plasma membrane of human T lymphocytes and monocytes [18,19]. The central domain (residues 421–730) contains two internal lysine residues (K^{562} and K^{687}) that are the sites of post-translational acylation, required for LtxA activation [9]. The repeat domain (residues 731–900) contains the typical repeated amino acid sequence of the RTX family with the C-terminal domain (residues 901–1055), and is believed to play a role in secretion [17].

Recent findings suggest that recirculating and resident memory T cells in gingival tissue play an important role in the maintenance of periodontal homeostasis [20]. In an experimental rat periodontal disease model, antigen-specific CD4 T lymphocytes were required for bone resorption [21]. Hence, the investigation of the LtxA effect on T lymphocytes is important for our understanding of how *Aa* causes periodontal disease. In our previous studies, the Jurkat cell line, subclone Jn.9, served as a model to study LtxA interaction with T lymphocytes' cell membrane. Jn.9 cells express cell-surface LFA-1 and are susceptible to LtxA-induced toxicity [22]. LtxA toxicity requires the presence of the β_2 integrin LFA-1(LFA-1, CD11a/CD18 or α_L/β_2) and cholesterol on the surface of Jn.9 cells [18,23,24]. LFA-1 is a native ligand for intercellular adhesion molecule (ICAM-1) located on vascular endothelial cells [25]. In immunocytes, LFA-1/ICAM-1 binding is one of the molecular mechanisms for leukocyte adhesion and migration to the site of infection [26]. LFA-1 is constantly endocytosed and then rapidly recycled back to the plasma membrane through vesicular transport [27,28] using the "long-loop" of recycling involving GTPase Rab11A-positive endosomes [29]. Also, LFA-1 activity is regulated by the ability of these receptors to switch between active and inactive conformations [25].

In the proposed mechanism of LtxA interaction with the Jn.9 cells membrane, the initial binding of the toxin with the membrane elevates cytosolic Ca^{2+} independent of the toxin binding to LFA-1. Ca^{2+} elevation involves the activation of calpain and talin cleavage, and the subsequent clustering of LFA-1 in lipid rafts on the membrane [24]. LtxA binds to the extracellular domains of LFA-1 subunits, CD11a and CD18. The toxin then transverses the cell membrane, binds to the cytoplasmic tails of LFA-1, and causes activation of LFA-1 [23]. Following from the results of the liposomal study, LtxA adopts a U-shaped conformation in the membrane, with the N- and C-terminal domains residing outside of the membrane [30].

After binding to the LFA-1 subunits, LtxA is quickly internalized into the cytosol, where it is found in vesicular structures [23]. Since LtxA binds to LFA-1, there is a possibility that LtxA could be using an integrin endocytic trafficking pathway to gain access to the target cell cytosol. The mechanism of LtxA uptake and the pathway of intracellular toxin trafficking has not been investigated. Here, we examined the components of the cytosol of LtxA-treated cells for co-localization of the toxin and the CD11a subunit of LFA-1 with different organelle markers. LtxA association with endosomal and lysosomal markers suggests a receptor-mediated endocytic process that may culminate in the delivery of the toxin to lysosomes. Additionally, the toxin can be redirected to the plasma membrane due to the LFA-1 receptor Rab11A-mediated recycling. This study provides new insight into convergent mechanisms of LFA-1 and LtxA trafficking, and the ability of LtxA to function in acidic environments.

2. Results

2.1. LtxA Does Not Damage Host Cell Membrane When Entering the Cell

The membrane damaging properties of LtxA have been documented [31,32]. Therefore, the first question we asked was whether the initial steps of LtxA interaction with the cells result in the plasma membrane damage. The green-fluorescent impermeable nucleic acid stain YO-PRO®-1 is used to detect early membrane damage as it permeates cells immediately after membrane destabilization [33]. Propidium iodide (PI) is used to identify late cell death in which the integrity of the plasma and nuclear membranes significantly decreases, allowing PI to penetrate the membranes and intercalate into nucleic acids [34]. To study the effect on membrane permeability, we first incubated Jn.9 cells with 20 nM LtxA at different times over a 10 h time period, and then flow cytometry analysis of LtxA-treated cells was performed to determine YO-PRO®-1 and PI internalization. The YO-PRO®-1 membrane permeabilization assay showed no evidence of plasma membrane damage in LtxA-treated Jn.9 cells at least within first 3 h of treatment (Figure 1A,B). However, our flow cytometry data demonstrated that 20 nM LtxA-DY488 became internalized with Jn.9 cells 30 min after the toxin was added and internalization steadily increased over time (Figure 1A,B). Lymphocytes are known to be moderately susceptible to LtxA and are killed by apoptosis [35]. The staining of Jn.9 cells with PI was observed after 10 h of treatment with LtxA, suggesting that cells are in the late apoptotic stage (Figure 1B). Hence, our data indicate that LtxA is quickly internalized by Jn.9 cells but the toxin does not rupture the plasma membrane when it enters the host cells.

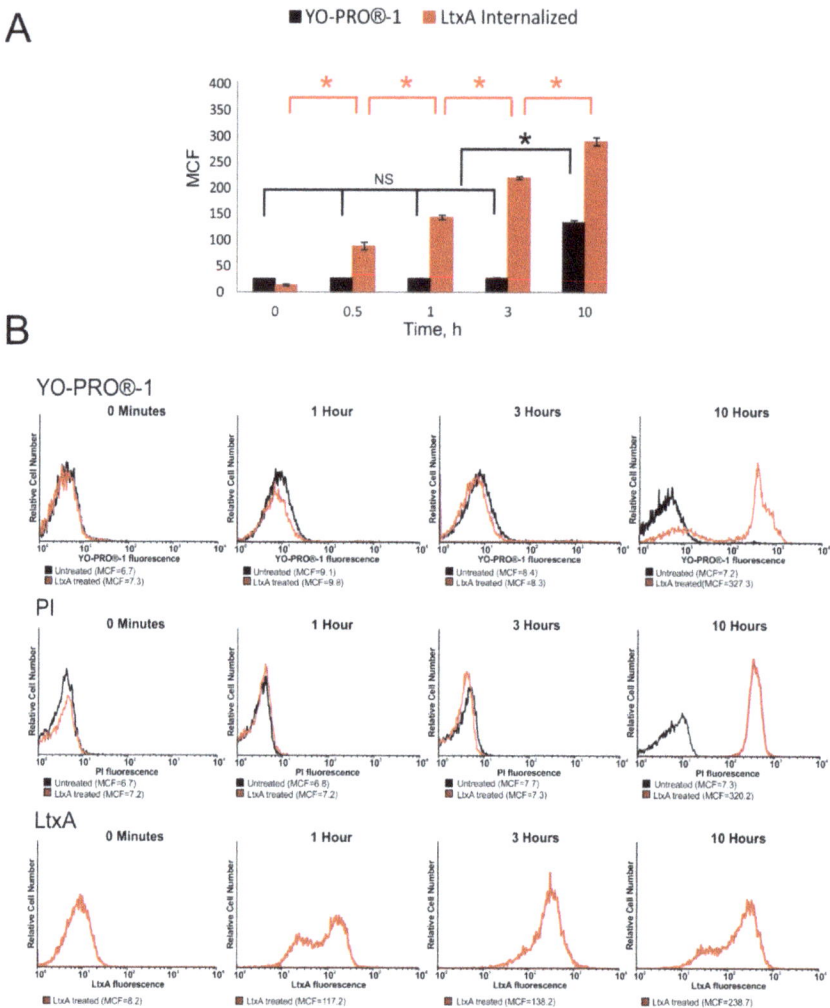

Figure 1. Damage to the plasma membrane in Jn.9 cells by LtxA. Flow cytometry analysis was used to detect YO-PRO®-1, PI and LtxA internalization with Jn.9 cells over time. Cells (1×10^6) were incubated with 0.1 µM YO-PRO®-1/ 1.5 µM PI alone or after treatment with 20 nM LtxA at indicated times at 37 °C. Another set of cells was treated with 20 nM LtxA-DY488 at different times. The extracellular fluorescence of the cells was quenched with 0.025% trypan blue [23] and the intracellular fluorescence was determined. (**A**). Uptake of YO-PRO®-1 (black) and internalization of LtxA-DY488 (red) at various times, presented as mean channel fluorescence (MCF). The data shown are the results of three independent experiments. Error bars indicate ± SEM, * $p \leq 0.05$. (**B**). Top and Middle: Flow cytometry histograms showing YO-PRO®-1 and PI dyes uptake by LtxA-treated cells (red line) vs. the dyes uptake by untreated Jn.9 cells (black line) at different times. Bottom: Flow cytometry histograms showing LtxA-DY488 internalized with Jn.9 cells. The data shown are representative of three independent experiments.

2.2. LtxA Uptake is Diminished by Dynamin Inhibitors

We hypothesized that LtxA could get access to the cytosol of Jn.9 cells through endocytic uptake. The exposure of cells to cold temperatures is used for the nonspecific inhibition of endocytosis [36]. Therefore, we treated Jn.9 cells with fluorescent-labeled LtxA in ice-cold medium and analyzed the toxin entry to cells by flow cytometry and confocal microscopy. We demonstrated that cold temperatures affected the binding of and slowed down internalization of the toxin with Jn.9 cells (Figure 2A, Figure S1). We then set up an experiment employing a set of chemical and pharmacological inhibitors of endocytosis (Table 1) to define the mechanism of the toxin uptake by the cells. The effect of dynamin- and clathrin-mediated endocytosis inhibitors on transferrin uptake is well established [37,38]. To confirm the efficiency and select the inhibitors' concentrations for our study, the internalization of transferrin conjugated to Alexa Fluor®555 and LtxA-DY650 by Jn.9 cells was followed using confocal microscopy Figure S2. At 10 µM Dynasore, 10 µM Dynole 34-2 and 5 µM Pitstop 2, the inhibitory effect on transferrin uptake was observed. First, we wanted to identify whether GTPase dynamin activity is essential for LtxA uptake. The LtxA-DY650 internalization in the presence of dynamin inhibitor 10 µM Dynasore was evaluated by live confocal imaging (Figure S3) and flow cytometry analysis (Figure 2C). To confirm our results, we performed flow cytometry analysis in cells treated with another dynamin inhibitor, 10 µM Dynole 34-2, which blocks the GTPase activity of dynamin [37,39]. Fluorescent-labeled toxin internalization was significantly reduced in cells pre-treated with dynamin-inhibitors. Cells pretreated with 10 µM Dynasore and Dynole 34-2 for 20 min internalized much less LtxA (Figure 2C). However, the inactive control for Dynole 34-2, Dynole 31-2, did not inhibit the toxin internalization. The inhibitors affecting the clathrin-mediated endocytic pathway, such as potassium-depleted medium [40] and 5 µM Pitstop 2 [41], did not change the efficiency of LtxA internalization with Jn.9 cells (Figure 2B,C). Collectively, these data suggest that LtxA internalization with Jn.9 cells is dynamin-dependent and predominantly clathrin-independent. Next, we evaluated the toxicity of LtxA on Jn.9 cells containing the above inhibitors. However, we identified some toxic effect of endocytosis inhibitors on Jn.9 cells. After 18 h of treatment with the 2 nM toxin, we observed some decrease in LtxA toxicity on Jn.9 cells pretreated with 10 µM Dynasore and 10 µM Dynole 34-2 (Figure S4), suggesting that these compounds could attenuate LtxA intoxication.

Table 1. Chemical inhibition of LtxA uptake.

Compound	Mode of Action	Effect on Internalization
10 µM Dynasore *	Blocks GTPase activity of dynamin [37]	Inhibits
10 µM Dynole 34-2 *	Blocks GTPase activity of dynamin [39]	Inhibits
10 µM Dynole 31-2 *	Inactive derivative of Dynole 34-2	No effect
5 µM Pitstop 2 *	Interferes with binding of proteins to the N-terminal domain of clathrin [41]	No effect
K^+-depletion	Inhibits clathrin mediated endocytosis [40]	No effect

* To measure LtxA internalization inhibition, Jn.9 cells were preincubated with 5–10 µM inhibitors for 20 min in serum free medium. The 0.5–1 mM chemical stocks were prepared in dimethyl sulfoxide (DMSO) and were added in the 1 µl volume to 1 ml of cells. No adverse effect of DMSO alone on Jn.9 cells was observed.

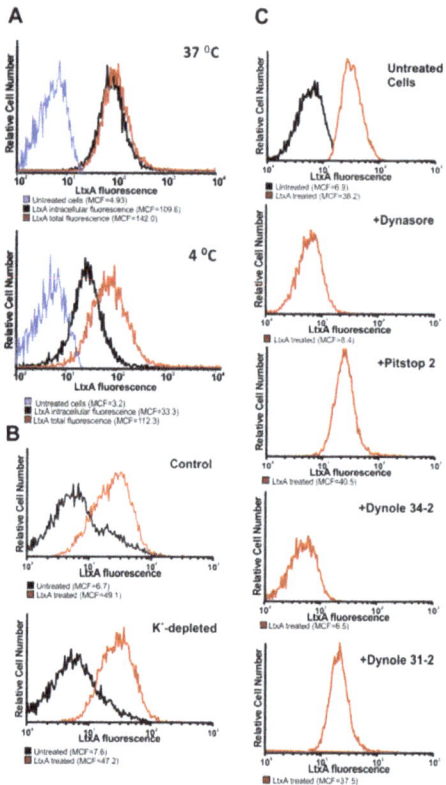

Figure 2. Effect of endocytosis inhibitors on LtxA internalization. (**A**). Flow cytometry analysis of LtxA internalization with Jn.9 cells at different temperatures. The cells were treated with LtxA-DY488 for 30 min on ice or 37 °C. In a set of cells, the total cell-associated fluorescence was measured by flow cytometry analysis (shown in red). In another set of cells, the extracellular fluorescence was quenched (0.025% trypan blue) [42] and intracellular fluorescence (red peak) was determined by flow cytometry analysis. (**B**). Flow cytometry analysis of LtxA internalization with Jn.9 cells in K$^+$-free buffer. Jn.9 cells (1 × 10^6) were incubated in K$^+$-containing (top) or K$^+$-free buffer (bottom), and then 20 nM LtxA-DY488 was added for 30 min. Flow cytometry analysis to determine the amount of internalized toxin (red peak) was performed as described in Figure 2A. (**C**). Flow cytometry analysis of LtxA-DY488 internalization with Jn.9 cells pretreated with chemical inhibitors. Jn.9 cells (1 × 10^6) were preincubated with 5–10 μM endocytosis inhibitors for 20 min in serum free medium, and then were treated with 20 nM LtxA-DY488 for 30 min at 37 °C. The extracellular fluorescence was quenched 0.025% trypan blue, and intracellular fluorescence (red peak) was determined by flow cytometry analysis.

2.3. LtxA and CD11a Are Found in Early and Recycling Endosomes

In our imaging studies, LtxA was found in vesicular structures after entry into Jn.9 cells [23]. The co-distribution of LtxA and LFA-1 heterodimer components on the surface of target cell membranes indicates that LtxA could intrude into the cytosol as individual LtxA molecules or as part of an LtxA/LFA-1 complex. In order to characterize LtxA-containing endocytic vesicles, Jn.9 cells were treated with fluorescent-labeled LtxA for 30 min and were used to perform immunocytochemistry experiments with endocytic pathway markers, including GTPase Rab5 and Rab11A. Our imaging studies demonstrated the abundant colocalization of LtxA, early endosome membrane protein Rab5 and CD11a, suggesting toxin uptake through receptor-mediated endocytosis. Figure 3 and Figure S5 show confocal images of Jn.9 cells with a co-localization of LtxA, CD11a, and Rab5 after treatment of the cells with LtxA-DY650 for 30 min at 37 °C.

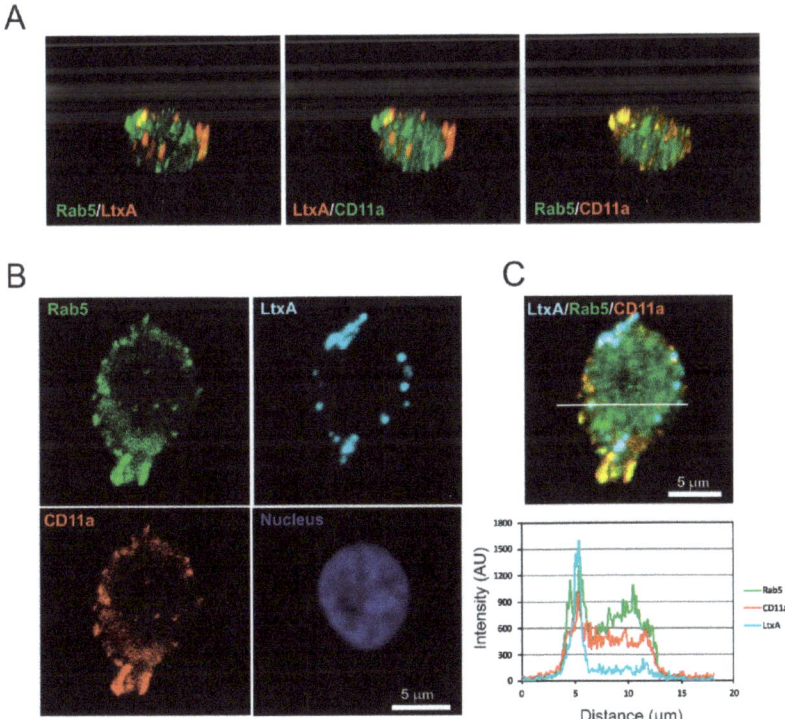

Figure 3. LtxA localization in early endosomes of Jn.9 cells. The cells were treated with 20 nM LtxA for 30 min at 37 °C. (**A**). 3D confocal images showing the distribution of LtxA, CD11a and Rab5. LtxA is pseudo colored in red and CD11a is in red or green (pseudo colored), as indicated on images. The 3D images were reconstructed from seventeen confocal planes using Nikon Elements AR 4.30.01 software. Bounding box dimensions are: width 14.19 µm; height 17.30 µm; depth 5.20 µm. (**B**). Localization of LtxA-DY650 is shown in cyan, CD11a recognized with mouse Alexa Fluor™ 594 clone HI111 is shown in red, and Rab5, recognized by rabbit anti-Rab5 antibody followed by staining with anti-rabbit IgG Alexa Fluor®488, is shown in green. The nucleus was stained with Hoechst dye and is shown in blue. (**C**). Top: Merged image "B" showing colocalization of LtxA DY650 (cyan), CD11a (red) and Rab5 (green). Bottom: Intensity profiles for LtxADY650 (cyan), CD11a (red) and Rab5 (green) across the line depicted in the image above. The degree of overlap in the LtxA-containing area was estimated with the Pearson's correlation coefficient in the LtxA-containing area of 0.78 for LtxA and Rab5, 0.68 for LtxA and CD11a, and of 0.88 for CD11a and Rab5. Representative cells are shown. Additional data are shown in Figure S5.

LFA-1 is exocytosed via GTPase Rab11A-mediated recycling [43] a process that involves trafficking through the perinuclear recycling compartment (PNRC), before reaching the plasma membrane. We found co-localization of CD11a and LtxA with Rab11A, a marker of recycling endosomes in approximately 1/3 of LtxA-containing spots (Figure 4 and Figure S6). The interaction of CD11a and LtxA with Rab11A in recycling suggests that after entering the early endosome a significant amount of LtxA is redirected back to the membrane in the LFA-1 recycling turnover. Alternatively, the release of

LtxA into PNRC can provide access to the nuclear membrane for LtxA. Indeed, in our imaging studies we often observed the toxin surrounding nuclei (Figure S7).

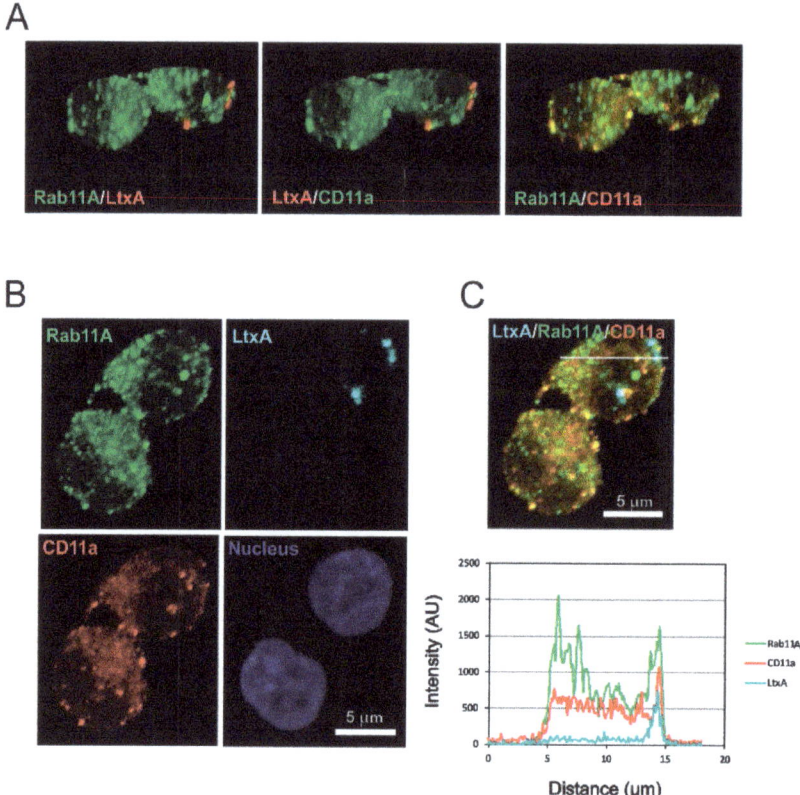

Figure 4. LtxA localization in Rab11A-positive endosomes of Jn.9 cells. The cells were treated with 20 nM LtxA for 30 min at 37 °C. (**A**). 3D confocal images showing the distribution of LtxA, CD11a and Rab11A. LtxA is pseudo colored in red and CD11a is in red or green (pseudo colored), as indicated on images. The 3D images were reconstructed from seventeen confocal planes using Nikon Elements AR 4.30.01 software. Bounding box dimensions are: width 22.58 μm; height 16.47 μm; depth 5.20 μm. (**B**). Localization of LtxA-DY650 is shown in cyan, CD11a recognized with mouse Alexa Fluor™ 594 clone HI111 is shown in red, and Rab11A, recognized by rabbit anti-Rab11A antibody followed by staining with anti-rabbit IgG Alexa Fluor®488, is shown in green. The nucleus was stained with Hoechst dye and is shown in blue. (**C**). Top: Merged image "B" showing co-localization of LtxA DY650 (cyan), CD11a (red) and Rab11A (green). Bottom: Intensity profiles for LtxADY650 (cyan), CD11a (red) and Rab11A (green) across the line depicted in the image above. The degree of overlap in the LtxA-containing area was estimated with the Pearson's correlation coefficient of 0.75 for LtxA and Rab11A, 0.72 for LtxA and CD11a, and of 0.76 for CD11a and Rab11A. Representative cells are shown. Additional data are shown in Figure S6.

2.4. LtxA and CD11a Are Found in Late Endosomes and Lysosomes

At later timepoints, Jn.9 cells treated with fluorescent-labeled LtxA were used in immunocytochemistry experiments with the endocytic pathway markers GTPases Rab7 and Lamp1. After 1 h of treatment with LtxA-DY650, LtxA was associated with the late endosome membrane protein Rab7 (Figure 5 and Supplemental Figure S8). Colocalization was detected in approximately 1/10 of LtxA-containing spots. Colocalization of LtxA with lysosomal marker Lamp1 after 2 h of treatment with LtxA-DY650 indicated that the toxin trafficking culminates in its delivery to the lysosomes, where LtxA was found separated from CD11a (Figure 6 and Figure S9).

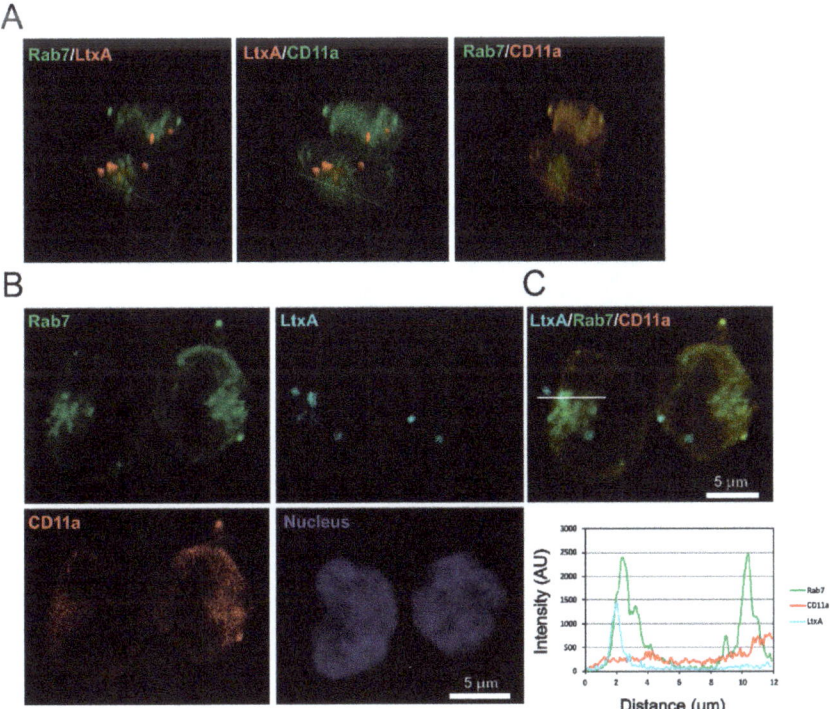

Figure 5. LtxA localization in Rab7-positive endosomes of Jn.9 cells. The cells were treated with 20 nM LtxA for 1 h at 37 °C. (**A**). 3D confocal images showing the distribution of LtxA, CD11a and Rab7. LtxA is pseudo colored in red and CD11a is in red or green (pseudo colored), as indicated on images. The 3D images were reconstructed from seventeen confocal planes using Nikon Elements AR 4.30.01 software. Bounding box dimensions are: width 22.17 μm; height 19.37 μm; depth 5.20 μm. (**B**). Localization of LtxA-DY650 is shown in cyan, CD11a recognized with mouse Alexa Fluor™ 594 clone HI111 is shown in red, and Rab7, recognized by rabbit anti-Rab7 antibody followed by staining with anti-rabbit IgG Alexa Fluor®488, is shown in green. The nucleus was stained with Hoechst dye and is shown in blue. (**C**). Top: Merged image "B" showing colocalization of LtxA DY650 (cyan), CD11a (red) and Rab7 (green). Bottom: Intensity profiles for LtxADY650 (cyan), CD11a (red) and Rab7 (green) across the line depicted in the image above. The degree of overlap in the LtxA-containing area was estimated with the Pearson's correlation coefficient of 0.88 for LtxA and Rab7, 0.03 for LtxA and CD11a, and of 0.13 for CD11a and Rab7. Representative cells are shown. Additional data are shown in Supplementary data Figure S8.

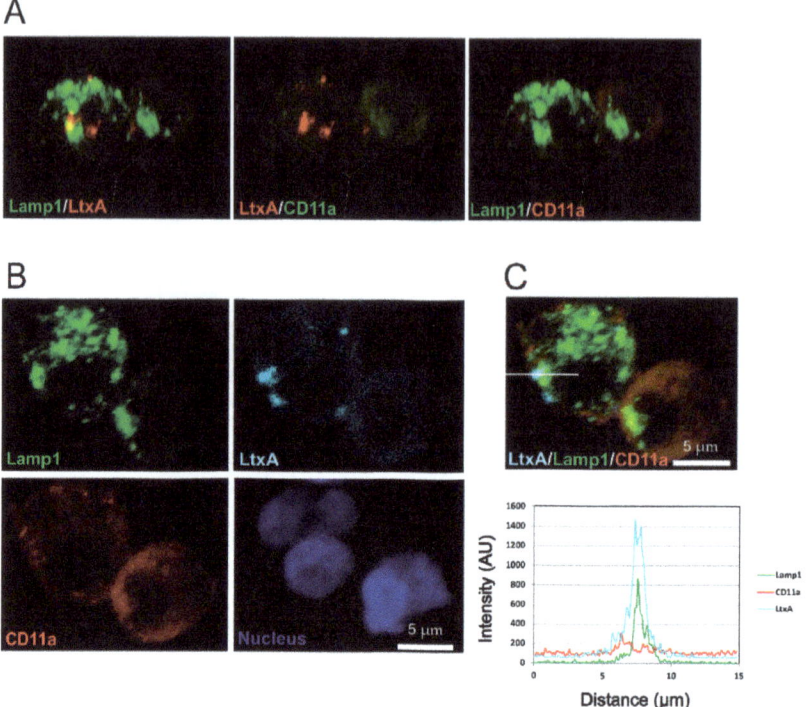

Figure 6. LtxA localization in lysosomes of Jn.9 cells. The cells were treated with 20 nM LtxA for 2 h at 37 °C. (**A**). 3D confocal images showing the distribution of LtxA, CD11a and Lamp1. LtxA is pseudo colored in red and CD11a is in red or green (pseudo colored), as indicated on images. The 3D images were reconstructed from seventeen confocal planes using Nikon Elements AR 4.30.01 software. Bounding box dimensions are: width 25.17 µm; height 19.37 µm; depth 5.20 µm. (**B**). Localization of LtxA-DY650 is shown in cyan, CD11a recognized with mouse Alexa Fluor™ 594 clone HI111 is shown in red, and Lamp1, recognized by rabbit anti-Lamp1 antibody followed by staining with anti-rabbit IgG Alexa Fluor®488, is shown in green. The nucleus was stained with Hoechst dye and is shown in blue. (**C**). Top: Merged image "B" showing colocalization of LtxA DY650 (cyan), CD11a (red) and Lamp1 (green). Bottom: Intensity profiles for LtxADY650 (cyan), CD11a (red) and Lamp1 (green) across the line depicted in the image above. The degree of overlap in the LtxA-containing area was estimated with the Pearson's correlation coefficient of 0.72 for LtxA and Lamp1, 0.15 for LtxA and CD11a, and of 0.11 for CD11a and Lamp1. Representative cells are shown. Additional data are shown in Supplementary data Figure S9.

2.5. Rab5 siRNA Knockdown limits LtxA Toxicity

Irrespective of routes of internalization, endocytic cargoes are trafficked to early endosomes, where Rab5 GTPases is the key player in subsequent trafficking events [44]. We investigated the impact of Rab5a downregulation on LtxA uptake and toxicity on cells (Figure 7). Western blot analysis 24 h after transfection with Rab5a siRNA confirmed that Rab5a was significantly downregulated ($\geq 90\%$) in Jn.9 cells compare to scrambled siRNA transfected cells. When transfected cells were treated with 20 nM LtxA for 18 h, the toxic effect of the toxin on Rab5a downregulated cells was 30% less than on control cells (Figure 7A). Internalization of LtxA was analyzed by flow cytometry after 30 min of treatment with 20 nM LtxA-DY488. No significant variations in the amount of internal fluorescence were detected in cells transfected with Rab5a siRNA (mean channel fluorescence (MCF) 28.2 ± 0.6) and cells using scrambled siRNA (MCF 29.8 ± 0.6) (Figure 7B). Our results suggest that the abolishment of Rab5a function does not affect LtxA internalization, but affects cytotoxicity.

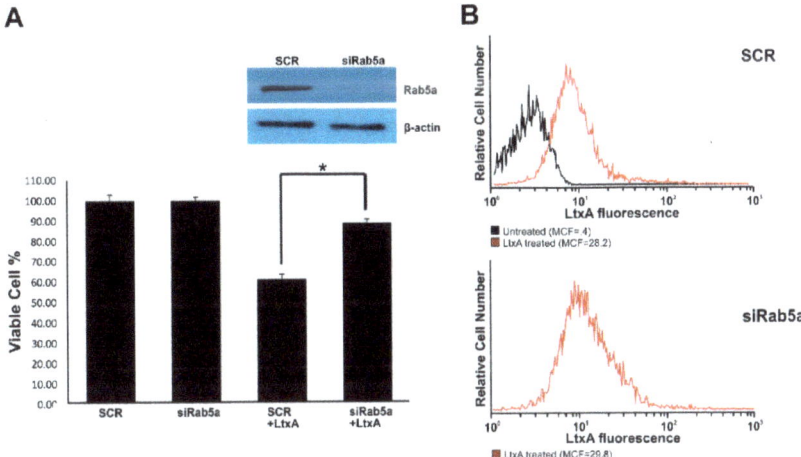

Figure 7. Modulation of Rab5a function in Jn.9 cells. A. Jn.9 cells (1×10^6 cells) were transfected with siRNA control (SCR) or with siRNA against Rab5a and collected 24 h post-transfection for Rab5a expression analysis by Western blotting. The cell viability testing was performed by trypan blue assay after 18 h of treatment with 20 nM LtxA. (**A**). representative expression of Rab5a protein was shown for 24 h of siRNA treatment. The Rab5a protein expression (inset) was analyzed in extracts obtained from 1×10^6 Jn.9 cells by Western blot, β-actin served as a loading control. Error bars indicate ±SEM, * $p \leq 0.05$ compared with siRNA SCR-treated cells. The experiment was performed three independent times. (**B**). Jn.9 cells (1×10^6 cells) were transfected with siRNA control (SCR) or with siRNA against Rab5a, then were collected 24 h post-transfection and treated with 20 nM LtxA-DY488 for 30 min at 37 °C. The extracellular fluorescence of the cells was quenched (0.025% trypan blue) [42,45] and intracellular cell fluorescence (red peak) was determined by flow cytometry analysis. No residual fluorescence was detected in 0.1% Triton X-100 permeabilized cells after the trypan blue treatment. Untreated cells (black) served as a negative control. Representative flow cytometry histograms are shown.

2.6. LtxA Causes Lysosomal Damage in Jn.9 Cells

We detected LtxA in Jn.9 lysosomes, and therefore we wanted to see whether LtxA was able to cause lysosomal damage in the cells. We have probed the effect of LtxA on lysosomal integrity in the cells using lysosomal dye, LysoTracker®Green DND-26. We followed changes in lysosomal properties of the cells after the addition of 20 nM LtxA to the cells by live cell confocal imaging. No changes in LysoTracker staining intensity were detected within the first 90 min of treatment and about 15% decrease in the intensity was identified in Jn.9 cells after 2 h of treatment (Figure 8A), which may indicate lysosomal damage due to lysosomal membrane permeabilization or lysosome alkalization. In order to assess if LtxA causes the rupture of lysosomes, we identified the intensity of Lamp1 staining in the presence and absence of toxin. Similar Lamp1 staining intensity in both conditions would indicate that this is likely because of a rise in pH in intact lysosomes. A decrease in Lamp1 intensity would suggest that change in lysosomal pH is due to lysosomal rupture (Figure 8B).

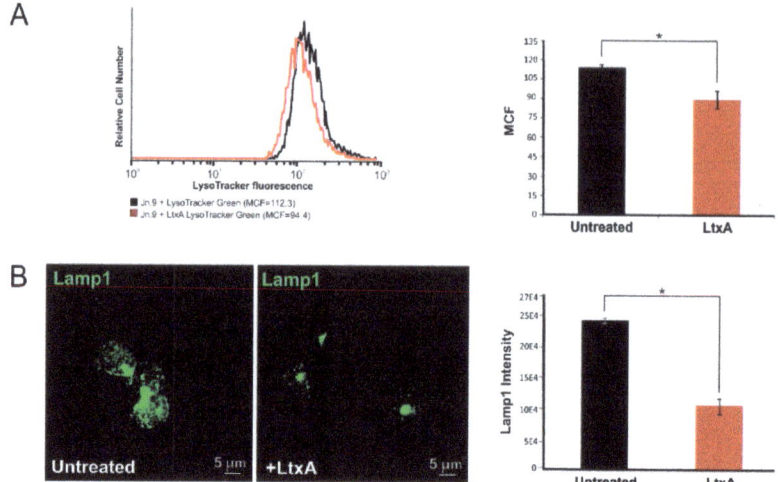

Figure 8. Lysosomal damage by LtxA. Jn.9 cells (1×10^6) were incubated in presence or absence of 20 nM LtxA for 2 h at 37 °C. (**A**). LtxA-treated and untreated cells were stained with 100 nM LysoTracker® Green DND-26 for 15 min at 37 °C. The LysoTracker® Green DND-26 intensity was evaluated by flow cytometry analysis. Representative flow cytometry histograms are shown on the left. The fluorescence of LtxA treated cells is shown in red, and untreated cells in black. The mean channel fluorescence (MCF) of LysoTracker® Green DND-26 in LtxA-treated vs. untreated cells is presented on the right. (**B**). Average fluorescence intensity of Lamp1 staining in Jn.9 cells was evaluated by confocal microscopy. The intensities of Lamp1 staining in 39 LtxA-treated cells and 44 untreated were analyzed and shown on the right. Error bars indicate ± SEM of three independent experiments. * $p \leq 0.05$.

2.7. LtxA is Active in Lipid Bilayer Membranes at a Low pH

Pore formation by LtxA was studied in detail at a neutral pH [32,46]. In lipid bilayer membranes formed by asolectin, LtxA forms cation-selective channels with a single-channel conductance of approximately 1.2 nS in 1 M KCl (pH 6.0) [46]. Since LtxA is found in endocytic vesicles, we asked whether LtxA is also able to form ion-permeable channels and damage membranes at an acidic pH. To address this, we performed lipid bilayer experiments with wildtype LtxA at different pH-values ranging from pH 3.5 to pH 10.0. LtxA formed ion-permeable channels in 1 M KCl solutions under all these conditions (pH 3.5, 4.7, 7.5, 8.5 and 10.0). However, because the membranes became very fragile at very low and very high pH values (3.7 and 10.0) it was not possible to record too many single-channel events under these conditions. At the other pH values, the membranes were rather stable, and a sufficient number of single-channel events could be recorded in the experiments. Figure 9 shows a single channel recording of LtxA in 1 M KCl, 10 mM MES-KOH, pH 4.7. The channel had a somewhat reduced lifetime at this pH as compared with a neutral pH [46]. Figure 9B,C shows a histogram obtained from 47 LtxA channels recorded under these conditions. A fit of the histogram with a Gaussian function yielded an average single-channel conductance of 1.1 ± 0.3 nS, somewhat smaller than that at pH 6.0 (G = 1.2 ± 0.3 nS) [46]. Again, we found that the single-channel distribution was quite broad, similar to the conditions at pH 6.0 (Figure 9B,C, Table 2).

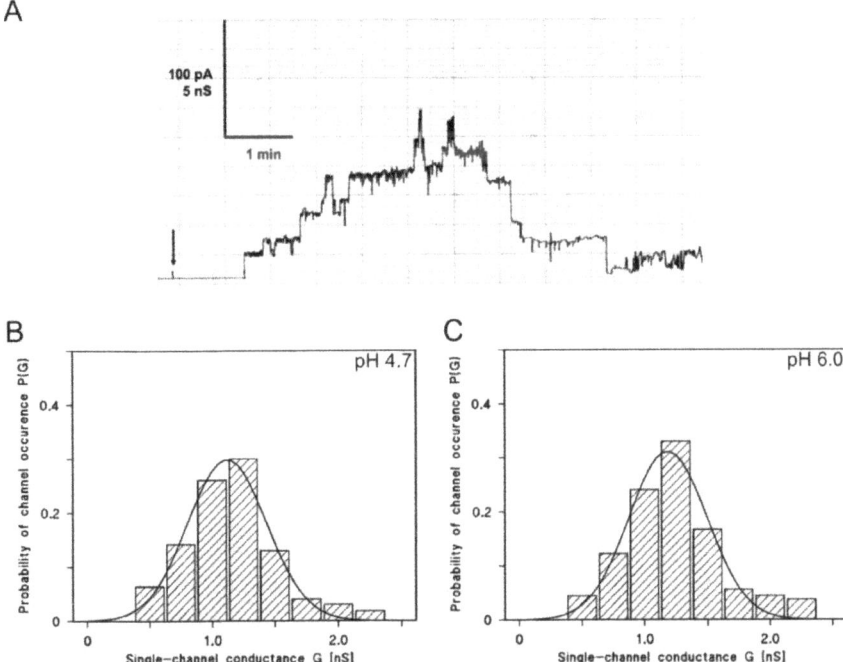

Figure 9. Pore-forming activity of LtxA in asolectin/*n*-decane membranes at different pH values. (**A**). Single-channel recording of LtxA in an asolectin/n-decane membrane at pH 4.7. Current recording of an asolectin/n-decane membrane, performed in the presence of 10 nM LtxA added to the cis-side of the membrane. The aqueous phase contained 1 M KCl, 10 mM MES-KOH, pH 4.7. The applied membrane potential was 20 mV at the cis-side (indicated by an arrow), at 20 °C. (**B**). Histogram of the probability P (G) of an occurrence of a given conductivity unit observed for LtxA with membranes formed of 1% asolectin dissolved in *n*-decane in a salt solution at pH 4.7. The histogram was calculated by dividing the number of fluctuations with a given conductance unit by the total number of conductance fluctuations. The average conductance was 1.1 ± 0.31 nS for 47 conductance steps derived from nine individual membranes. The value was calculated from a Gaussian distribution of all conductance fluctuations (solid line). The aqueous phase contained 1 M KCl, 10 mM MES-KOH, pH 4.7 and 10 nM LtxA; the applied membrane potential was 20 mV at 20 °C. (**C**). Histogram of the probability P(G) for the occurrence of a given conductivity unit observed for LtxA with membranes formed of 1% asolectin dissolved in n-decane in a salt solution at pH 6.0. The average conductance was 1.20 ± 0.31 nS for 95 conductance steps derived from 17 individual membranes. The aqueous phase contained 1 M KCl, 10 mM MES, pH 6.0 and about 10 nM LtxA; the applied membrane potential was 20 mV at 20 °C.

We also studied the effect of high pH values on channel formation, mediated by LtxA. Ion-permeable channels were also observed at these conditions. The average single channel conductances at pH 7.5, 8.5 and 10 are shown in Table 2. The influence of the aqueous pH was rather small on the conductance of the LtxA channel, despite a possible shift of the selectivity of the LtxA channel from being slightly cation selective at pH 6.0 to a higher selectivity for potassium ions over chloride.

No residual fluorescence was detected in 0.1% Triton X-100 permeabilized cells after the trypan blue treatment. Untreated cells (blue or black) served as a negative control. Representative flow cytometry histograms are shown.

Table 2. Influence of the aqueous pH on the conductance of channels formed by LtxA.

Salt and Buffer	pH	G * ± SD (nS)	Number of Events (n)
1 M KCl, 10 mM MES-KOH	3.7	1.0 ± 0.21	12
1 M KCl, 10 mM MES-KOH	4.7	1.1 ± 0.31	47
1 M KCl, 10 mM MES-KOH	6.0	1.2 ± 0.30	95
1 M KCl, 10 mM Tris-HCl	7.5	1.2 ± 0.24	39
1 M KCl, 10 mM Tris-HCl	8.5	1.3 ± 0.29	53
1 M KCl, 10 mM Tris-HCl	10	1.2 ± 0.26	14

* The LtxA conductance (G ± variance/SD) in each 1 M KCl solution was either taken from Gaussian distributions (see Figure 9) or directly from the statistics of single-channel data (n number of single events). To analyze the conductance in each case, n channels were reconstituted in asolectin/n-decane membranes at 20 mV voltage at 20 °C. The number of events analyzed at pH 3.7 and 10 was low due to the instability of the lipid bilayers at extreme pH values.

3. Discussion

Leukocytes need to rapidly move from blood vessels to tissues upon inflammation or infection. A crucial mechanism regulating this process is the subcellular trafficking of adhesion molecules, primarily integrins [47]. Integrins undergo constant endo/exocytic turnover, necessary for the dynamic regulation of cell adhesion. Bacterial toxins have developed a number of schemes to cross the membrane in order to enter the cell. LtxA evolved the strategy to target specifically β_2 integrin LFA-1 on leukocytes' surface [22]. This binding is required for toxin internalization [23].

We here report that LtxA is delivered to the cytosol of Jn.9 cells through endocytic trafficking. Historically, endocytic pathways are classified as either clathrin-dependent or clathrin-independent. The large GTPase dynamin [48] is hypothesized to be directly involved in closing off endocytic vesicles from the plasma membrane. The key players in the formation of clathrin-coated vesicles are dynamin [48] and adaptor proteins [49]. The studies with *Mannheimia haemolytica* LktA, another RTX leukotoxin, show that LktA is internalized in a *dynamin-2* and *clathrin-dependent* manner [50]. The following LktA-trafficking events involve the toxin binding to the mitochondria and interaction with cyclophilin D, a mitochondrial chaperone protein, in bovine lymphoblastoid cells [51].

Our data indicate that LtxA enters Jn.9 cells using a clathrin-independent mechanism (or predominantly uses this pathway). Our results correlate with the finding that LFA-1 is internalized through a clathrin-independent, cholesterol-dependent pathway and this process is essential for cell migration [52]. In this scenario, non-clathrin-coated lipid raft microdomains form 50–100 nm flask-shaped vesicles in the plasma membrane regions rich in lipid rafts [53]. Lipid-raft dependent endocytosis was shown to be dynamin-dependent [54] and may involve caveolae formation. Thus, we hypothesize that LtxA/LFA-1 is endocytosed through caveolae-mediated endocytosis.

Bacterial toxins often piggyback existing endocytic trafficking pathways [55,56] to deliver active proteins to subcellular targets. The small GTPases Rab are essential regulators of intracellular membrane trafficking and exist in an inactive GDP-bound form and an active GTP-bound form [57]. The co-localization experiments with Rab5, Rab7, Lamp1 revealed that LtxA can follow the degradation pathway process that culminates in the delivery of the toxin to lysosomes. Rab5 localizes to early endosomes where it is involved in the recruitment of Rab7 and the maturation of these compartments to late endosomes [58]. Impaired Rab5a function affects endo- and exocytosis rates and, conversely, Rab5 overexpression increases the release efficacy [59]. Therefore, the termination of Rab5 function blocks the movement of proteins downstream of the endocytic pathway. Downregulation of Rab5a decreased LtxA toxicity, suggesting that further toxin trafficking is required for intoxication by LtxA. LFA-1 was suggested to undergo endocytic recycling through the long-Rab11A-dependent pathway with a transitional step at PNRC [29]. Here we, for the first time, demonstrated CD11a localization in Rab11A-containing endocytic vesicles. Extensive colocalization of CD11a and Rab11A was found in Jn.9 cells which were not treated with LtxA (Figure S10). While some LtxA follows LFA-1 in its recycling turnover, a portion of LtxA is separated from LFA-1 and the toxin proceeds to late endosomes and lysosomes. A proposed model of LtxA trafficking in lymphocytes is shown in Figure 10.

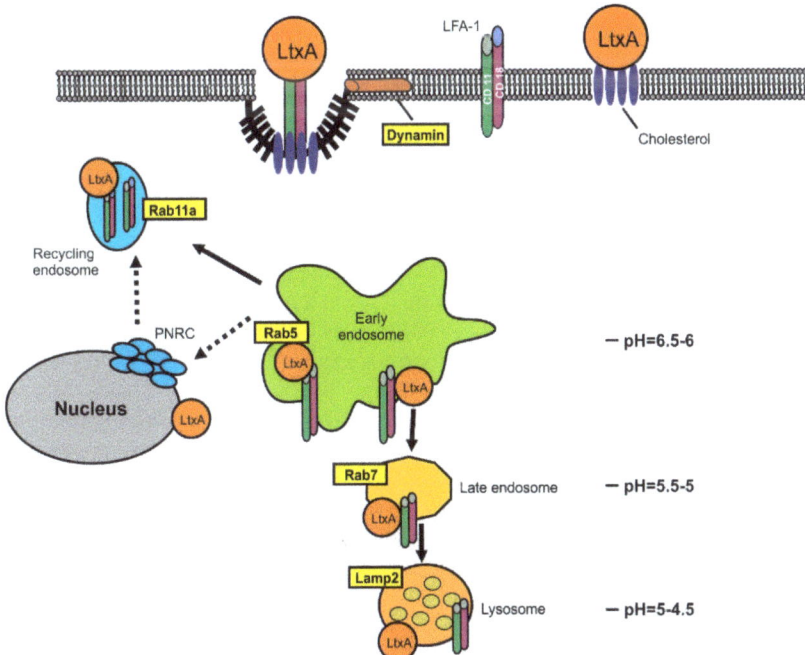

Figure 10. Proposed mechanism of LtxA entry and trafficking in human lymphocytes. LtxA binds to cholesterol and LFA-1 on the surface of Jn.9 cell. LtxA/LFA-1 complex internalization is dynamin-dependent. Internalized LtxA/LFA-1 complexes are quickly transported to early endosomes. The small GTPase Rab5 regulates membrane binding and fusion in the early endocytic pathway. The interruption of Rab5 expression in Jn.9 cells results in the abolishment of the LtxA activity. LFA-1 undergoes endocytic recycling through the long-Rab11A-dependent pathway with a transitional step at PNRC [29]. While some LtxA follows LFA-1 in its recycling turnover, a portion of LtxA is separated from LFA-1 and the toxin proceeds to late endosomes and lysosomes. The ability of LtxA to damage lipid membranes at a low pH may cause endocytic vesicles and lysosomal rupture and release of the toxin to the cytosol.

Interaction between integrins and their β-integrin ligands typically leads to enhanced cell survival and several immunological changes [60,61]. Our experiment using cell impermeable dye, YO-PRO®-1, serves to demonstrate that LtxA gains access to the Jn.9 cell cytosol without evidence of plasma membrane damage. Our study and others suggest that LtxA could accumulate in the lysosomes and alter lysosomal pH [62,63]. Damage to lysosomes by LtxA in human and rat monocytes cells [62,64] and in human erythroleukemia cells [62] was reported. In our previous study, treatment with 100 ng/mL LtxA led to cytosol acidification in K562 cells expressing LFA-1, presumably due to the leakage of lysosomal content, as was identified using a pH-sensitive indicator pHrodo®. This process correlated with the disappearance of lysosomes in the cytosol, as determined by both acridine orange and LysoTracker®Red DND-99 staining. Similarly, using LysoTracker®Red DND-99 dye, lysosomal damage was detected in malignant monocytes (THP-1 cells) as early as 15 min after treatment with LtxA, and reached 70% after 2 h of treatment (unpublished data). In these cells, LtxA was shown to localize to the lysosome where it induces active cathepsin D release [64]. Here, we demonstrate that

LtxA causes changes in lysosomal pH in T lymphocytes, however, to a leser extent. As the Lysotracker dye is sensitive to luminal pH, the decrease in the dye staining could have resulted from either a rise in lysosomal pH or a decrease in the number of lysosomes. To distinguish between these possibilities, cells were stained for lysosomal marker Lamp1. The clear decrease in Lamp1 staining, combined with the decrease in the Lysotracker signal, forms a strong argument that the toxin decreased the number of lysosomes. As the transcription factor EB (TFEB) feedback systems try to increase lysosomal biogenesis [65], the most likely explanation for this is that the toxin has ruptured the lysosomes and overridden the TFEB pathways. The pore-forming properties of LtxA are well established [32,46]. Therefore, we propose that LtxA can cause permeabilization of the lysosomal membrane, and possibly other intracellular organelles after the toxin is released from lysosomes.

LtxA was reported to cause different cellular responses leading to cell death in LFA-1-expressing cells. Kelk et al. reported that LtxA lyses healthy monocytes by the activation of inflammatory caspase 1 and causes release of IL-1b and IL-18. In contrast to myeloid cells, LtxA uses a "slow mode" of lymphocyte killing. The killing of malignant lymphocytes requires Fas receptors and caspase 8 in both T and B lymphocytes [66]. In B lymphocytes (JY cells), LtxA caused loss of the mitochondrial membrane potential, cytochrome c release, reactive oxygen species release, and activation of caspases 3,7,9 [24]. One possible explanation for the cell death mechanism induced by LtxA is the degree of lysosomal damage caused by the toxins in the cell. The extent of lysosomal rupture will determine morphological outcomes following lysosomal membrane permeabilization. Extensive lysosomal injury may lead to necrotic cell death, while less substantial damage to lysosomes may instigate several apoptotic pathways, which can be attenuated by the inhibition of lysosomal cathepsins [66–69].

The planar lipid bilayer assay is a highly sensitive method that allows the characterization of the membrane damaging activity of RTX-toxins in different physical conditions [70]. A current model proposes that RTX-toxins form cation-selective channels with a diameter of 0.6–2.6 nm in artificial membranes formed of lipid mixtures such as the asolectin/n-decane membrane [46]. It was demonstrated that the membrane-damaging activity of LtxA in artificial bilayers did not require the presence of the receptor [71]. In the endocytic pathway, subsequent acidification may initiate proteolysis and conformational changes, resulting in the ability of toxins and viruses to cross the endocytic vesicle membrane, since drugs that interfere with the endosomal pH are able to block the infection [72,73]. In this study, we used this method to observe and compare the pore formation of LtxA at different pH. We demonstrated that LtxA is functional in acidic pH found in endocytic vesicles and lysosomes, which may result in their damage. RTX toxins are intrinsically disordered proteins, therefore changes in pH may affect their secondary structure and consequently change their activity [74]. Further investigation is required to improve our understanding of the intracellular events leading to LtxA-induced cytolysis.

In conclusion, our results show that LtxA enters the cytosol of Jurkat cells without evidence of plasma membrane damage, utilizing receptor-mediated endocytic mechanisms. In our studies, colocolization between LtxA/CD11a was demonstrated on the plasma membrane [23] and in the early steps of LtxA endocytic trafficking. Our results suggest that LtxA can accompany LFA-1 in its recycling pathway; however, the toxin molecules can apparently dissociate from the receptor in an acidic environment of endocytic vesicles and independently follow the degradative pathway. LtxA delivery to the terminal point of this route results in the lysosomal membrane rupture.

4. Materials and Methods

4.1. Antibodies and Chemicals

The following primary antibodies were used; CD11a Alexa Fluor™ 594 clone HI111 (Biolegend, San Diego, CA), rabbit polyclonal anti-Rab5, anti-Rab11A, anti-Rab7, or anti-Lamp1 antibody (Abcam, Cambridge, UK), anti-beta-actin antibody (AnaSpec, Fremont, CA) (1:1000), and anti-LtxA monoclonal antibody 107A3A3 [75] in hybridoma supernatants (1:10 dilution). The following secondary antibodies were used: goat anti-rabbit IgG Alexa Fluor®488 (1:1000); horseradish peroxidase (HRP)-conjugated goat anti-mouse IgG (Fc) or (HRP)-goat anti-rabbit (Pierce, Rockford, IL) (1:10,000). Transferrin labeled with Alexa Fluor®555 was from Invitrogen (Waltham, MA, USA). Dynamin inhibitor Dynole 34-2 and its inactive control, Dynole 31-2, were purchased from SigmaAldrich (St. Louis, MO), Dynasore and Pitstop 2 (Abcam, Cambridge, UK). The inhibitors were used in the following concentrations: 10 µM Dynole 34-2; 10 µM Dynole 31-2; 10 µM Dynasore; 5 µM Pitstop 2.

4.2. Cell Culture

Jn.9, a subclone of Jurkat cells [76] was utilized in this study. The cells were cultivated in RPMI 1640 medium containing 10% FBS, 0.1 mM MEM non-essential amino acids, 1x MEM vitamin solution, and 2 mM L-glutamine, and 0.5 µg/mL gentamicin at 37 °C under 5% CO_2.

4.3. LtxA Purification and Labeling

Aa strain JP2 [77] was grown on solid AAGM medium [78] for 48 h at 37 °C in 10% CO_2 atmosphere. The colony was then inoculated in 1.5 L of liquid AAGM medium and the culture was incubated for 18 h. The toxin was purified from cell culture supernatants as described previously [79]. Purified LtxA was labeled with DyLight™ 650 (LtxA-DY650) or DyLight™ 488 (LtxA-DY488) using DyLight™ Amine-Reactive dyes (Pierce). The toxin was purified after labeling using a Zeba™ Spin Desalting column (40 K MWCO, Thermo Fisher™ Scientific), according to previously published protocol [23].

4.4. Immunofluorescence

For LtxA trafficking studies, 1×10^6 of Jn.9 cells were incubated with 20 nM LtxA-DY650 for 15 min to 2 h at 37 °C in the growth medium. The cells were then washed with PBS, fixed with 2% paraformaldehyde for 10 min, washed twice with PBS, and permeabilized with 0.2% Triton X-100 for 20 min. The cells were subsequently blocked with 4% BSA for 30 min at 37 °C, incubated with primary antibody for 18 h at 4 °C, washed, and incubated with secondary antibody conjugated to Alexa Fluor 488 for 1 h at 37 °C. The nuclei were stained with 1 µg/ml Hoechst 33342 (Molecular Probes™, Eugene, OR) for 15 min at 37 °C. Samples were mounted in Cytoseal mounting medium (Electron Microscopy Sciences, Hatfield, PA) and images captured with a Nikon A1R laser scanning confocal microscope (Nikon Instruments Inc., Melville, NY) with a PLAN APO VC 60 × water (NA 1.2) objective at 18 °C. Data were analyzed using Nikon Elements AR 4.30.01 software. For co-distribution analyses, the Pearson's' coefficient of 0.55 was used as a cut off and was identified using circular ROIs. A Z-stack series consisting of seventeen individual planes 0.33 µm apart were assembled in 3D animations using Nikon Elements AR 4.30.01 software. Maximum intensity projection and standard LUT adjustment were used for the images' presentation.

For live imaging of LtxA uptake, Jn.9 cells were washed with in the serum free medium and were placed to attach for 20 min in ibiTreat 60 µ-dishes (Ibidi, Madison, WI) coated with poly-L-lysine (Sigma St. Louis, MO, USA). After floating cells were removed, the attached cells were pretreated with specific inhibitor, if necessary, and 20 nM LtxA-DY650 or 1 µM transferrin labeled with Alexa Fluor®555 was added. The cells were examined using a Nikon A1R laser scanning confocal microscope with a 60× water objective at different intervals of treatment at 37 °C.

4.5. Inhibitors

Chemicals stocks were prepared in DMSO and were added in the 1 µl volume to 1 ml of cells. To measure LtxA internalization inhibition, Jn.9 cells (1×10^6 cells) were pre-incubated with 5–10 µM inhibitors for 20 min in the serum free medium at 37 °C and then 20 nM LtxA-488 was added for 30 min. The effect of intracellular K^+-depletion was evaluated using previously published protocol [80]. Pelleted Jn.9 cells (1×10^6 cells) were incubated in 2 ml hypotonic medium (RPMI/water, 1:1) for 5 min, followed by incubation in isotonic K^+-free buffer (50 mM Hepes and 100 mM NaCl at pH 7.4) for 40 min at 37 °C, and then 20 nM LtxA-488 was added for 30 min. The toxin internalization assay was performed as described in the "*Flow cytometry*" section. Live imaging of LtxA uptake was performed as described in the "*Immunofluorescence*" section. For cytotoxicity evaluation, the cells were treated with 2 nM LtxA and cell viability was evaluated as described in the "*Cytotoxicity assay*" section. The cells treated with specific inhibitors alone served as a control

4.6. Flow Cytometry

YO-PRO®-1 and PI internalization was investigated using Membrane permeability/dead cell apoptosis kit (Invitrogen, Carlsbad, CA) according to the manufacture's protocol. Jn.9 cells (1×10^6) were treated with 20 nM LtxA at 37 °C in Jn.9 culture medium at indicated times, washed with PBS and then treated with 0.1 µM YO-PRO®-1 or 1.5 µM PI, followed by flow cytometry analysis. To detect internalized LtxA, Jn.9 cells (1×10^6 cells) were incubated with 20 nM LtxA-DY488 for the specified time on ice or at 37 °C in Jn.9 culture medium, washed with PBS, and total cell-associated fluorescence was analyzed. To quench the extracellular fluorescence, LtxA-DY488-treated cells were incubated with 0.025% trypan blue (Sigma, St. Louis, MO) for 20 min as described previously [42,45]. To quench the intracellular fluorescence cells were permeabilized using 0.1% Triton X-100 (SigmaArdrich, St. Louis, MO) for 10 min and then subjected to 0.025% trypan blue treatment. Fluorescence was measured using a BD LSR II flow cytometer (BD Biosciences). Ten thousand events were recorded per sample, and MCF values were determined using WinList™7.0 software (Verity Software House). No residual fluorescence was detected in 0.1% Triton X-100 permeabilized cells after the trypan blue treatment. Samples that were not treated with LtxA or LtxA-DY488 served as a control.

For lysosomal staining analysis, Jn.9 cells were incubated with 20 nM LtxA for 2 h at 37 °C in the growth medium. Then 100 nM LysoTracker® Green DND-26 (Life Technologies, Carlsbad, CA, USA) was added to LtxA-treated and control cells for 15 min.

4.7. Protein Analyses

The protein concentration was determined by absorption at 280 nm on A1 NanoDrop spectrophotometer (Thermo Fisher Scientific, Waltham, MA). Proteins were resolved on 4% to 20% SDS-PAGE and visualized by staining with GelCode blue stain reagent (Pierce, Rockford, IL). The Western blot analysis was performed as described previously [70].

4.8. siRNA

The validated Silencer®Select siRNA targeting human Rab5a (ID s11678) and Silencer® Select Negative Control #2 siRNA (catalog# 4390846) were synthesized by Life Technology (Carlsbad, CA, USA). Jn.9 cells were transfected with lipofectamine 2000 (Life Technologies, Carlsbad, CA, USA) according to the manufacturer's instructions. For each transfection, 5 µl of the 20 µM siRNA stocks were added to 400 µl of Jn.9 cells grown to 90% confluency. Rab5a levels in 1×10^6 Jn.9 cells were confirmed by Western blot analysis 24 h after transfection. β-actin served as a loading control.

4.9. Cytotoxicity Assay

For toxicity tests, 2–20 nM LtxA was added to 1×10^6 Jn.9 cells in growth medium and incubated for 18 h at 37 °C. The cell membrane permeability was determined with trypan blue assay using Vi-cell Cell Viability Analyzer (Beckman Coulter, Miami, FL). All reactions were run in duplicate; the assay was performed three independent times. Untreated cells were used as controls.

4.10. Planar Lipid Bilayers

Lipid bilayer measurements have been described previously in detail [81]. In short, A Teflon chamber, containing two 5 mL compartments connected by a small circular hole with a surface area of about 0.4 mm^2, were filled with 1 M KCl, 10 mM MES, pH 6.0. Black lipid bilayer membranes were created by painting onto the hole solutions of 1% (w/v) asolectin (phospholipids from soybean,

Sigma-Aldrich) in *n*-decane. The temperature was maintained at 20 °C during all experiments. The current across the membrane was measured with a pair of Ag/AgCl electrodes with salt bridges switched in series with a voltage source and current amplifier Keithley 427 (Keithley Instruments, INC. Cleveland, OH). The amplified signal was recorded by a strip chart recorder (Rikadenki Electronics GmbH, Freiburg, Germany).

4.11. Statistical Analysis

The statistical analyses were performed using either Student's test or one-way analysis of variance using SigmaPlot® (Systat Software, Inc. Chicago, IL, USA). The following statistical criteria were applied: $p < 0.001$, $p < 0.05$, and $p < 0.01$.

Supplementary Materials: The following are available online at http://www.mdpi.com/2076-0817/9/2/74/s1, Figure S1: "Confocal imaging of LtxA and CD11a in Jn.9 cells"; Figure S2: "Effect of inhibitors on transferrin uptake by Jn.9 cells"; Figure S3: "Effect of 10 µM Dynasore on LtxA uptake by Jn.9 cells."; Figure S4 "LtxA toxicity on Jn.9 cells"; Figure S5 "Localization of LtxA in early endosomes of Jn.9 cells"; Figure S6: "Localization of LtxA in Rab11A-positive endosomes of Jn.9 cells."; Figure S7: "Localization of LtxA around nuclear membrane of Jn.9 cells"; Figure S8: "Images of late endosomes in Jn.9 cells"; Figure S9: "Images of lysosomes in Jn.9 cells". Figure S10: "Confocal imaging of CD11a trafficking in Jn.9 cells".

Author Contributions: Conceptualization, E.T.L. and N.B.; data curation, N.M.G. and N.B.; formal analysis, N.M.G., A.D., R.B., J.L. and N.B.; funding acquisition, E.T.L. and N.B.; investigation, N.M.G., A.G., S.A.F. and R.B.; methodology, K.B.-B., C.H.M. and R.B.; project administration, N.B.; software, A.D.; supervision, N.B.; writing—review and editing, N.B., K.B.-B., and C.H.M. All authors have read and agreed to the published version of the manuscript.

Funding: This work was supported by the United States National Institute of Health grants R01DE009517 (ETL and NB), R01DE022465 (KBB).

Acknowledgments: The authors thank Juan Reyes-Reveles (JRRDesign Inc.) for technical assistance.

Conflicts of Interest: The authors declare no conflict of interest.

References

1. Linhartova, I.; Bumba, L.; Masin, J.; Basler, M.; Osicka, R.; Kamanova, J.; Prochazkova, K.; Adkins, I.; Hejnova-Holubova, J.; Sadilkova, L.; et al. RTX proteins: a highly diverse family secreted by a common mechanism. *FEMS Microbiol. Rev.* **2010**, *34*, 1076–1112. [CrossRef] [PubMed]
2. Goni, F.M.; Ostolaza, H.E. coli alpha-hemolysin: a membrane-active protein toxin. *Braz. J. Med. Biol. Res.* **1998**, *31*, 1019–1034. [CrossRef]
3. Ostolaza, H.; Soloaga, A.; Goni, F.M. The binding of divalent cations to Escherichia coli alpha-haemolysin. *Eur. J. Biochem.* **1995**, *228*, 39–44. [CrossRef] [PubMed]
4. Soloaga, A.; Veiga, M.P.; Garcia-Segura, L.M.; Ostolaza, H.; Brasseur, R.; Goni, F.M. Insertion of Escherichia coli alpha-haemolysin in lipid bilayers as a non-transmembrane integral protein: prediction and experiment. *Mol. Microbiol.* **1999**, *31*, 1013–1024. [CrossRef] [PubMed]
5. Boehm, D.F.; Welch, R.A.; Snyder, I.S. Domains of Escherichia coli hemolysin (HlyA) involved in binding of calcium and erythrocyte membranes. *Infect. Immun.* **1990**, *58*, 1959–1964. [CrossRef] [PubMed]
6. Coote, J.G. Structural and functional relationships among the RTX toxin determinants of gram-negative bacteria. *FEMS Microbiol. Rev.* **1992**, *8*, 137–161. [CrossRef] [PubMed]
7. Stanley, P.; Packman, L.C.; Koronakis, V.; Hughes, C. Fatty acylation of two internal lysine residues required for the toxic activity of Escherichia coli hemolysin. *Science* **1994**, *266*, 1992–1996. [CrossRef]
8. Stanley, P.; Koronakis, V.; Hughes, C. Acylation of Escherichia coli hemolysin: a unique protein lipidation mechanism underlying toxin function. *Microbiol. Mol. Biol. Rev.* **1998**, *62*, 309–333. [CrossRef]
9. Balashova, N.V.; Shah, C.; Patel, J.K.; Megalla, S.; Kachlany, S.C. Aggregatibacter actinomycetemcomitans LtxC is required for leukotoxin activity and initial interaction between toxin and host cells. *Gene* **2009**, *443*, 42–47. [CrossRef]
10. Osickova, A.; Balashova, N.; Masin, J.; Sulc, M.; Roderova, J.; Wald, T.; Brown, A.C.; Koufos, E.; Chang, E.H.; Giannakakis, A.; et al. Cytotoxic activity of Kingella kingae RtxA toxin depends on post-translational acylation of lysine residues and cholesterol binding. *Emerg. Microbes Infect.* **2018**, *7*, 178. [CrossRef]

11. Mazzone, A.; Ricevuti, G. Leukocyte CD11/CD18 integrins: biological and clinical relevance. *Haematologica* **1995**, *80*, 161–175. [PubMed]
12. Fine, D.H.; Patil, A.G.; Loos, B.G. Classification and diagnosis of aggressive periodontitis. *J. Periodontol.* **2018**, *89* (Suppl. 1), S103–S119. [CrossRef] [PubMed]
13. Loe, H.; Brown, L.J. Early onset periodontitis in the United States of America. *J. Periodontol.* **1991**, *62*, 608–616. [CrossRef] [PubMed]
14. Welch, R.A. Pore-forming cytolysins of gram-negative bacteria. *Mol. Microbiol.* **1991**, *5*, 521–528. [CrossRef]
15. Haubek, D.; Johansson, A. Pathogenicity of the highly leukotoxic JP2 clone of Aggregatibacter actinomycetemcomitans and its geographic dissemination and role in aggressive periodontitis. *J. Oral Microbiol.* **2014**, *6*. [CrossRef]
16. Brogan, J.M.; Lally, E.T.; Poulsen, K.; Kilian, M.; Demuth, D.R. Regulation of Actinobacillus actinomycetemcomitans leukotoxin expression: Analysis of the promoter regions of leukotoxic and minimally leukotoxic strains. *Infect. Immun.* **1994**, *62*, 501–508. [CrossRef]
17. Lally, E.T.; Golub, E.E.; Kieba, I.R.; Taichman, N.S.; Rosenbloom, J.; Rosenbloom, J.C.; Gibson, C.W.; Demuth, D.R. Analysis of the Actinobacillus actinomycetemcomitans leukotoxin gene. Delineation of unique features and comparison to homologous toxins. *J. Biol. Chem.* **1989**, *264*, 15451–15456.
18. Brown, A.C.; Balashova, N.V.; Epand, R.M.; Epand, R.F.; Bragin, A.; Kachlany, S.C.; Walters, M.J.; Du, Y.; Boesze-Battaglia, K.; Lally, E.T. Aggregatibacter actinomycetemcomitans leukotoxin utilizes a cholesterol recognition/amino acid consensus site for membrane association. *J. Biol. Chem.* **2013**, *288*, 23607–23621. [CrossRef]
19. Brown, A.C.; Koufos, E.; Balashova, N.; Boesze-Battaglia, K.; Lally, E.T. Inhibition of LtxA Toxicity by Blocking Cholesterol Binding With Peptides. *Mol. Oral Microbiol.* **2016**, *31*, 94–105. [CrossRef]
20. Mahanonda, R.; Champaiboon, C.; Subbalekha, K.; Sa-Ard-Iam, N.; Yongyuth, A.; Isaraphithakkul, B.; Rerkyen, P.; Charatkulangkun, O.; Pichyangkul, S. Memory T cell subsets in healthy gingiva and periodontitis tissues. *J. Periodontol.* **2018**, *89*, 1121–1130. [CrossRef]
21. Li, Y.; Messina, C.; Bendaoud, M.; Fine, D.H.; Schreiner, H.; Tsiagbe, V.K. Adaptive immune response in osteoclastic bone resorption induced by orally administered Aggregatibacter actinomycetemcomitans in a rat model of periodontal disease. *Mol. Oral Microbiol.* **2010**, *25*, 275–292. [CrossRef] [PubMed]
22. Lally, E.T.; Kieba, I.R.; Sato, A.; Green, C.L.; Rosenbloom, J.; Korostoff, J.; Wang, J.F.; Shenker, B.J.; Ortlepp, S.; Robinson, M.K.; et al. RTX toxins recognize a b2 integrin on the surface of human target cells. *J. Biol. Chem.* **1997**, *272*, 30463–30469. [CrossRef] [PubMed]
23. Nygren, P.; Balashova, N.; Brown, A.C.; Kieba, I.; Dhingra, A.; Boesze-Battaglia, K.; Lally, E.T. Aggregatibacter actinomycetemcomitans leukotoxin causes activation of lymphocyte function-associated antigen 1. *Cell. Microbiol.* **2019**, *21*, e12967. [CrossRef] [PubMed]
24. Fong, K.P.; Pacheco, C.M.; Otis, L.L.; Baranwal, S.; Kieba, I.R.; Harrison, G.; Hersh, E.V.; Boesze-Battaglia, K.; Lally, E.T. Actinobacillus actinomycetemcomitans leukotoxin requires lipid microdomains for target cell cytotoxicity. *Cell. Microbiol.* **2006**, *8*, 1753–1767. [CrossRef]
25. Kinashi, T. Intracellular signalling controlling integrin activation in lymphocytes. *Nat. Rev. Immunol.* **2005**, *5*, 546–559. [CrossRef]
26. Li, N.; Yang, H.; Wang, M.; Lu, S.; Zhang, Y.; Long, M. Ligand-specific binding forces of LFA-1 and Mac-1 in neutrophil adhesion and crawling. *Mol. Biol. Cell* **2018**, *29*, 408–418. [CrossRef]
27. Tohyama, Y.; Katagiri, K.; Pardi, R.; Lu, C.; Springer, T.A.; Kinashi, T. The critical cytoplasmic regions of the a_L/b_2 integrin in Rap1-induced adhesion and migration. *Mol. Biol. Cell* **2003**, *14*, 2570–2582. [CrossRef]
28. Fabbri, M.; Fumagalli, L.; Bossi, G.; Bianchi, E.; Bender, J.R.; Pardi, R. A tyrosine-based sorting signal in the b_2 integrin cytoplasmic domain mediates its recycling to the plasma membrane and is required for ligand-supported migration. *EMBO J.* **1999**, *18*, 4915–4925. [CrossRef]
29. Caswell, P.T.; Norman, J.C. Integrin trafficking and the control of cell migration. *Traffic* **2006**, *7*, 14–21. [CrossRef]
30. Brown, A.C.; Boesze-Battaglia, K.; Balashova, N.V.; Mas Gomez, N.; Speicher, K.; Tang, H.Y.; Duszyk, M.E.; Lally, E.T. Membrane localization of the Repeats-in-Toxin (RTX) Leukotoxin (LtxA) produced by Aggregatibacter actinomycetemcomitans. *PLoS ONE* **2018**, *13*, e0205871. [CrossRef]

31. Brown, A.C.; Boesze-Battaglia, K.; Du, Y.; Stefano, F.P.; Kieba, I.R.; Epand, R.F.; Kakalis, L.; Yeagle, P.L.; Epand, R.M.; Lally, E.T. Aggregatibacter actinomycetemcomitans leukotoxin cytotoxicity occurs through bilayer destabilization. *Cell. Microbiol.* **2012**, *14*, 869–881. [CrossRef]
32. Lear, J.D.; Furblur, U.G.; Lally, E.T.; Tanaka, J.C. Actinobacillus actinomycetemcomitans leukotoxin forms large conductance, voltage-gated ion channels when incorporated into planar lipid bilayers. *Biochim. Biophys. Acta* **1995**, *1238*, 34–41. [CrossRef]
33. Kumaresan, A.; Kadirvel, G.; Bujarbaruah, K.M.; Bardoloi, R.K.; Das, A.; Kumar, S.; Naskar, S. Preservation of boar semen at 18 degrees C induces lipid peroxidation and apoptosis like changes in spermatozoa. *Anim. Reprod. Sci.* **2009**, *110*, 162–171. [CrossRef] [PubMed]
34. Vermes, I.; Haanen, C.; Steffens-Nakken, H.; Reutelingsperger, C. A novel assay for apoptosis. Flow cytometric detection of phosphatidylserine expression on early apoptotic cells using fluorescein labelled Annexin V. *J. Immunol. Methods* **1995**, *184*, 39–51. [CrossRef]
35. Mangan, D.F.; Taichman, N.S.; Lally, E.T.; Wahl, S.M. Lethal effects of Actinobacillus actinomycetemcomitans leukotoxin on human T lymphocytes. *Infect. Immun.* **1991**, *59*, 3267–3272. [CrossRef]
36. Chang, C.C.; Wu, M.; Yuan, F. Role of specific endocytic pathways in electrotransfection of cells. *Mol. Ther. Methods Clin. Dev.* **2014**, *1*, 14058. [CrossRef]
37. Kirchhausen, T.; Macia, E.; Pelish, H.E. Use of dynasore, the small molecule inhibitor of dynamin, in the regulation of endocytosis. *Methods Enzymol.* **2008**, *438*, 77–93. [CrossRef]
38. Dutta, D.; Williamson, C.D.; Cole, N.B.; Donaldson, J.G. Pitstop 2 is a potent inhibitor of clathrin-independent endocytosis. *PLoS ONE* **2012**, *7*, e45799. [CrossRef]
39. Hill, T.A.; Gordon, C.P.; McGeachie, A.B.; Venn-Brown, B.; Odell, L.R.; Chau, N.; Quan, A.; Mariana, A.; Sakoff, J.A.; Chircop, M.; et al. Inhibition of dynamin mediated endocytosis by the dynoles–synthesis and functional activity of a family of indoles. *J. Med. Chem.* **2009**, *52*, 3762–3773. [CrossRef]
40. Larkin, J.M.; Brown, M.S.; Goldstein, J.L.; Anderson, R.G. Depletion of intracellular potassium arrests coated pit formation and receptor-mediated endocytosis in fibroblasts. *Cell* **1983**, *33*, 273–285. [CrossRef]
41. Dutta, D.; Donaldson, J.G. Search for inhibitors of endocytosis: Intended specificity and unintended consequences. *Cell. Logist.* **2012**, *2*, 203–208. [CrossRef]
42. Maldonado, R.; Wei, R.; Kachlany, S.C.; Kazi, M.; Balashova, N.V. Cytotoxic effects of Kingella kingae outer membrane vesicles on human cells. *Microb. Pathog.* **2011**, *51*, 22–30. [CrossRef]
43. Samuelsson, M.; Potrzebowska, K.; Lehtonen, J.; Beech, J.P.; Skorova, E.; Uronen-Hansson, H.; Svensson, L. RhoB controls the Rab11-mediated recycling and surface reappearance of LFA-1 in migrating T lymphocytes. *Sci. Signal.* **2017**, *10*. [CrossRef]
44. Naslavsky, N.; Weigert, R.; Donaldson, J.G. Convergence of non-clathrin- and clathrin-derived endosomes involves Arf6 inactivation and changes in phosphoinositides. *Mol. Biol. Cell* **2003**, *14*, 417–431. [CrossRef] [PubMed]
45. Parker, H.; Chitcholtan, K.; Hampton, M.B.; Keenan, J.I. Uptake of *Helicobacter pylori* outer membrane vesicles by gastric epithelial cells. *Infect. Immun.* **2010**, *78*, 5054–5061. [CrossRef]
46. Balashova, N.; Giannakakis, A.; Brown, A.C.; Koufos, E.; Benz, R.; Arakawa, T.; Tang, H.Y.; Lally, E.T. Generation of a recombinant Aggregatibacter actinomycetemcomitans RTX toxin in Escherichia coli. *Gene* **2018**, *672*, 106–114. [CrossRef]
47. Bretscher, M.S. On the shape of migrating cells–a 'front-to-back' model. *J. Cell Sci.* **2008**, *121*, 2625–2628. [CrossRef] [PubMed]
48. Bashkirov, P.V.; Akimov, S.A.; Evseev, A.I.; Schmid, S.L.; Zimmerberg, J.; Frolov, V.A. GTPase cycle of dynamin is coupled to membrane squeeze and release, leading to spontaneous fission. *Cell* **2008**, *135*, 1276–1286. [CrossRef] [PubMed]
49. Pearse, B.M.; Bretscher, M.S. Membrane recycling by coated vesicles. *Annu. Rev. Biochem.* **1981**, *50*, 85–101. [CrossRef] [PubMed]
50. Aulik, N.A.; Hellenbrand, K.M.; Kisiela, D.; Czuprynski, C.J. Mannheimia haemolytica leukotoxin binds cyclophilin D on bovine neutrophil mitochondria. *Microb. Pathog.* **2011**, *50*, 168–178. [CrossRef] [PubMed]
51. Atapattu, D.N.; Albrecht, R.M.; McClenahan, D.J.; Czuprynski, C.J. Dynamin-2-dependent targeting of mannheimia haemolytica leukotoxin to mitochondrial cyclophilin D in bovine lymphoblastoid cells. *Infect. Immun.* **2008**, *76*, 5357–5365. [CrossRef] [PubMed]

52. Fabbri, M.; Di Meglio, S.; Gagliani, M.C.; Consonni, E.; Molteni, R.; Bender, J.R.; Tacchetti, C.; Pardi, R. Dynamic partitioning into lipid rafts controls the endo-exocytic cycle of the alphaL/beta2 integrin, LFA-1, during leukocyte chemotaxis. *Mol. Biol. Cell* **2005**, *16*, 5793–5803. [CrossRef] [PubMed]
53. Anderson, R.G. The caveolae membrane system. *Annu. Rev. Biochem.* **1998**, *67*, 199–225. [CrossRef] [PubMed]
54. Oh, P.; McIntosh, D.P.; Schnitzer, J.E. Dynamin at the neck of caveolae mediates their budding to form transport vesicles by GTP-driven fission from the plasma membrane of endothelium. *J. Cell Biol.* **1998**, *141*, 101–114. [CrossRef]
55. Atapattu, D.N.; Czuprynski, C.J. Mannheimia haemolytica leukotoxin binds to lipid rafts in bovine lymphoblastoid cells and is internalized in a dynamin-2- and clathrin-dependent manner. *Infect. Immun.* **2007**, *75*, 4719–4727. [CrossRef]
56. Chinnapen, D.J.; Chinnapen, H.; Saslowsky, D.; Lencer, W.I. Rafting with cholera toxin: endocytosis and trafficking from plasma membrane to ER. *FEMS Microbiol. Lett.* **2007**, *266*, 129–137. [CrossRef]
57. Zhen, Y.; Stenmark, H. Cellular functions of Rab GTPases at a glance. *J. Cell Sci.* **2015**, *128*, 3171–3176. [CrossRef]
58. Huotari, J.; Helenius, A. Endosome maturation. *EMBO J.* **2011**, *30*, 3481–3500. [CrossRef]
59. Rubino, M.; Miaczynska, M.; Lippe, R.; Zerial, M. Selective membrane recruitment of EEA1 suggests a role in directional transport of clathrin-coated vesicles to early endosomes. *J. Biol. Chem.* **2000**, *275*, 3745–3748. [CrossRef]
60. Damiano, J.S.; Cress, A.E.; Hazlehurst, L.A.; Shtil, A.A.; Dalton, W.S. Cell adhesion mediated drug resistance (CAM-DR): role of integrins and resistance to apoptosis in human myeloma cell lines. *Blood* **1999**, *93*, 1658–1667. [CrossRef]
61. de la Fuente, M.T.; Casanova, B.; Moyano, J.V.; Garcia-Gila, M.; Sanz, L.; Garcia-Marco, J.; Silva, A.; Garcia-Pardo, A. Engagement of alpha4beta1 integrin by fibronectin induces in vitro resistance of B chronic lymphocytic leukemia cells to fludarabine. *J. Leukoc. Biol.* **2002**, *71*, 495–502. [PubMed]
62. Balashova, N.; Dhingra, A.; Boesze-Battaglia, K.; Lally, E.T. Aggregatibacter actinomycetemcomitans leukotoxin induces cytosol acidification in LFA-1 expressing immune cells. *Mol. Oral Microbiol.* **2016**, *31*, 106–114. [CrossRef] [PubMed]
63. DiFranco, K.M.; Kaswala, R.H.; Patel, C.; Kasinathan, C.; Kachlany, S.C. Leukotoxin kills rodent WBC by targeting leukocyte function associated antigen 1. *Comp. Med.* **2013**, *63*, 331–337. [PubMed]
64. DiFranco, K.M.; Gupta, A.; Galusha, L.E.; Perez, J.; Nguyen, T.V.; Fineza, C.D.; Kachlany, S.C. Leukotoxin (Leukothera(R)) targets active leukocyte function antigen-1 (LFA-1) protein and triggers a lysosomal mediated cell death pathway. *J. Biol. Chem.* **2012**, *287*, 17618–17627. [CrossRef] [PubMed]
65. Nnah, I.C.; Wang, B.; Saqcena, C.; Weber, G.F.; Bonder, E.M.; Bagley, D.; De Cegli, R.; Napolitano, G.; Medina, D.L.; Ballabio, A.; et al. TFEB-driven endocytosis coordinates MTORC1 signaling and autophagy. *Autophagy* **2019**, *15*, 151–164. [CrossRef] [PubMed]
66. DiFranco, K.M.; Johnson-Farley, N.; Bertino, J.R.; Elson, D.; Vega, B.A.; Belinka, B.A., Jr.; Kachlany, S.C. LFA-1-targeting Leukotoxin (LtxA; Leukothera(R)) causes lymphoma tumor regression in a humanized mouse model and requires caspase-8 and Fas to kill malignant lymphocytes. *Leuk. Res.* **2015**, *39*, 649–656. [CrossRef]
67. Kagedal, K.; Johansson, U.; Ollinger, K. The lysosomal protease cathepsin D mediates apoptosis induced by oxidative stress. *FASEB J.* **2001**, *15*, 1592–1594. [CrossRef]
68. Kagedal, K.; Zhao, M.; Svensson, I.; Brunk, U.T. Sphingosine-induced apoptosis is dependent on lysosomal proteases. *Biochem. J.* **2001**, *359*, 335–343. [CrossRef]
69. Kirkegaard, T.; Jaattela, M. Lysosomal involvement in cell death and cancer. *Biochim. Biophys. Acta* **2009**, *1793*, 746–754. [CrossRef]
70. Barcena-Uribarri, I.; Benz, R.; Winterhalter, M.; Zakharian, E.; Balashova, N. Pore forming activity of the potent RTX-toxin produced by pediatric pathogen Kingella kingae: Characterization and comparison to other RTX-family members. *Biochim. Biophys. Acta* **2015**, *1848*, 1536–1544. [CrossRef]
71. Lear, J.D.; Karakelian, D.; Furblur, U.; Lally, E.T.; Tanaka, J.C. Conformational studies of Actinobacillus actinomycetemcomitans leukotoxin: partial denaturation enhances toxicity. *Biochim. Biophys. Acta* **2000**, *1476*, 350–362. [CrossRef]
72. Friebe, S.; van der Goot, F.G.; Burgi, J. The Ins and Outs of Anthrax Toxin. *Toxins* **2016**, *8*, 69. [CrossRef] [PubMed]

73. Lemichez, E.; Bomsel, M.; Devilliers, G.; vanderSpek, J.; Murphy, J.R.; Lukianov, E.V.; Olsnes, S.; Boquet, P. Membrane translocation of diphtheria toxin fragment A exploits early to late endosome trafficking machinery. *Mol. Microbiol.* **1997**, *23*, 445–457. [CrossRef] [PubMed]
74. O'Brien, D.P.; Hernandez, B.; Durand, D.; Hourdel, V.; Sotomayor-Perez, A.C.; Vachette, P.; Ghomi, M.; Chamot-Rooke, J.; Ladant, D.; Brier, S.; et al. Structural models of intrinsically disordered and calcium-bound folded states of a protein adapted for secretion. *Sci. Rep.* **2015**, *5*, 14223. [CrossRef]
75. DiRienzo, J.M.; Tsai, C.C.; Shenker, B.J.; Taichman, N.S.; Lally, E.T. Monoclonal antibodies to leukotoxin of Actinobacillus actinomycetemcomitans. *Infect. Immun.* **1985**, *47*, 31–36. [CrossRef]
76. Schneider, U.; Schwenk, H.U.; Bornkamm, G. Characterization of EBV-genome negative "null" and "T" cell lines derived from children with acute lymphoblastic leukemia and leukemic transformed non-Hodgkin lymphoma. *Int. J. Cancer* **1977**, *19*, 621–626. [CrossRef]
77. Tsai, C.C.; Shenker, B.J.; DiRienzo, J.M.; Malamud, D.; Taichman, N.S. Extraction and isolation of a leukotoxin from Actinobacillus actinomycetemcomitans with polymyxin B. *Infect. Immun.* **1984**, *43*, 700–705. [CrossRef]
78. Fine, D.H.; Furgang, D.; Kaplan, J.; Charlesworth, J.; Figurski, D.H. Tenacious adhesion of Actinobacillus actinomycetemcomitans strain CU1000 to salivary-coated hydroxyapatite. *Arch. Oral Biol.* **1999**, *44*, 1063–1076. [CrossRef]
79. Diaz, R.; Ghofaily, L.A.; Patel, J.; Balashova, N.V.; Freitas, A.C.; Labib, I.; Kachlany, S.C. Characterization of leukotoxin from a clinical strain of Actinobacillus actinomycetemcomitans. *Microb. Pathog.* **2006**, *40*, 48–55. [CrossRef]
80. Altankov, G.; Grinnell, F. Fibronectin receptor internalization and AP-2 complex reorganization in potassium-depleted fibroblasts. *Exp. Cell Res.* **1995**, *216*, 299–309. [CrossRef]
81. Benz, R.; Janko, K.; Boos, W.; Lauger, P. Formation of large, ion-permeable membrane channels by the matrix protein (porin) of Escherichia coli. *Biochim. Biophys. Acta* **1978**, *511*, 305–319. [CrossRef]

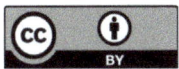

© 2020 by the authors. Licensee MDPI, Basel, Switzerland. This article is an open access article distributed under the terms and conditions of the Creative Commons Attribution (CC BY) license (http://creativecommons.org/licenses/by/4.0/).

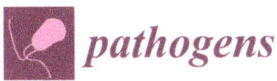

Article

The Cell-Cycle Regulatory Protein p21$^{CIP1/WAF1}$ Is Required for Cytolethal Distending Toxin (Cdt)-Induced Apoptosis

Bruce J. Shenker [1,*], Lisa M. Walker [1], Ali Zekavat [1], Robert H. Weiss [2] and Kathleen Boesze-Battaglia [3]

1. Department of Pathology, University of Pennsylvania School of Dental Medicine, Philadelphia, PA 19104, USA; lism@dental.upenn.edu (L.M.W.); seyed20@upenn.edu (A.Z.)
2. Department of Medicine, University of California at Davis School of Medicine, Sacramento, CA 95616, USA; rhweiss@ucdavis.edu
3. Department of Biochemistry, University of Pennsylvania School of Dental Medicine, Philadelphia, PA 19104, USA; battagli@upenn.edu
* Correspondence: shenker@upenn.edu; Tel.: +1-215-898-5959

Received: 14 November 2019; Accepted: 28 December 2019; Published: 2 January 2020

Abstract: The *Aggregatibacter actinomycetemcomitans* cytolethal distending toxin (Cdt) induces lymphocytes to undergo cell-cycle arrest and apoptosis; toxicity is dependent upon the active Cdt subunit, CdtB. We now demonstrate that p21$^{CIP1/WAF1}$ is critical to Cdt-induced apoptosis. Cdt induces increases in the levels of p21$^{CIP1/WAF1}$ in lymphoid cell lines, Jurkat and MyLa, and in primary human lymphocytes. These increases were dependent upon CdtB's ability to function as a phosphatidylinositol (PI) 3,4,5-triphosphate (PIP3) phosphatase. It is noteworthy that Cdt-induced increases in the levels of p21$^{CIP1/WAF1}$ were accompanied by a significant decline in the levels of phosphorylated p21$^{CIP1/WAF1}$. The significance of Cdt-induced p21$^{CIP1/WAF1}$ increase was assessed by preventing these changes with a two-pronged approach; pre-incubation with the novel p21$^{CIP1/WAF1}$ inhibitor, UC2288, and development of a p21$^{CIP1/WAF1}$-deficient cell line (Jurkat^{p21-}) using clustered regularly interspaced short palindromic repeats (CRISPR)/cas9 gene editing. UC2288 blocked toxin-induced increases in p21$^{CIP1/WAF1}$, and Jurkat^{WT} cells treated with this inhibitor exhibited reduced susceptibility to Cdt-induced apoptosis. Likewise, Jurkat^{p21-} cells failed to undergo toxin-induced apoptosis. The linkage between Cdt, p21$^{CIP1/WAF1}$, and apoptosis was further established by demonstrating that Cdt-induced increases in levels of the pro-apoptotic proteins Bid, Bax, and Bak were dependent upon p21$^{CIP1/WAF1}$ as these changes were not observed in Jurkat^{p21-} cells. Finally, we determined that the p21$^{CIP1/WAF1}$ increases were dependent upon toxin-induced increases in the level and activity of the chaperone heat shock protein (HSP) 90. We propose that p21$^{CIP1/WAF1}$ plays a key pro-apoptotic role in mediating Cdt-induced toxicity.

Keywords: *Aggregatibacter actinomycetemcomitans*; cytolethal distending toxin; lymphocytes; apoptosis; virulence

1. Introduction

The cytolethal distending toxin (Cdt) is a putative virulence factor that is produced by a wide range of human pathogens capable of colonizing mucocutaneous tissue, resulting in disease characterized by persistent infection and inflammation (reviewed in References [1,2]). In general, Cdts are heterotrimeric complexes encoded by an operon of three genes designated *cdtA*, *cdtB*, and *cdtC* which encode three polypeptides: CdtA, CdtB, and CdtC with molecular masses of 23–30, 28–32, and 19–20 kDa, respectively [3–13]. Analyses of subunit structure and function indicate that the heterotrimeric holotoxin functions as an AB_2 toxin; the cell binding unit (B) is responsible for toxin association with the cell surface and is composed of subunits CdtA and CdtC. These subunits deliver the active subunit (A), CdtB, to intracellular compartments. Cdt binding and CdtB internalization are both dependent upon toxin binding to target cell cholesterol in the context of cholesterol-rich membrane microdomains (reviewed in Reference [14]).

Cdt B internalization leads to irreversible cell-cycle arrest and eventually apoptotic cell death. These toxic effects were originally attributable to CdtB's ability to function as a DNase, thereby causing DNA damage which in turn leads to G2/M arrest and death [9,15–23]. Over the past several years, our studies suggested an alternative paradigm to account for *Aggregatibacter actinomycetemcomitans* Cdt-mediated toxicity which is based upon a novel molecular mode of action for CdtB. In this regard, we demonstrated that, in addition to exhibiting DNase activity, CdtB is a potent lipid phosphatase capable of converting the signaling lipid phosphatidylinositol (PI)-3,4,5-triphosphate (PIP3) to PI-3,4-diphosphate [24–28]. Moreover, our investigations demonstrated that the ability of CdtB to function as a PIP3 phosphatase enables this toxin subunit to intoxicate cells via blockade of the PI-3K signaling pathway. Indeed, we demonstrated that the toxic effects of Cdt on lymphocytes, macrophages, and mast cells results in PI-3K signaling blockade characterized by decreases in PIP3, leading to concomitant reductions in the phosphorylation status of downstream targets: Akt and GSK3β. Additionally, we demonstrated that the induction of both G2/M arrest and apoptosis is dependent upon CdtB-mediated PI-3K blockade.

In order to more accurately define the molecular mechanisms that link CdtB-mediated PI-3K blockade with G2/M arrest and apoptosis, we investigated the role of the cyclin-dependent kinase inhibitor known as CDK-interacting protein 1 (Cip1) and wild-type p53-activated fragment 1 (WAF1) ($p21^{CIP1/WAF1}$). $P21^{CIP1/WAF1}$ was originally identified as a negative regulator of the cell cycle, as well as a tumor suppressor. However, recent studies demonstrated additional functions for $p21^{CIP1/WAF1}$ that are associated with regulation of a number of cellular processes including cell differentiation, migration, senescence, and apoptosis [29–33]. Thus, it is not surprising that several investigators demonstrated an association between $p21^{CIP1/WAF1}$ expression and exposure to Cdt [16,34–37]. It should be noted, however, that these studies did not provide any information as to whether the $p21^{CIP1/WAF1}$ levels were mechanistically linked to and/or required for Cdt toxicity. In this study, we investigated the relationship between lymphocyte exposure to *A. actinomycetemcomitans* Cdt, altered $p21^{CIP1/WAF1}$ levels, and induction of toxicity. We now report that Cdt-treated human lymphocytes exhibit dose-dependent increases in levels of $p21^{CIP1/WAF1}$ and the chaperone HSP90 within 4–16 h of exposure to the toxin. To study the biologic consequence of these increases, we employed a two-pronged approach to modify the ability of Cdt to alter expression of $p21^{CIP1/WAF1}$: gene editing and pharmacologic intervention. Additionally, these interventions were assessed for their ability to alter cell susceptibility to Cdt toxicity. Our results indicate a requisite role for $p21^{CIP1/WAF1}$ in Cdt-induced apoptosis.

2. Results

2.1. Cdt Induces Elevations in Lymphocyte Levels of $p21^{CIP1/WAF1}$

Cdt derived from *A. actinomycetemcomitans*, *Haemophilus ducreyi*, and *Helicobacter hepaticus* were shown to induce increases in $p21^{CIP1/WAF1}$ within 24–48 h in several cell lines including fibroblasts, lymphocytes, enterocytes, and hepatocytes [16,34–38]. Likewise, we now demonstrate that *A. actinomyetemcomitans* Cdt induces increases in $p21^{CIP1/WAF1}$ levels in Jurkat cells in a time- and dose-dependent manner. Jurkat cells were treated with varying amounts of Cdt (0–400 pg/mL) for 4, 8, and 16 h and then analyzed by Western blot to assess total $p21^{CIP1/WAF1}$ levels (Figure 1A,B). Analysis indicates that a small, but consistent, increase in $p21^{CIP1/WAF1}$ was detected within 4 h in cells exposed to the highest concentration of Cdt (400 pg/mL). Following an 8-h exposure, significant increases of nine- and 18-fold were observed in cells exposed to 100 and 400 pg/mL Cdt, respectively. After a 16-h exposure, the relative levels of $p21^{CIP1/WAF1}$ remained elevated; cells treated with 25, 100, and 400 pg/mL Cdt exhibited three-, six-, and seven-fold increases, respectively.

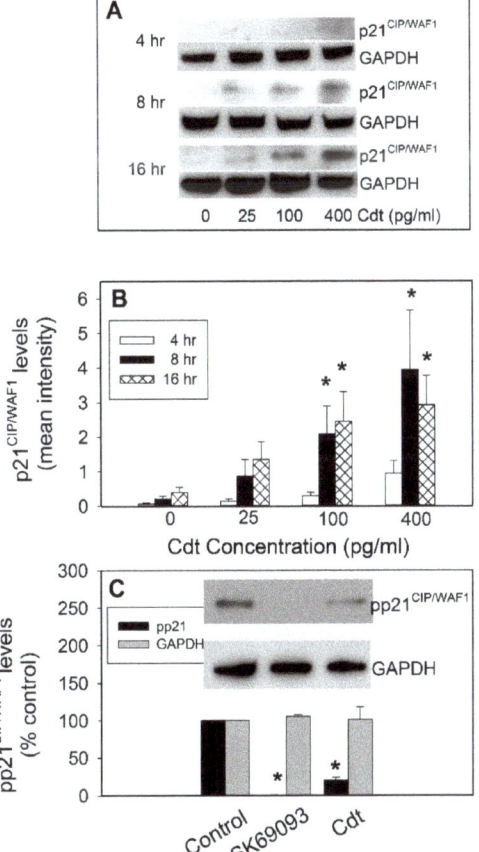

Figure 1. Effect of cytolethal distending toxin (Cdt) on p21$^{CIP1/WAF1}$ levels in Jurkat cells. Jurkat cells were exposed to 0–400 pg/mL Cdt for 4, 8, and 16 h; cells were then harvested, and extracts were fractionated by SDS-PAGE and analyzed by Western blot for the presence of p21$^{CIP1/WAF1}$. Panel (**A**) shows representative Western blots of p21$^{CIP1/WAF1}$ for cells treated with each dose of toxin at 4, 8, and 16 h; glyceraldehyde 3-phosphate dehydrogenase (GAPDH) served as a gel loading control. Panel (**B**) shows the results from multiple blots which were analyzed by digital densitometry; the value of relative intensity obtained from digital densitometry is presented as the mean ± standard error of the mean (SEM) of four experiments. Panel (**C**) shows the relative levels of pp21$^{CIP1/WAF1}$ in cells treated with 50 pg/mL Cdt or 0.5 μM GSK690693 for 16 h expressed as a percentage observed in control (medium only) cells. A representative blot is shown along with compiled results from three experiments: results are expressed as the percentage (mean ± SEM) of pp21$^{CIP1/WAF1}$ observed in control cells; * indicates statistical significance ($p < 0.05$) when compared to untreated cells.

To verify that the effects of Cdt on p21$^{CIP1/WAF1}$ levels were not unique to the Jurkat cell line, the cutaneous T-cell lymphoma line, MyLa, was also assessed for altered p21$^{CIP1/WAF1}$ levels when exposed to the same doses of Cdt. As shown in Figure 2A,B, MyLa cells treated with 0–400 pg/mL Cdt for 16 h exhibited significant increases in p21$^{CIP1/WAF1}$ levels: 4.5- (100 pg/mL Cdt) and 5.7-fold (400 pg/mL Cdt) over control levels. In addition to lymphoid cell lines, p21$^{CIP1/WAF1}$ levels were assessed in primary human lymphocytes (HPBMCs). As shown in Figure 2A,B, exposure to 25 pg/mL Cdt resulted in a detectable but not statistically significant increase in p21$^{CIP1/WAF1}$. Significant increases in p21$^{CIP1/WAF1}$ levels were observed in the presence of 100 and 400 pg/mL Cdt leading to 361% ± 82% and 673% ± 185% over that observed in untreated control cells.

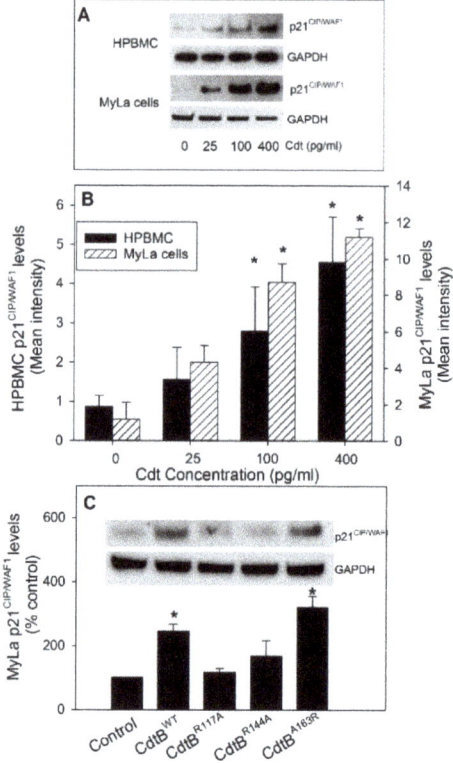

Figure 2. Effect of Cdt on p21$^{CIP1/WAF1}$ levels in primary human lymphocytes (HPBMCs) and MyLa cells. HPBMC and MyLa cells were treated with 0–400 pg/mL Cdt for 16 h. The cells were harvested, and extracts were fractionated by SDS-PAGE and analyzed by Western blot for the presence of p21$^{CIP1/WAF1}$. Panel (**A**) shows representative Western blots, and panel (**B**) shows results from four experiments assessed by digital densitometry; results (intensity) are expressed as the mean ± SEM. Panel (**C**) shows the effect of 50 pg/mL of Cdt containing wild-type CdtB (CdtB^{WT}) or CdtB containing mutations (CdtB^{R117A}, CdtB^{R144A}, and CdtB^{A163R}) on p21$^{CIP1/WAF1}$ levels in MyLa cells. A representative Western blot is shown, as well as results from four experiments that were analyzed by digital densitometry; results are expressed as a percentage of p21$^{CIP1/WAF1}$ levels observed in control (untreated) cells; * indicates statistical significance ($p < 0.05$) when compared to untreated cells.

As noted earlier, we previously demonstrated that Cdt toxicity in lymphocytes (both primary and cell lines), macrophages, and mast cells is dependent upon PIP3 phosphatase activity exhibited by the active Cdt subunit, CdtB [24–28]. We generated and previously reported on the characterization of the enzymatic and toxic activities of Cdts containing targeted mutations within the CdtB subunit [24]. In each instance, we observed that the retention of lipid phosphatase activity, and not DNase activity, was a requisite for both Cdt-induced cell-cycle arrest and apoptosis in lymphocytes, as well as the induction of pro-inflammatory responses in macrophages. Therefore, we next determined the requirement for PIP3 phosphatase activity in Cdt-induced increases in the levels of p21$^{CIP1/WAF1}$. Cdt containing CdtB mutant proteins that were previously described were employed [24]: CdtB^{A163R} retains lipid phosphatase activity, lacks DNase activity, and is toxic; CdtB^{R144A} exhibits low lipid phosphatase activity, exhibits increased DNase activity and is not toxic; CdtB^{R117A} exhibits low lipid phosphatase activity, retains DNase activity, and is not toxic. As shown in Figure 2C, elevations in p21$^{CIP1/WAF1}$ levels were only observed when MyLa cells were treated with toxin containing the active wild-type subunit, CdtB^{WT} (2.5-fold increase), or the CdtB mutant, CdtB^{A163R} (3.2-fold increase) [24]. Cells exposed to CdtB mutant proteins that we previously demonstrated to be deficient in phosphatase activity and lack toxicity (CdtB^{R144A} and CdtB^{R117A}) did not exhibit significant changes in levels of p21$^{CIP1/WAF1}$: 1.2-fold and 1.7 fold, respectively. It is noteworthy that we previously reported that *A. actinomycetemcomitans* Cdt-induced cell-cycle arrest and apoptosis in human lymphocytes does not involve activation of the DNA damage response (DDR) [24,39]. These observations were confirmed as we now demonstrate that Cdt containing CdtB^{WT}, as well as the other CdtB mutant proteins employed in this study, does not induce phosphorylation of the histone H2AX, a commonly employed indicator of DDR activation due to DNA damage (Figure S1, Supplementary Materials).

The biologic activity of p21$^{CIP1/WAF1}$ is governed by post-translational modifications such as phosphorylation; therefore, we also assessed Cdt-treated Jurkat cells for changes in phosphorylation status (T145; (pp21$^{CIP1/WAF1}$)) (Figure 1C). Baseline levels of p21$^{CIP1/WAF1}$ were very low, but detectable; as described above, these levels increased at 8–16 h in the presence of Cdt (see above). In contrast, the relative amount present as phosphorylated p21$^{CIP1/WAF1}$ (pp21$^{CIP1/WAF1}$) significantly declined in the presence of Cdt. Cells treated with 50 pg/mL Cdt for 16 h exhibited a reduction in the amount of pp21$^{CIP1/WAF1}$ to 20.6% ± 3.4% of the amount observed in untreated control cells. Interestingly, the PI-3K signaling pathway exhibits cross-talk with other regulatory pathways; specifically, p21$^{CIP1/WAF1}$ was shown to be a downstream target of activated Akt (pAkt) [40]. Furthermore, we showed that Cdt-treated cells exhibit reduced levels of pAkt (reduced kinase activity) [24]. These observations, along with our current findings that toxin-treated cells also exhibit reduced levels of pp21$^{CIP1/WAF1}$, are consistent with the proposed molecular mode of action for CdtB which involves PIP3 phosphatase activity leading to PI-3K signaling blockade. To further support our findings and provide additional "proof-of-principle" evidence for a relationship between pAkt and p21$^{CIP1/WAF1}$, we employed GSK690693, an Akt inhibitor [41]. Jurkat cells treated for 16 h with 0.5 μM GSK690693, exhibited a reduction in pp21$^{CIP1/WAF1}$ to 0.7% ± 0.3% of that observed with untreated cells (Figure 1C).

2.2. Blockade of Cdt-Induced Increases in p21$^{CIP1/WAF1}$ Results in Reduced Jurkat Cell Susceptibility to Cdt Toxicity

We next extended our investigation to address the biological significance of Cdt-induced increases in p21$^{CIP1/WAF1}$ by utilizing a two-pronged approach: pharmacologic modulation and altered expression using gene editing. The novel inhibitor of p21$^{CIP1/WAF1}$, UC2288, was demonstrated to reduce p21$^{CIP1/WAF1}$ levels [42]; therefore, we firstly employed UC2288 as a potential inhibitor of Cdt toxicity by virtue of its ability to block increases in p21$^{CIP1/WAF1}$. As shown in Figure 3A, pre-treatment of Jurkat^{WT} cells with UC2288 (2.5–10 μM) resulted in reduced Cdt-induced apoptosis in the presence of the highest concentration of the inhibitor (10 μM); interestingly, this is the same concentration reported to be effective in other studies [42]. Untreated control cells exhibited 7.7% ± 1.1% terminal deoxynucleotidyl transferase (TdT)-mediated dUTP nick end labeling (TUNEL)-positive cells and, in the presence of 50 pg/mL Cdt, the percentage of TUNEL-positive cells increased to 35.0% ± 1.9%. Pre-treatment of cells with UC2288 reduced the percentage of TUNEL-positive cells to 19.7% ± 1.4%. Two inactive analogues of UC2288 were employed: UC1770 and UC1472; neither of these altered Cdt-induced apoptosis, as the percentage of TUNEL-positive cell was not reduced below 31% when cells were treated with equivalent concentrations of these analogues. The ability of UC2288 to block Cdt-induced increases in p21$^{CIP1/WAF1}$ levels was also confirmed (Figure 3B). Results are expressed as a percentage of p21$^{CIP1/WAF1}$ levels observed in cells exposed to toxin alone (100%); the latter represents almost a five-fold increase over control cells (medium only). Pre-treatment with 10 μM UC2288 resulted in a significant reduction of p21$^{CIP1/WAF1}$ levels to 24.7% of that observed with cells treated with toxin alone.

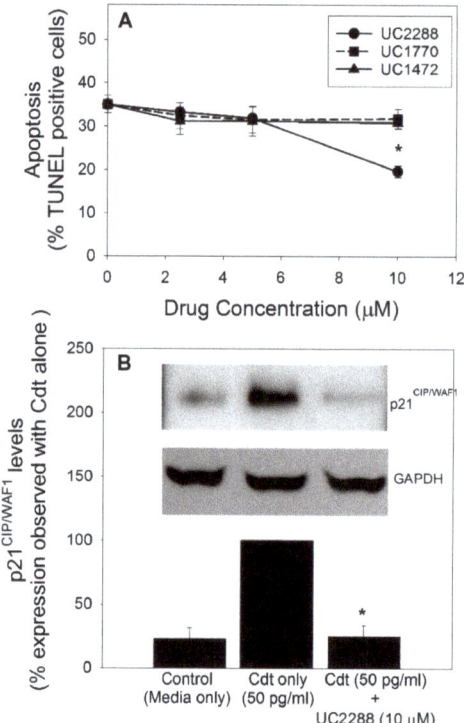

Figure 3. Effect of UC2288 on Cdt-induced apoptosis and on p21$^{CIP1/WAF1}$ levels. Jurkat^{WT} cells were pre-incubated with 0–10 µM UC2288 or its inactive analogues UC1770 and UC1472 for 30 min. Cdt (50 pg/mL) was added to the cell cultures, and the cells were harvested 24 h later and analyzed for apoptosis using the TUNEL assay as described (panel (**A**)). Results are expressed as a percentage of apoptotic cells versus drug concentration; the mean ± SEM for four experiments is plotted. Panel (**B**) shows the effect of UC2288 on Cdt-induced p21$^{CIP1/WAF1}$ levels at 16 h. A representative blot is shown along with results from four experiments. Western blots were analyzed by digital densitometry; the data are expressed as a percentage of the p21$^{CIP1/WAF1}$ levels observed in cells treated with Cdt alone; * indicates statistical significance ($p < 0.05$) when compared to untreated cells.

To confirm our observations with UC2288 and to better understand the biological significance of Cdt-induced elevations in p21$^{CIP1/WAF1}$ levels, we utilized CRISPR/Cas9 gene editing to establish a stable Jurkat cell line deficient in p21$^{CIP1/WAF1}$ expression (Jurkat^{p21-}). As shown in Figure 4A, Jurkat^{p21-} cells were unable to express p21$^{CIP1/WAF1}$ when challenged with either Cdt or etoposide for 16 h; in contrast, Jurkat^{WT} cells exhibited clear elevations in this protein when challenged with either agent under identical conditions. As noted above, we established that Cdt-induced toxicity is dependent on the CdtB subunit's ability to function as a PIP3 phosphatase, thereby mediating blockade of the PI-3K signaling pathway [26,27]. Therefore, we next verified that Jurkat^{p21-} cells remained susceptible to toxin-induced signaling blockade. Specifically, cells were assessed after 2 and 4 h of exposure to Cdt for changes in the phosphorylation status of two downstream PI-3K signaling targets: Akt and GSK3β. Jurkat^{WT} and Jurkat^{p21-} cells were treated with 50 pg/mL Cdt and then analyzed by Western blot for the presence of Akt, pAkt, GSK3β, and pGSK3β at 0, 2, and 4 h. Figure 4B shows representative immunoblots indicating that the levels of both pAkt and pGSK3β were reduced at 2 and 4 h in both Jurkat^{WT} and Jurkat^{p21-}; in contrast, the total amount of these proteins (Akt and GSK3β) remained unchanged. In previous studies, we reported that decreases in pAkt and pGSK3β within Jurkat^{WT} cells were statistically significant with levels of pAkt reduced to 48.7% ± 9.3% (2 h) and 45.5% ± 11.6% (4 h) relative to untreated control cells; likewise, pGSK3β levels were reduced to 55.7% ± 6.0% and 47.6% ± 6.1% of control values at 2 and 4 h, respectively [24]. Figure 4C shows similar compiled results from multiple experiments for Jurkat^{p21-} cells. Akt and GSK3β levels remained relatively constant for the 4-h period. In contrast, pAkt levels were reduced to 56.4% ± 19% (2 h) and to 34.8% ± 16.7% (4 h); pGSK3β levels were reduced to 59.7% ± 22.7% (2 h) and 49.5% ± 21.7% (4 h).

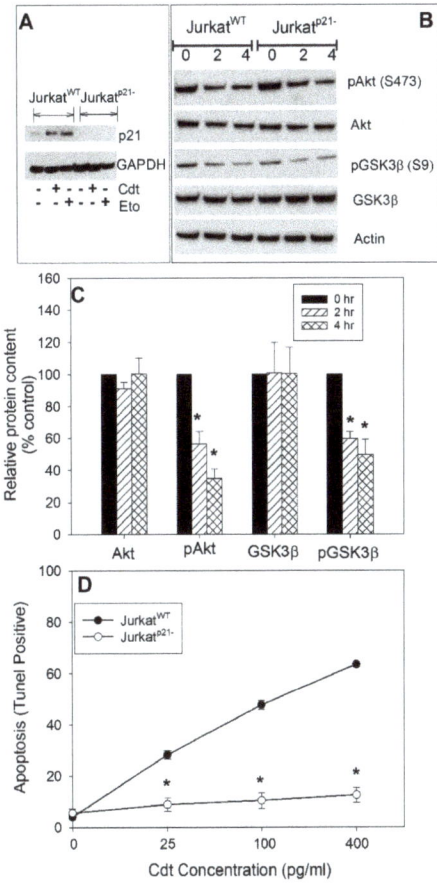

Figure 4. Analysis of Jurkat^{p21-} cells. CRISPR/Cas9 gene editing was employed to produce a Jurkat^{p21-} cell line. Panel (**A**) shows the results of p21$^{CIP1/WAF1}$ analysis by Western blot of both Jurkat^{WT} and Jurkat^{p21-} cells at 16 h following exposure to either Cdt (50 pg/mL) or etoposide (Eto; 50 µM); GAPDH is shown as a gel loading control. Panels (**B,C**) show the effect of Cdt on PI-3K signaling targets. Jurkat^{WT} and Jurkat^{p21-} cells were treated with medium alone (0) or with Cdt (50 pg/mL) for 2 or 4 h and then analyzed by Western blot for the expression of Akt, pAkt (S473), GSK3β, and pGSK3β (S9), as well as actin which served as a loading control. Representative blots are shown in panel (**B**), and the results of three experiments for Jurkat^{p21-} cells are shown in panel (**C**). Data are plotted as the percentage of protein expressed in untreated control cells; the mean ± SEM is shown and * indicates statistical significance ($p < 0.05$) when compared to untreated cells. Panel (**D**) shows the effect of Cdt on apoptosis (TUNEL-positive) in Jurkat^{WT} and Jurkat^{p21-} cells. The percentage of apoptotic cells was determined at 24 h and is plotted versus Cdt concentration; the mean ± SEM is shown for three experiments; * indicates statistical significance ($p < 0.01$) when compared to untreated cells.

Jurkat^{WT} and Jurkat^{p21-} cells were next assessed and compared for their susceptibility to Cdt-induced apoptosis using the TUNEL assay (Figure 4D) following a 24-h treatment with toxin. Consistent with our previous findings, Jurkat^{WT} cells exhibit dose-dependent apoptosis; the percentages of TUNEL-positive were 4.2% ± 0.9% (0 Cdt), 28.3% ± 1.6% (25 pg/mL Cdt), 47.7% ± 1.7% (100 pg/mL Cdt), and 63.5% ± 0.9% (400 pg/mL Cdt). In contrast, Jurkat^{p21-} cells were resistant to Cdt-induced apoptosis; cells incubated with 0–400 pg/mL toxin exhibited 5.7% ± 1.7%, 8.9% ± 2.6%, 10.5% ± 3.0%, and 12.6% ± 3.0% apoptotic cells. It is noteworthy that Jurkat^{p21-} cells retained the capacity to undergo apoptotic cell death as they remained sensitive to paclitaxel (Figure S2, Supplementary Materials).

Previously, we demonstrated that Cdt-induced apoptosis involves the intrinsic apoptotic pathway and, in particular, development of the mitochondrial permeability transition (MPT) [39,43]. Therefore, we assessed and compared Jurkat^{WT} and Jurkat^{p21-} for expression of pro-apoptotic members of the Bcl-2 protein family in response to Cdt. Treatment of Jurkat^{WT} cells with 50 pg/mL Cdt resulted in significant increases in both Bid and Bax at 8 hrs (Figure 5A); Bid levels increased by 498.3% ± 290.5% relative to control cells and Bax levels increased by 637.0% ± 274.7%. A consistent, but not statistically significant, increase was observed for Bak to 160% ± 38.0%. In comparison, Cdt failed to induce increases in the levels of any of the three pro-apoptotic proteins in Jurkat^{p21-} cells; relative to untreated cells, Bid, Bax, and Bak expression levels were 73.2% ± 7.5%, 94.2% ± 10.5%, and 80.4% ± 20.4%, respectively.

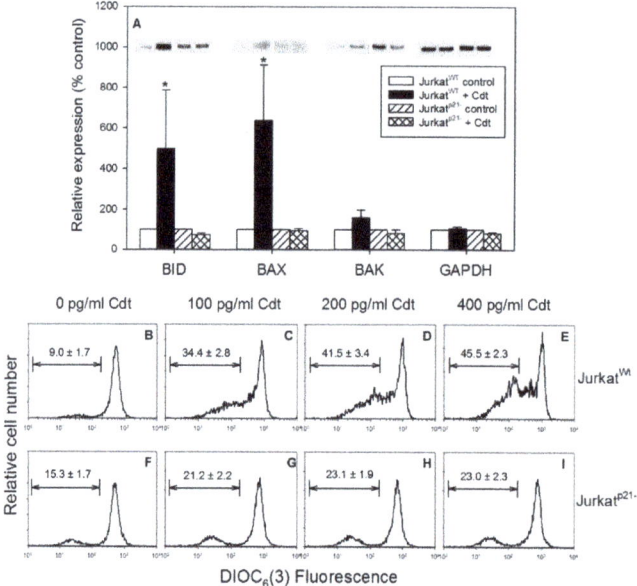

Figure 5. Effect of Cdt on the expression of pro-apoptotic Bcl-2 family members, as well as on the ΔΨm. Panel (**A**): Jurkat^{WT} and Jurkat^{p21-} cells were incubated with medium or 50 pg/mL Cdt for 8 h. Cells were then analyzed by Western blot for Bid, Bax, Bak, and GAPDH (loading control). Representative blots are shown on top for Bid, Bax, Bak, and GAPDH for Jurkat^{WT} cells exposed to medium and Cdt-treated, as well as for Jurkat^{p21-} cells exposed to medium and Cdt-treated. Western blots were analyzed by digital densitometry; results represent the levels of protein expressed as a percentage of that observed in respective control cells. The mean ± SEM for five experiments is shown; * indicates statistical significance ($p < 0.05$) when compared to untreated cells. Panels (**B–I**) show the effect of Cdt (0–400 pg/mL) on the ΔΨm in both Jurkat^{WT} (panels (**B–E**)) and Jurkat^{p21-} cells (panels (**F–I**)). ΔΨm was determined using DIOC$_6$(3), and the percentage of cells exhibiting a reduction the membrane potential was determined using the analytical gate indicated; the numbers represent the mean ± SEM of three experiments, each performed in duplicate.

Cdt was also assessed for its ability to induce the MPT in both Jurkat^{WT} and Jurkat^{P21-} cells by measuring a decline in the mitochondrial transmembrane potential ($\Delta\Psi$m) using the fluorochrome DIOC$_6$(3) [39,43]. As shown in Figure 5B–E, Jurkat^{WT} cells treated with 0–400 pg/mL Cdt exhibited a dose-dependent increase in the percentage of cells exhibiting a decline in the $\Delta\Psi$m, with 9% in control cells versus 34.4%, 41.5%, and 45.5% in cells exposed to 100, 200, and 400 pg/mL Cdt. In contrast, Jurkat^{P21-} did not exhibit a significant change in the $\Delta\Psi$m; 15.3% of control cells exhibited reduced $\Delta\Psi$m, and Cdt treatment resulted in a slight, but not statistically significant increase to 21.2%, 23.1%, and 23% in the presence of 100, 200, and 400 pg/mL Cdt, respectively (Figure 5 F–I).

2.3. Cdt-Induced Increases in p21$^{CIP1/WAF1}$ Levels and Induction of Apoptosis Are Blocked by the Chaperone HSP90

The intracellular levels of p21$^{CIP1/WAF1}$ are controlled transcriptionally, as well as post-translationally, by the proteasome. Experiments were carried out to account for the mode of Cdt-induced increases in p21$^{CIP1/WAF1}$. We firstly addressed the effect of Cdt on p21$^{CIP1/WAF1}$ messenger RNA (mRNA) levels in Jurkat cells. As shown in Figure 6A, p21$^{CIP1/WAF1}$ mRNA levels were marginally elevated at high toxin doses within 4 h and declined in the presence of the same doses of Cdt at 16 h; however, these changes were not statistically significant. It should also be noted that *A. actinomycetemcomitans* Cdt-induced increases in lymphocyte p21$^{CIP1/WAF1}$ levels were previously shown to be p53-independent [35]. These findings were confirmed as we demonstrate that Cdt-induced p21$^{CIP1/WAF1}$ increases were observed in the presence of the p53 inhibitor, pifithrin-α (Figure S3, Supplementary Materials); this inhibitor also failed to block Cdt-induced apoptosis. Similar results were observed with Molt-4 cells (data not shown). On the post-translational side, the chaperone HSP90 was shown to stabilize p21$^{CIP1/WAF1}$ and prevent its degradation by the proteasome [44–46]. Jurkat cells were assessed for changes in the levels of HSP90 by Western blot following 4 and 8 h of exposure to Cdt (Figure 6B,C). Untreated cells exhibited detectable levels of HSP90 at both time points. Exposure of Jurkat cells to Cdt for 4 h resulted in 1.5- (25 pg/mL), 2.0- (100 pg/mL), and 1.9-fold (400 pg/mL) increases in HSP90 levels. Treatment with the same doses of Cdt for 8 h resulted in increases of 1.6-, 1.5-, and 3.6- fold. The dependence of Cdt-induced increases in HSP90 on CdtB-associated PIP3 phosphatase activity was also assessed (Figure 6D). Jurkat cells treated with Cdt containing the active CdtB subunits CdtB^{WT} and CdtB^{A163R} exhibited increased HSP90 levels of 5.1-fold and 4.6-fold over levels observed in control cells, respectively. The HSP90 levels in cells treated with the PIP3 phosphatase-inactive CdtB units, CdtB^{R117A} and CdtB^{R144A}, did not change.

The relationship between HSP90 and Cdt-induced increases in p21$^{CIP1/WAF1}$ levels, as well as the induction of apoptosis, was demonstrated by employing geldanamycin (GM), an inhibitor of HSP90 ATPase activity [47]. As shown in Figure 6E, GM was assessed for its ability to inhibit HSP90 and in turn Cdt-induced apoptosis. Jurkat cells were pre-treated with medium or GM (0–5 µM) for 1 h, followed by the addition of medium or Cdt (50 pg/mL). Cells were assessed for apoptosis (TUNEL-positive) 24 h later (Figure 6E). Cells treated with medium exhibited 6.2% ± 1.8% TUNEL-positive cells; in comparison, cells treated with 50 pg/mL Cdt exhibited 63.7% ± 8.8% TUNEL-positive cells. Pre-treatment of cells with GM followed by the addition of toxin resulted in a dose-dependent reduction in apoptosis. In the presence of 1.25, 2.5, and 5 µM GM, the percentage of TUNEL-positive cells was reduced to 21.6% ± 0.7%, 16.4% ± 1.7%, and 8.7% ± 2.3%. It should be noted that GM alone exhibited low levels of toxicity (net 5–10% over untreated cells).

In addition to evaluating the effects of GM on Cdt-induced apoptosis, Jurkat cells were also assessed for p21$^{CIP1/WAF1}$ levels by Western blot (Figure 6F). Untreated Jurkat cells contained marginally detectable levels of p21$^{CIP1/WAF1}$; cells treated with diluent (DMSO) or GM (2.5 µM) exhibited slight increases in p21$^{CIP1/WAF1}$ to 1.2 ± 1.0 and 1.1 ± 0.98, respectively. Cells exposed to Cdt alone exhibited a significant increase in p21$^{CIP1/WAF1}$ levels to 2.4 ± 1.0; pretreatment of cells with 2.5 µM GM reduced p21$^{CIP1/WAF1}$ to near baseline levels (0.56 ± 0.19).

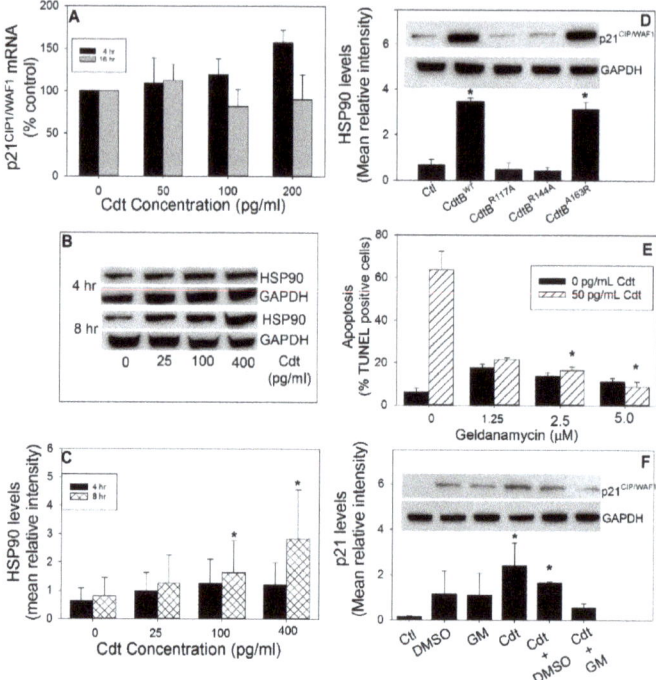

Figure 6. Cdt-induced increases in p21$^{CIP1/WAF1}$ and induction of apoptosis are dependent upon HSP90. Panel (**A**) shows the effects of Cdt on p21$^{CIP1/WAF1}$ messenger RNA (mRNA) by RT-PCR. Jurkat cells were incubated with 50 pg/mL Cdt for 4 and 16 h. RNA extraction, complementary DNA (cDNA) synthesis, RT-PCR, and changes in mRNA were calculated as previously described [28]. Results are the mean of three experiments plotted as a percentage of mRNA levels observed in control cells (time 0). Panels (**B**,**C**) show the results of experiments that assess the effect of Cdt on HSP90 levels. Jurkat cells were treated with Cdt (0–400 pg/mL) for 4 and 8 h, and the cell extracts were assessed by Western blot. Panel (**B**) shows a representative Western blot with GAPDH as a loading control. Panel (**C**) shows the results of four experiments; Western blots were analyzed by digital densitometry, and the results are plotted as the mean intensity ± SEM. Panel (**D**) shows Western blot analysis of the effect of 50 pg/mL Cdt containing CdtB^{WT} or CdtB containing mutations (CdtB^{R117A}, CdtB^{R144A}, and CdtB^{A163R}) on HSP90 levels in Jurkat cells. A representative Western blot is shown, as well as results from three experiments that were analyzed by digital densitometry; results are expressed as the mean intensity ± SEM; * indicates statistical significance ($p < 0.05$) when compared to untreated cells. The effects of geldanamycin D (GM) on Cdt-induced apoptosis are shown in panel (**E**). Jurkat cells were incubated with 0–5 μM GM for 60 min, followed by the addition of medium and 50 pg/mL Cdt, before being analyzed for apoptosis (TUNEL assay) 24 h later. The percentage of TUNEL-positive cells is plotted as the mean ± SEM of four experiments. Panel (**F**) shows the effects of GM on Cdt-induced increases in Jurkat cell p21$^{CIP1/WAF1}$ level. Jurkat cells were treated with medium or Cdt (50 pg/mL) in the presence of DMSO (vehicle) or 2.5 μM GM for 16 h. Cells were analyzed by Western blot and digital densitometry for the levels of p21$^{CIP1/WAF1}$. A representative blot and the results from three experiments is shown; results are plotted as the mean ± SEM of three experiments; * indicates statistical significance ($p < 0.05$) when compared to untreated cells.

3. Discussion

3.1. Functional Significance of Cdt-induced Increases in the Levels of p21$^{CIP1/WAF1}$

We now report that *A. actinomycetemcomitans* Cdt induces intracellular increases of p21$^{CIP1/WAF1}$ in human lymphocyte cell lines, as well as primary HPBMCs. These observations are consistent with those of other investigators who also demonstrated similar increases in response to Cdt derived from either *A. actinomycetemcomitans* or *Haemophilus ducreyi* [16,18,35,36]. P21$^{CIP1/WAF1}$ increases were observed in a murine B-cell hybridoma cell line, fibroblasts, the Hep-2 carcinoma cell line, and a gingival squamous cell carcinoma cell line, Ca9-22. These investigators did not demonstrate the biological significance of the observed Cdt-dependent changes in cellular levels of p21$^{CIP1/WAF1}$. As noted earlier, increases in p21$^{CIP1/WAF1}$ levels are typically observed in response to cell stress or following DNA damage. The binding of p21$^{CIP1/WAF1}$ to cyclins and their CDK binding partner (e.g., CDK1 or CDK2) results in inhibition of the kinase complex, resulting in cell-cycle arrest (reviewed in References [29,31–33]). It is generally accepted that p21$^{CIP1/WAF1}$ regulates both cell-cycle arrest, i.e., checkpoint activation, and apoptosis. Collectively, the actions of p21$^{CIP1/WAF1}$ promote cell survival and provide time for cells to undergo DNA repair before completing the cell cycle. However, it is becoming increasingly clear that the role of p21$^{CIP1/WAF1}$ in regulating apoptosis is more complex than originally thought [30,48]. For example, several investigators demonstrated that pro-apoptotic agents induce increases in p21$^{CIP1/WAF1}$ and, furthermore, over-expression of p21$^{CIP1/WAF1}$ enhances apoptosis [49–52]. Likewise, cells and animals deficient in p21$^{CIP1/WAF1}$ expression exhibit reduced susceptibility to apoptotic cell death [53,54].

In the current study, we employed a combination of gene editing (CRISPR/cas9) and pharmacologic intervention to assess the functional consequence of Cdt-induced increases in p21$^{CIP1/WAF1}$. Collectively, our observations indicate that Cdt-induced apoptosis is dependent upon increased levels of p21$^{CIP1/WAF1}$. Jurkat^{p21-} cells failed to exhibit apoptotic death following treatment with Cdt. Nonetheless, Jurkat^{p21-} cells retained their susceptibility to other pro-apoptotic agents such as paclitaxel. Additionally, we employed the novel p21$^{CIP1/WAF1}$ inhibitor UC2288 whose structure is based upon sorafenib, another inhibitor of p21$^{CIP1/WAF1}$. UC2288 is a new-generation inhibitor that exhibits greater selectivity with higher potency to attenuate p21$^{CIP1/WAF1}$ levels [41,55]. Similar to our findings with Jurkat^{p21-} cells, Jurkat^{WT} cells treated with Cdt in the presence of 10 μM UC2288 also failed to exhibit increased levels of p21$^{CIP1/WAF1}$; moreover, the drug suppressed Cdt-induced apoptosis. It should also be noted that the effective dose of UC2288 used in this study was identical to that employed in other studies [41,55].

Our results demonstrate a pivotal role for p21$^{CIP1/WAF1}$ in Cdt-induced apoptosis (Figure 7); these observations encompass a non-conventional role for p21$^{CIP1/WAF1}$ as it proposes a pro-apoptotic function when increases in this regulatory protein are commonly thought to, at least initially, serve a pro-survival role. It is well established that the pleiotropic effects of p21$^{CIP1/WAF1}$ are regulated by post-transcriptional modification. For example, phosphorylation of p21$^{CIP1/WAF1}$ is known to alter its function which includes a shift in the balance between its pro- and anti-apoptotic effects [29,31,56,57]. In this regard, p21$^{CIP1/WAF1}$ was shown to serve as a downstream target for phosphorylation (pp21$^{CIP1/WAF1}$ (T-145)) by pAkt, the active form of Akt [58,59]. Consistent with these findings is our observation that Cdt-induced increases in p21$^{CIP1/WAF1}$ were not only associated with the induction of apoptosis but also accompanied by a substantial shift in the distribution of pp21$^{CIP1/WAF1}$ levels relative to untreated cells. It is noteworthy that, in addition to inducing p21$^{CIP1/WAF1}$ increases, we previously established that treatment of lymphocytes with *A. actinomycetemcomitans* Cdt results in blockade of the PI-3K signaling cascade and, furthermore, Cdt toxicity is dependent upon perturbation of these early signaling events. Cdt-mediated PI-3K blockade is the result of potent lipid phosphatase activity, specifically PIP3 phosphatase activity, associated with the active Cdt subunit, CdtB [26]. Cells exposed to Cdt exhibit PI-3K signaling blockade within 2 h; this is characterized by PIP3 depletion and reduced Akt activity [24,27,28]. It is important to note that Jurkat^{p21-} cells retained their susceptibility to Cdt-induced PI-3K signaling blockade but were unable to undergo apoptosis due to their inability to produce p21$^{CIP1/WAF1}$. We propose that depletion of pAkt in Cdt-treated cells limits phosphorylation of p21$^{CIP1/WAF1}$ (Figure 7); this relationship is further supported by our finding that the Akt inhibitor, GSK690693, also depletes Jurkat^{WT} cells of pp21$^{CIP1/WAF1}$. Collectively, these findings support a critical pro-apoptotic role for non-phosphorylated p21$^{CIP1/WAF1}$ in mediating Cdt-induced cell death.

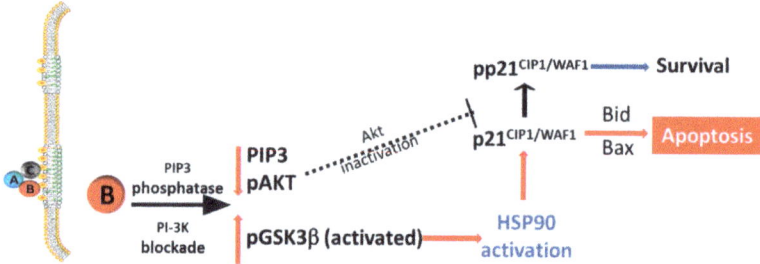

Figure 7. Overview of the proposed mechanism via which Cdt induces p21$^{CIP1/WAF1}$-dependent apoptosis. Based upon the data presented in this paper, the proposed pathway of Cdt-induced p21$^{CIP1/WAF1}$-dependent apoptosis is shown with red arrows. The dotted line shows the proposed relationship between Akt and the putative downstream target, p21$^{CIP1/WAF1}$.

Finally, the link between increased p21$^{CIP1/WAF1}$ levels and the onset of apoptosis was established in experiments in which we assessed the ability of Cdt to alter the expression of pro-apoptotic members of the Bcl-2 family. In previous studies, we, and others, established that Cdt-induced apoptosis involves development of the mitochondrial permeability transition state characterized by a decrease in the transmembrane potential and an increase in production of reactive oxygen species [43,60,61]; these events were followed by activation of the caspase cascade. Of particular relevance to our current study were our previous findings that over-expression of Bcl-2 blocked Cdt-induced apoptosis [39]. In this context, the pro-apoptotic requirement for p21$^{CIP1/WAF1}$ in Cdt-induced apoptosis is further supported by our current observation that the toxin induces p21$^{CIP1/WAF1}$-dependent upregulation of the pro-apoptotic proteins Bid, Bax, and Bak. P21$^{CIP1/WAF1}$-dependency was demonstrated by the observation that the levels of these proteins were not altered in Cdt-treated Jurkat^{p21-} cells. Moreover, Jurkat^{p21-} cells also failed to exhibit changes in the $\Delta\Psi$m as we observed with Cdt-susceptible cells. It is noteworthy that Gogada et al. [62] demonstrated that p21$^{CIP1/WAF1}$ played a critical role in circumin-induced apoptosis by altering mitochondrial permeability, thereby facilitating the release of cytochrome c.

3.2. Cdt Toxicity Requires HSP90-Dependent Increases in the Levels of p21$^{CIP1/WAF1}$

Eukaryotic cell-cycle progression and cell survival are regulated at multiple checkpoints involving a number of critical regulatory proteins. One such regulatory protein is p21$^{CIP1/WAF1}$ which functions as a cyclin-dependent kinase inhibitor [29]. Elevated levels of p21$^{CIP1/WAF1}$ are critical to its function; typically, p21$^{CIP1/WAF1}$ is expressed at low levels under normal growth conditions as an unstable protein with a short half-life. It is well established that p21$^{CIP1/WAF1}$ can be upregulated via a number of p53-dependent and -independent mechanisms (reviewed in Reference [31]). Likewise, Cdt-induced p21$^{CIP1/WAF1}$ increases were reported to be both p53-dependent and -independent (reviewed in Reference [1]); these findings led others to propose that the role of p53 with respect to Cdt is dependent upon both the specific target cell and the source of toxin. Of particular relevance to this study, Sato et al. [35] demonstrated that *A. actinomycetemcomitans* Cdt-treated lymphocytes exhibit p53-independent increases in p21$^{CIP1/WAF1}$. We confirmed these observations by demonstrating that *A. actinomycetemcomitans* Cdt-treated lymphocytes exhibited increases in p21$^{CIP1/WAF1}$ and apoptosis when pre-exposed to the p53 inhibitor pifithrin-α.

Stress and/or DNA damage are known to induce increases in p21$^{\text{CIP1/WAF1}}$ levels as a result of elevated transcription, RNA stability and/or decreased proteasomal degradation (reviewed in References [29,33]). Cdt-induced increases in p21$^{\text{CIP1/WAF1}}$ were not accompanied by significant changes in mRNA levels. These findings led us to explore the possibility that the observed increases were instead due to protein stabilization and reduced proteasomal degradation. It is in this context that we considered the role of the heat shock protein HSP90 in both Cdt-induced increases in p21$^{\text{CIP1/WAF1}}$ and toxicity. As noted above, p21$^{\text{CIP1/WAF1}}$ is typically expressed at low levels as an unstable protein with a short half-life in normally growing cells. HSP90 is known to function as a chaperone that is critical to stabilizing proteins involved in several cellular processes [46]. In particular, HSP90 was shown to be recruited to p21$^{\text{CIP1/WAF1}}$ where it binds via the WAF1/CIP1 stabilizing protein 39 (WISp39). The complex of HSP90, WISp39, and p21$^{\text{CIP1/WAF1}}$ was reported to stabilize and protect the cell-cycle inhibitor from proteasomal degradation [44,45].

We extended these observations to Cdt-induced stress in lymphocytes by firstly assessing toxin-treated Jurkat cells for changes in both WISp39 and HSP90. Jurkat cells constitutively express WISp39, and we observed that exposure to Cdt did not result in further increases (data not shown). In contrast, Cdt-treated cells exhibited significant increases in HSP90 levels within 4 h, prior to the peak elevation in p21$^{\text{CIP1/WAF1}}$. It should also be noted that the ability of CdtB to alter HSP90 levels, as demonstrated for p21$^{\text{CIP1/WAF1}}$, was found to be dependent upon PIP3 phosphatase activity, since toxin-containing CdtB subunit mutants that lacked phosphatase activity were unable to induce increases in HSP90 levels. To further investigate the relationship between HSP90, p21$^{\text{CIP1/WAF1}}$, and apoptosis, we employed the HSP90 inhibitor, GM. Specifically, our observations demonstrate that cells pre-treated with GM prior to exposure to Cdt prevented toxin induces increases in p21$^{\text{CIP1/WAF1}}$; moreover, these cells exhibited decreased susceptibility to toxin-induced apoptosis, demonstrating a linkage between HSP90, changes in p21$^{\text{CIP1/WAF1}}$ levels, and toxicity.

4. Conclusions

In summary, this study advances our understanding of the molecular events leading to *A. actinomycetemcomitans* Cdt-mediated toxicity in lymphocytes. We previously demonstrated that Cdt toxicity is dependent upon PI-3K signaling blockade in lymphocytes, mast cells, and macrophages [2,24–26,28,63,64]. A key to impairment of this signaling pathway is the ability of the active Cdt subunit, CdtB, to function as a PIP3 phosphatase. Our current observations utilized both pharmacologic and gene editing approaches to demonstrate that toxin-induced apoptosis is also dependent upon increased levels of p21$^{\text{CIP1/WAF1}}$. Furthermore, toxin-induced increases in this critical regulatory protein are dependent upon HSP90. Moreover, the timeline for these and previous observations suggest a sequence in which the earliest events involve: Cdt binding to membrane cholesterol via CdtC and CdtB, internalization of CdtB, and depletion of PIP3, leading to a concomitant decrease in pAkt (loss of activity), increased expression/activation of HSP90, increased levels of p21$^{\text{CIP1/WAF1}}$, and increased levels of pro-apoptotic Bcl-2 family proteins [28,65]. We propose that the ability of Cdt to impair lymphocyte proliferation and promote cell death therefore compromises the host response to Cdt-producing organisms. Our observations are of particular significance, as Cdts are produced by not only *A. actinomycetemcomtans*, but also by over 30 γ- and ε- Proteobacteria [1,2]. Therefore, we further propose that the action of this putative virulence factor contributes to the pathogenesis of a range of diseases leading to persistent infection by Cdt-producing pathogens. Our current findings not only contribute to a greater understanding of the molecular events critical to Cdt toxicity, but also provide avenues for developing novel approaches to attenuating the immunoinhibitory effects of the toxin.

5. Materials and Methods

5.1. Reagents and Antibodies

We previously reported on the construction and expression of the plasmids which contain the *cdt* genes for the holotoxin (pUCAacdtABC^{his}), as well as those constructs containing CdtB mutations [10]. The histidine-tagged holotoxin was isolated by nickel affinity chromatography as previously described [66]. All antibodies were obtained from commercial sources as indicated. UC2288 was provided by RH Weiss), GM was purchased from Thermofisher Scientific (Waltham, MA, USA), and GSK690962 was purchased from Cayman Chemical (Ann Arbor, MI, USA).

5.2. Culture Conditions and CRISPR/cas9-Mediated Genome Editing

Two human lymphoid cell lines were employed in these studies: the T-cell leukemia cell line Jurkat (E6-1) and the cutaneous T-cell lymphoma cell line, MyLa2059. Cells were maintained as previously described [10]. Jurkat^{WT} cells were cultured in Roswell Park Memorial Institute (RPMI) 1640 supplemented with fetal bovine serum (FBS) (10%), glutamine (2 mM), 4-(2-hydroxyethyl)-1-piperazineethanesulfonic acid (HEPES) (10 mM), penicillin (100 U/mL), and streptomycin (100 µg/mL). MyLa2059 cells were maintained in the same medium containing 20% FBS. Human peripheral blood mononuclear cells (HPBMCs) were prepared and incubated as described previously [67]; blood was obtained using an Institutional Review Board-approved protocol, and all donors provided written consent.

To generate p21$^{CIP1/WAF1}$-deficient Jurkat cells (Jurkat^{P21-}), we utilized CRISPR/cas9 technology (Santa Cruz Biotechnology; Santa Cruz, CA, USA) as previously described [68]. Cells were transfected (Amaxa Nucleofector system; Lonza, Basel) with a pool of three plasmids, each encoding the Cas9 nuclease and a p21$^{CIP1/WAF1}$-specific 20-nt guide RNA (gRNA). Cells were co-transfected with a pool of three plasmids each containing a homology-directed DNA repair (HDR) template; this corresponded to sites generated by the p21$^{CIP1/WAF1}$ CRISPR/cas9 knockout plasmids. HDR plasmids insert the puromycin resistance gene that facilitates selection of stable knockout cells. Cells were firstly incubated for a five-day period following transfection and then for an additional seven days in incubation in puromycin (5 µg/mL). Limiting dilution of surviving cells was utilized to clone cells; clones were expanded and assessed by Western blot analysis for both the presence of p21$^{CIP1/WAF1}$ their ability to increase p21$^{CIP1/WAF1}$ levels in response to Cdt or etoposide. Clones determined to be deficient in p21$^{CIP1/WAF1}$ were then cloned a second time using limiting dilution (Figure 4A). Jurkat^{P21-} cell lines were maintained in medium containing puromycin (1 µg/mL); experiments were conducted in medium without puromycin.

5.3. Assessment of Apoptosis

Jurkat^{WT} and Jurkat^{P21-} cells were challenged with Cdt or medium (control) for 24 h, and apoptosis was assessed by measuring DNA fragmentation (In Situ Cell Death Detection Kit; Sigma Aldrich, St. Louis, MI, USA) [43]. Briefly, after 24 h of incubation, the cells were re-suspended in freshly prepared 4% formaldehyde and permeabilized with 0.1% Triton X-100 for 2 min at 4 °C; then, they were washed and stained with a solution containing FITC-labeled nucleotide and terminal deoxynucleotidyl transferase (TdT). Flow cytometry was employed to measure FITC fluorescence with a laser at 488 nm to excite the fluorochrome; fluorescence emission was measured through a 530/30-nm bandpass filter.

To measure development of the permeability phase transition, Jurkat cells were incubated for 18 h in medium alone or containing Cdt under conditions described above. Changes in the transmembrane potential ($\Delta\Psi_m$) were determined using 4 nM 3,3′-dihexyloxacarbocyanine (DIOC$_6$(3); Thermofisher) [39,43]. Cells were stained for 15 min (37 °C) with the fluorochrome and fluorescence measured following excitation with a laser at 488 nm (250 mW), and emission was monitored through a 530/30-nm bandpass filter; at least 10,000 cells were analyzed per sample.

5.4. Western Blot Analysis

Cells were incubated with and without Cdt as described above; following the indicated incubation period, cells were solubilized in 20 mM Tris-HCl buffer (pH7.5) containing 150 mM NaCl, 1 mM EDTA, 1% NP-40, 1% sodium deoxycholate, and a protease inhibitor cocktail (ThermoFisher Scientific; Waltham, MA, USA). Samples (30 µg) were fractionated on 12% SDS-PAGE and then blotted onto PVDF membranes; the membranes were blocked with BLOTTO and then incubated with one of the following primary antibodies (Cell Signaling Technology; Danvers, MA, USA) for 18 h at 4 °C [12]: anti-Akt, anti-pAkt (S473), anti-GSK3β, anti-pGSK3β (S9), or anti-GAPDH; anti-p21$^{CIP1/WAF1}$, anti-pp21$^{CIP1/WAF1}$, and anti-HSP90 antibodies were also employed (Abcam; Cambridge, MA, USA). The membranes were incubated with goat anti-rabbit immunoglobulin conjugated to horseradish peroxidase (Southern Biotech Technology; Birmingham, AL, USA) after they were blocked and washed. The Western blots were developed using chemiluminescence and analyzed by digital densitometry (Li-Cor Biosciences; Lincoln, NE, USA) as previously described [25].

5.5. Statistical Analysis

The mean ± standard error of the mean was calculated for replicate experiments. Significance was determined using a Student's *t*-test using SigmaPlot Software (Systat; San Jose, CA); a *p*-value of less than 0.05 was considered to be statistically significant.

Supplementary Materials: The following are available online at http://www.mdpi.com/2076-0817/9/1/38/s1: Figure S1: Effect of Cdt containing CdtB^{WT} or one of the CdtB mutants on phosphorylation of H2AX; Figure S2: Susceptibility of Jurkat^{p21-} cells paclitaxel; Figure S3: Effect of pifithrin-α (PFT) on Cdt-induced increases in p21$^{CIP1/WAF1}$ and apoptosis.

Author Contributions: Conceptualization, B.J.S., K.B.-B., and R.H.W.; methodology, B.J.S., L.M.W., A.Z., and K.B.-B.; validation, L.M.W. and A.Z.; formal analysis, B.J.S., L.M.W., A.Z., and K.B.-B.; investigation, L.M.W. and A.Z.; resources, B.J.S., R.H.W., and K.B.-B.; data curation, L.M.W. and A.Z.; writing—original draft preparation, B.J.S.; writing—review and editing, R.H.W. and K.B.-B.; supervision, B.J.S. and K.B.-B.; project administration, B.J.S. and K.B.-B.; funding acquisition, B.J.S. and K.B.-B. All authors have read and agreed to the published version of the manuscript.

Funding: This research was funded by the National Institutes of Health grants DE0006014 and DE023071.

Acknowledgments: The authors wish to acknowledge the expertise and assistance of the Flow Cytometry Core Facility at the University of Pennsylvania School of Dental Medicine.

Conflicts of Interest: The authors declare no conflict of interest.

References

1. Jinadasa, R.N.; Bloom, S.E.; Weiss, R.S.; Duhamel, G.E. Cytolethal distending toxin: A conserved bacterial genotoxin that blocks cell cycle progression, leading to apoptosis of a broad range of mammalian cell lineages. *Microbiology* **2011**, *157 Pt 7*, 1851–1875. [CrossRef]
2. Scuron, M.D.; Boesze-Battaglia, K.; Dlakic, M.; Shenker, B.J. The Cytolethal Distending Toxin Contributes to Microbial Virulence and Disease Pathogenesis by Acting as a Tri-Perditious Toxin. *Front. Cell. Infect. Microbiol.* **2016**, *6*, 168. [CrossRef]
3. De Rycke, J.; Oswald, E. Cytolethal distending toxin (CDT): A bacterial weapon to control host cell proliferation? *FEMS Microbiol. Lett.* **2001**, *203*, 141–148. [CrossRef]
4. Elwell, C.; Chao, K.; Patel, K.; Dreyfus, L. Escherichia coli CdtB mediates cytolethal distending toxin cell cycle arrest. *Infect. Immun.* **2001**, *69*, 3418–3422. [CrossRef]
5. Mao, X.; DiRienzo, J.M. Functional studies of the recombinant subunits of a cytolethal distending holotoxin. *Cell Microbiol.* **2002**, *4*, 245–255. [CrossRef] [PubMed]
6. Sansaricq, P.A.; Mao, K.; DiRienzo, C.J. Expression of cytolethal distending toxin genes from actinobacillus actinomycetemcomitans in escherichia coli. *Penn Dent. J.* **2001**, *101*, 9. [PubMed]
7. Gargi, A.; Reno, M.; Blanke, S.R. Bacterial toxin modulation of the eukaryotic cell cycle: Are all cytolethal distending toxins created equally? *Front. Cell. Infect. Microbiol.* **2012**, *2*, 124. [CrossRef] [PubMed]

8. Lara-Tejero, M.; Galan, J.E. CdtA, CdtB, and CdtC form a tripartite complex that is required for cytolethal distending toxin activity. *Infect. Immun.* **2001**, *69*, 4358–4365. [CrossRef] [PubMed]
9. Nesic, D.; Hsu, Y.; Stebbins, C.E. Assembly and function of a bacterial genotoxin. *Nature* **2004**, *429*, 429–433. [CrossRef]
10. Shenker, B.J.; Besack, D.; McKay, T.; Pankoski, L.; Zekavat, A.; Demuth, D.R. Actinobacillus actinomycetemcomitans cytolethal distending toxin (Cdt): Evidence that the holotoxin is composed of three subunits: CdtA, CdtB, and CdtC. *J. Immunol.* **2004**, *172*, 410–417. [CrossRef]
11. Shenker, B.J.; Besack, D.; McKay, T.; Pankoski, L.; Zekavat, A.; Demuth, D.R. Induction of cell cycle arrest in lymphocytes by Actinobacillus actinomycetemcomitans cytolethal distending toxin requires three subunits for maximum activity. *J. Immunol.* **2005**, *174*, 2228–2234. [CrossRef]
12. Shenker, B.J.; McKay, T.; Datar, S.; Miller, M.; Chowhan, R.; Demuth, D. Actinobacillus actinomycetemcomitans immunosuppressive protein is a member of the family of cytolethal distending toxins capable of causing a G2 arrest in human T cells. *J. Immunol.* **1999**, *162*, 4773–4780. [PubMed]
13. Thelestam, M.; Frisan, T. Cytolethal distending toxins. *Rev. Physiol. Biochem. Pharmacol.* **2004**, *152*, 111–133. [PubMed]
14. Boesze-Battaglia, K.; Alexander, D.; Dlakic, M.; Shenker, B.J. A Journey of Cytolethal Distending Toxins through Cell Membranes. *Front. Cell. Infect. Microbiol.* **2016**, *6*, 81. [CrossRef] [PubMed]
15. Cortes-Bratti, X.; Frisan, T.; Thelestam, M. The cytolethal distending toxins induce DNA damage and cell cycle arrest. *Toxicon* **2001**, *39*, 1729–1736. [CrossRef]
16. Cortes-Bratti, X.; Karlsson, C.; Lagergard, T.; Thelestam, M.; Frisan, T. The Haemophilus ducreyi cytolethal distending toxin induces cell cycle arrest and apoptosis via the DNA damage checkpoint pathways. *J. Biol. Chem.* **2001**, *276*, 5296–5302. [CrossRef] [PubMed]
17. Frisan, T.; Cortes-Bratti, X.; Chaves-Olarte, E.; Stenerlow, B.; Thelestam, M. The Haemophilus ducreyi cytolethal distending toxin induces DNA double-strand breaks and promotes ATM-dependent activation of RhoA. *Cell Microbiol.* **2003**, *5*, 695–707. [CrossRef]
18. Frisk, A.; Lebens, M.; Johansson, C.; Ahmed, H.; Svensson, L.; Ahlman, K.; Lagergard, T. The role of different protein components from the Haemophilus ducreyi cytolethal distending toxin in the generation of cell toxicity. *Microb. Pathog.* **2001**, *30*, 313–324. [CrossRef]
19. Guerra, L.; Carr, H.S.; Richter-Dahlfors, A.; Masucci, M.G.; Thelestam, M.; Frost, J.A.; Frisan, T. A bacterial cytotoxin identifies the RhoA exchange factor Net1 as a key effector in the response to DNA damage. *PLoS ONE* **2008**, *3*, e2254. [CrossRef]
20. Lara-Tejero, M.; Galan, J.E. A bacterial toxin that controls cell cycle progression as a deoxyribonuclease I-like protein. *Science* **2000**, *290*, 354–357. [CrossRef]
21. Li, L.; Sharipo, A.; Chaves-Olarte, E.; Masucci, M.G.; Levitsky, V.; Thelestam, M.; Frisan, T. The Haemophilus ducreyi cytolethal distending toxin activates sensors of DNA damage and repair complexes in proliferating and non-proliferating cells. *Cell Microbiol.* **2002**, *4*, 87–99. [CrossRef] [PubMed]
22. Nesic, D.; Stebbins, C.E. Mechanisms of assembly and cellular interactions for the bacterial genotoxin CDT. *PLoS Pathog.* **2005**, *1*, e28. [CrossRef] [PubMed]
23. Belibasakis, G.N.; Mattsson, A.; Wang, Y.; Chen, C.; Johansson, A. Cell cycle arrest of human gingival fibroblasts and periodontal ligament cells by Actinobacillus actinomycetemcomitans: Involvement of the cytolethal distending toxin. *APMIS* **2004**, *112*, 674–685. [CrossRef] [PubMed]
24. Shenker, B.J.; Boesze-Battaglia, K.; Scuron, M.D.; Walker, L.P.; Zekavat, A.; Dlakic, M. The toxicity of the Aggregatibacter actinomycetemcomitans cytolethal distending toxin correlates with its phosphatidylinositol-3,4,5-triphosphate phosphatase activity. *Cell Microbiol.* **2016**, *18*, 223–243. [CrossRef] [PubMed]
25. Shenker, B.J.; Boesze-Battaglia, K.; Zekavat, A.; Walker, L.; Besack, D.; Ali, H. Inhibition of mast cell degranulation by a chimeric toxin containing a novel phosphatidylinositol-3,4,5-triphosphate phosphatase. *Mol. Immunol.* **2010**, *48*, 203–210. [CrossRef] [PubMed]
26. Shenker, B.J.; Dlakic, M.; Walker, L.P.; Besack, D.; Jaffe, E.; LaBelle, E.; Boesze-Battaglia, K. A novel mode of action for a microbial-derived immunotoxin: The cytolethal distending toxin subunit B exhibits phosphatidylinositol 3,4,5-triphosphate phosphatase activity. *J. Immunol.* **2007**, *178*, 5099–5108. [CrossRef] [PubMed]

27. Shenker, B.J.; Walker, L.P.; Zekavat, A.; Boesze-Battaglia, K. Lymphoid susceptibility to the Aggregatibacter actinomycetemcomitans cytolethal distending toxin is dependent upon baseline levels of the signaling lipid, phosphatidylinositol-3,4,5-triphosphate. *Mol. Oral Microbiol.* **2016**, *31*, 33–42. [CrossRef]
28. Shenker, B.J.; Walker, L.P.; Zekavat, A.; Dlakic, M.; Boesze-Battaglia, K. Blockade of the PI-3K signalling pathway by the Aggregatibacter actinomycetemcomitans cytolethal distending toxin induces macrophages to synthesize and secrete pro-inflammatory cytokines. *Cell Microbiol.* **2014**, *16*, 1391–1404. [CrossRef]
29. Warfel, N.A.; El-Deiry, W.S. p21WAF1 and tumourigenesis: 20 years after. *Curr. Opin. Oncol.* **2013**, *25*, 52–58. [CrossRef]
30. Abbas, T.; Dutta, A. p21 in cancer: Intricate networks and multiple activities. *Nat. Rev. Cancer* **2009**, *9*, 400–414. [CrossRef]
31. Karimian, A.; Ahmadi, Y.; Yousefi, B. Multiple functions of p21 in cell cycle, apoptosis and transcriptional regulation after DNA damage. *DNA Repair* **2016**, *42*, 63–71. [CrossRef] [PubMed]
32. Romanov, V.S.; Pospelov, V.A.; Pospelova, T.V. Cyclin-dependent kinase inhibitor p21(Waf1): Contemporary view on its role in senescence and oncogenesis. *Biochemistry* **2012**, *77*, 575–584. [PubMed]
33. Dutto, I.; Tillhon, M.; Cazzalini, O.; Stivala, L.A.; Prosperi, E. Biology of the cell cycle inhibitor p21(CDKN1A): Molecular mechanisms and relevance in chemical toxicology. *Arch. Toxicol.* **2015**, *89*, 155–178. [CrossRef] [PubMed]
34. Graillot, V.; Dormoy, I.; Dupuy, J.; Shay, J.W.; Huc, L.; Mirey, G.; Vignard, J. Genotoxicity of Cytolethal Distending Toxin (CDT) on Isogenic Human Colorectal Cell Lines: Potential Promoting Effects for Colorectal Carcinogenesis. *Front. Cell. Infect. Microbiol.* **2016**, *6*, 34. [CrossRef]
35. Sato, T.; Koseki, T.; Yamato, K.; Saiki, K.; Konishi, K.; Yoshikawa, M.; Ishikawa, I.; Nishihara, T. p53-independent expression of p21(CIP1/WAF1) in plasmacytic cells during G(2) cell cycle arrest induced by Actinobacillus actinomycetemcomitans cytolethal distending toxin. *Infect. Immun.* **2002**, *70*, 528–534. [CrossRef]
36. Yamamoto, K.; Tominaga, K.; Sukedai, M.; Okinaga, T.; Iwanaga, K.; Nishihara, T.; Fukuda, J. Delivery of cytolethal distending toxin B induces cell cycle arrest and apoptosis in gingival squamous cell carcinoma in vitro. *Eur. J. Oral Sci.* **2004**, *112*, 445–451. [CrossRef]
37. Pere-Vedrenne, C.; Prochazkova-Carlotti, M.; Rousseau, B.; He, W.; Chambonnier, L.; Sifre, E.; Buissonniere, A.; Dubus, P.; Megraud, F.; Varon, C.; et al. The Cytolethal Distending Toxin Subunit CdtB of Helicobacter hepaticus Promotes Senescence and Endoreplication in Xenograft Mouse Models of Hepatic and Intestinal Cell Lines. *Front. Cell. Infect. Microbiol.* **2017**, *7*, 268. [CrossRef]
38. Alaoui-El-Azher, M.; Mans, J.J.; Baker, H.V.; Chen, C.; Progulske-Fox, A.; Lamont, R.J.; Handfield, M. Role of the ATM-checkpoint kinase 2 pathway in CDT-mediated apoptosis of gingival epithelial cells. *PLoS ONE* **2010**, *5*, e11714. [CrossRef]
39. Shenker, B.J.; Demuth, D.R.; Zekavat, A. Exposure of lymphocytes to high doses of Actinobacillus actinomycetemcomitans cytolethal distending toxin induces rapid onset of apoptosis-mediated DNA fragmentation. *Infect. Immun.* **2006**, *74*, 2080–2092. [CrossRef]
40. Zhou, B.P.; Hung, M.C. Novel targets of Akt, p21(Cipl/WAF1), and MDM2. *Semin. Oncol.* **2002**, *29* (Suppl. 11), 62–70. [CrossRef]
41. Rhodes, N.; Heerding, D.A.; Duckett, D.R.; Eberwein, D.J.; Knick, V.B.; Lansing, T.J.; McConnell, R.T.; Gilmer, T.M.; Zhang, S.Y.; Robell, K.; et al. Characterization of an Akt kinase inhibitor with potent pharmacodynamic and antitumor activity. *Cancer Res.* **2008**, *68*, 2366–2374. [CrossRef] [PubMed]
42. Wettersten, H.I.; Hee Hwang, S.; Li, C.; Shiu, E.Y.; Wecksler, A.T.; Hammock, B.D.; Weiss, R.H. A novel p21 attenuator which is structurally related to sorafenib. *Cancer Biol. Ther.* **2013**, *14*, 278–285. [CrossRef] [PubMed]
43. Shenker, B.J.; Hoffmaster, R.H.; Zekavat, A.; Yamaguchi, N.; Lally, E.T.; Demuth, D.R. Induction of apoptosis in human T cells by Actinobacillus actinomycetemcomitans cytolethal distending toxin is a consequence of G2 arrest of the cell cycle. *J. Immunol.* **2001**, *167*, 435–441. [CrossRef] [PubMed]
44. Diehl, M.C.; Idowu, M.O.; Kimmelshue, K.; York, T.P.; Elmore, L.W.; Holt, S.E. Elevated expression of nuclear Hsp90 in invasive breast tumors. *Cancer Biol. Ther.* **2009**, *8*, 1952–1961. [CrossRef]
45. Jascur, T.; Brickner, H.; Salles-Passador, I.; Barbier, V.; El Khissiin, A.; Smith, B.; Fotedar, R.; Fotedar, A. Regulation of p21(WAF1/CIP1) stability by WISp39, a Hsp90 binding TPR protein. *Mol. Cell* **2005**, *17*, 237–249. [CrossRef]

46. Schopf, F.H.; Biebl, M.M.; Buchner, J. The HSP90 chaperone machinery. *Nat. Rev. Mol. Cell Biol.* **2017**, *18*, 345–360. [CrossRef]
47. Sugimoto, K.; Sasaki, M.; Isobe, Y.; Tsutsui, M.; Suto, H.; Ando, J.; Tamayose, K.; Ando, M.; Oshimi, K. Hsp90-inhibitor geldanamycin abrogates G2 arrest in p53-negative leukemia cell lines through the depletion of Chk1. *Oncogene* **2008**, *27*, 3091–3101. [CrossRef]
48. Gartel, A.L. The conflicting roles of the cdk inhibitor p21(CIP1/WAF1) in apoptosis. *Leuk. Res.* **2005**, *29*, 1237–1238. [CrossRef]
49. Ghanem, L.; Steinman, R. A proapoptotic function of p21 in differentiating granulocytes. *Leuk. Res.* **2005**, *29*, 1315–1323. [CrossRef]
50. Giordano, C.; Rovito, D.; Barone, I.; Mancuso, R.; Bonofiglio, D.; Giordano, F.; Catalano, S.; Gabriele, B.; Ando, S. Benzofuran-2-acetic ester derivatives induce apoptosis in breast cancer cells by upregulating p21(Cip/WAF1) gene expression in p53-independent manner. *DNA Repair* **2017**, *51*, 20–30. [CrossRef]
51. Kang, K.H.; Kim, W.H.; Choi, K.H. p21 promotes ceramide-induced apoptosis and antagonizes the antideath effect of Bcl-2 in human hepatocarcinoma cells. *Exp. Cell Res.* **1999**, *253*, 403–412. [CrossRef] [PubMed]
52. Lincet, H.; Poulain, L.; Remy, J.S.; Deslandes, E.; Duigou, F.; Gauduchon, P.; Staedel, C. The p21(cip1/waf1) cyclin-dependent kinase inhibitor enhances the cytotoxic effect of cisplatin in human ovarian carcinoma cells. *Cancer Lett.* **2000**, *161*, 17–26. [CrossRef]
53. Poole, A.J.; Heap, D.; Carroll, R.E.; Tyner, A.L. Tumor suppressor functions for the Cdk inhibitor p21 in the mouse colon. *Oncogene* **2004**, *23*, 8128–8134. [CrossRef] [PubMed]
54. Qiao, L.; McKinstry, R.; Gupta, S.; Gilfor, D.; Windle, J.J.; Hylemon, P.B.; Grant, S.; Fisher, P.B.; Dent, P. Cyclin kinase inhibitor p21 potentiates bile acid-induced apoptosis in hepatocytes that is dependent on p53. *Hepatology* **2002**, *36*, 39–48. [CrossRef] [PubMed]
55. Liu, R.; Wettersten, H.I.; Park, S.H.; Weiss, R.H. Small-molecule inhibitors of p21 as novel therapeutics for chemotherapy-resistant kidney cancer. *Future Med. Chem.* **2013**, *5*, 991–994. [CrossRef] [PubMed]
56. Child, E.S.; Mann, D.J. The intricacies of p21 phosphorylation: Protein/protein interactions, subcellular localization and stability. *Cell Cycle* **2006**, *5*, 1313–1319. [CrossRef]
57. Rossig, L.; Jadidi, A.S.; Urbich, C.; Badorff, C.; Zeiher, A.M.; Dimmeler, S. Akt-dependent phosphorylation of p21(Cip1) regulates PCNA binding and proliferation of endothelial cells. *Mol. Cell Biol.* **2001**, *21*, 5644–5657. [CrossRef]
58. Li, Y.; Dowbenko, D.; Lasky, L.A. AKT/PKB phosphorylation of p21Cip/WAF1 enhances protein stability of p21Cip/WAF1 and promotes cell survival. *J. Biol. Chem.* **2002**, *277*, 11352–11361. [CrossRef]
59. Zhou, B.P.; Liao, Y.; Xia, W.; Spohn, B.; Lee, M.H.; Hung, M.C. Cytoplasmic localization of p21Cip1/WAF1 by Akt-induced phosphorylation in HER-2/neu-overexpressing cells. *Nat. Cell Biol.* **2001**, *3*, 245–252. [CrossRef]
60. Liyanage, N.P.; Manthey, K.C.; Dassanayake, R.P.; Kuszynski, C.A.; Oakley, G.G.; Duhamel, G.E. Helicobacter hepaticus cytolethal distending toxin causes cell death in intestinal epithelial cells via mitochondrial apoptotic pathway. *Helicobacter* **2010**, *15*, 98–107. [CrossRef]
61. Ohara, M.; Hayashi, T.; Kusunoki, Y.; Nakachi, K.; Fujiwara, T.; Komatsuzawa, H.; Sugai, M. Cytolethal distending toxin induces caspase-dependent and -independent cell death in MOLT-4 cells. *Infect. Immun.* **2008**, *76*, 4783–4791. [CrossRef] [PubMed]
62. Gogada, R.; Amadori, M.; Zhang, H.; Jones, A.; Verone, A.; Pitarresi, J.; Jandhyam, S.; Prabhu, V.; Black, J.D.; Chandra, D. Curcumin induces Apaf-1-dependent, p21-mediated caspase activation and apoptosis. *Cell Cycle* **2011**, *10*, 4128–4137. [CrossRef] [PubMed]
63. Shenker, B.J.; Ali, H.; Boesze-Battaglia, K. PIP3 regulation as promising targeted therapy of mast-cell-mediated diseases. *Curr. Pharm. Des.* **2011**, *17*, 3815–3822. [CrossRef] [PubMed]
64. Shenker, B.J.; Ojcius, D.M.; Walker, L.P.; Zekavat, A.; Scuron, M.D.; Boesze-Battaglia, K. Aggregatibacter actinomycetemcomitans cytolethal distending toxin activates the NLRP3 inflammasome in human macrophages, leading to the release of proinflammatory cytokines. *Infect. Immun.* **2015**, *83*, 1487–1496. [CrossRef]
65. Boesze-Battaglia, K.; Brown, A.; Walker, L.; Besack, D.; Zekavat, A.; Wrenn, S.; Krummenacher, C.; Shenker, B.J. Cytolethal distending toxin-induced cell cycle arrest of lymphocytes is dependent upon recognition and binding to cholesterol. *J. Biol. Chem.* **2009**, *284*, 10650–10658. [CrossRef]

66. Shenker, B.J.; Hoffmaster, R.H.; McKay, T.L.; Demuth, D.R. Expression of the cytolethal distending toxin (Cdt) operon in Actinobacillus actinomycetemcomitans: Evidence that the CdtB protein is responsible for G2 arrest of the cell cycle in human T cells. *J. Immunol.* **2000**, *165*, 2612–2618. [CrossRef]
67. Shenker, B.J.; McArthur, W.P.; Tsai, C.C. Immune suppression induced by Actinobacillus actinomycetemcomitans. I. Effects on human peripheral blood lymphocyte responses to mitogens and antigens. *J. Immunol.* **1982**, *128*, 148–154.
68. Boesze-Battaglia, K.; Walker, L.P.; Dhingra, A.; Kandror, K.; Tang, H.Y.; Shenker, B.J. Internalization of the Active Subunit of the Aggregatibacter actinomycetemcomitans Cytolethal Distending Toxin Is Dependent upon Cellugyrin (Synaptogyrin 2), a Host Cell Non-Neuronal Paralog of the Synaptic Vesicle Protein, Synaptogyrin 1. *Front. Cell. Infect. Microbiol.* **2017**, *7*, 469. [CrossRef]

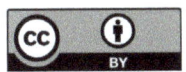

© 2020 by the authors. Licensee MDPI, Basel, Switzerland. This article is an open access article distributed under the terms and conditions of the Creative Commons Attribution (CC BY) license (http://creativecommons.org/licenses/by/4.0/).

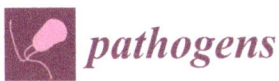

Article

Transcriptomic Analysis of *Aggregatibacter actinomycetemcomitans* Core and Accessory Genes in Different Growth Conditions

Natalia O. Tjokro [1,†], Weerayuth Kittichotirat [2,†], Annamari Torittu [3], Riikka Ihalin [3], Roger E. Bumgarner [4] and Casey Chen [1,*]

1. Division of Periodontology, Diagnostic Sciences, and Dental Hygiene, Herman Ostrow School of Dentistry, University of Southern California, 925 West 34th Street, Los Angeles, CA 90089, USA; tjokro@usc.edu
2. Systems Biology and Bioinformatics Research Group, Pilot Plant Development and Training Institute, King Mongkut's University of Technology Thonburi, Bangkok 10150, Thailand; weerayuth.kit@kmutt.ac.th
3. Department of Biochemistry, University of Turku, FI-20014 Turku, Finland; atorittu@abo.fi (A.T.); riikka.ihalin@utu.fi (R.I.)
4. Department of Microbiology, University of Washington, Seattle, WA 98109, USA; rogerb@uw.edu
* Correspondence: ccchen@usc.edu; Tel.: +1-213-740-7407
† These authors contributed equally to this work.

Received: 10 October 2019; Accepted: 29 November 2019; Published: 3 December 2019

Abstract: *Aggregatibacter actinomycetemcomitans* genome can be divided into an accessory gene pool (found in some but not all strains) and a core gene pool (found in all strains). The functions of the accessory genes (genomic islands and non-island accessory genes) are largely unknown. We hypothesize that accessory genes confer critical functions for *A. actinomycetemcomitans* in vivo. This study examined the expression patterns of accessory and core genes of *A. actinomycetemcomitans* in distinct growth conditions. We found similar expression patterns of island and non-island accessory genes, which were generally lower than the core genes in all growth conditions. The median expression levels of genomic islands were 29%–37% of the core genes in enriched medium but elevated to as high as 63% of the core genes in nutrient-limited media. Several putative virulence genes, including the cytolethal distending toxin operon, were found to be activated in nutrient-limited conditions. In conclusion, genomic islands and non-island accessory genes exhibited distinct patterns of expression from the core genes and may play a role in the survival of *A. actinomycetemcomitans* in nutrient-limited environments.

Keywords: *A. actinomycetemcomitans*; RNA-Seq; genomic islands; core genes; accessory genes; stress; nutrient limitation; differentially expressed genes

1. Introduction

Gram-negative facultative *A. actinomycetemcomitans* is an oral commensal bacterium and a major causative agent of periodontitis, as well as an occasional cause of extra-oral infections [1–4]. The species comprises genetically heterogeneous strains that display differential association with periodontal health, disease, or disease progression, suggesting a pattern of strain-dependent virulence potentials including an example of a well-characterized highly leukotoxic JP2 type [5–9]. Beyond disease-association, genetically distinct *A. actinomycetemcomitans* strains are expected to be phenotypically distinct, which has been observed but not fully investigated [7,8,10,11]. In the landmark study by Socransky et al. [12], the correlation analysis of subgingival bacterial species identified discrete bacterial complexes (each composed of different species), suggesting either niche-sharing or metabolic interdependence of the bacteria within the complexes. Interestingly, *A. actinomycetemcomitans* serotype a and serotype b strains have different patterns of microbial associations, which may be indicative of differences in phenotypes and preferred niches.

Comparative genomics by whole genome sequencing has identified five evolutionarily distinct clades among human strains of *A. actinomycetemcomitans*, which are separated from an *A. actinomycetemcomitans* strain isolated from a Rhesus monkey and strains of a closely related oral species *Aggregatibacter aphrophilus* [13,14]. The evolutionary divergence of *A. actinomycetemcomitans* is marked by the acquisitions of strain- and clade-specific accessory genes via horizontal gene transfer. Within *A. actinomycetemcomitans*, strains of different clades may differ by as much as 20% in their genomic content. Large scale genomic rearrangements have also been noted among *A. actinomycetemcomitans* strains of different clades [15].

Accessory genes, including those organized into genomic islands, accounted for 14.1%–23.2% of the *A. actinomycetemcomitans* genomes. A total of 387 genomic islands of 5 Kb or larger have been identified among 31 *A. actinomycetemcomitans* strains. With a few exceptions, such as the genomic island that carries genetic determinants for cytolethal distending toxins, the functions of these islands are largely unknown. As a first step to probe the functions of genomic islands and other non-island accessory genes, this study examined the patterns of gene expression of *A. actinomycetemcomitans* in different growth conditions. We compared the gene expression profiles of a wild type biofilm-forming *A. actinomycetemcomitans* D7S-1 in enriched trypticase soy broth with yeast extract (modified Trypticase Soy Broth, mTSB) and two nutrient-limited media (RPMI and keratinocyte medium) commonly used in co-cultures of bacteria and mammalian cells. We also examined the gene expression profiles of *A. actinomycetemcomitans* D7S-1 and its isogenic non-fimbriated mutant strain D7SS in mTSB. The results showed that genomic islands and non-island accessory genes exhibited similar patterns of gene expression, and exhibited lower levels of expression than core genes in all growth conditions. However, accessory genes, including genomic islands, were highly active in nutrient-limited media. A few virulence genes, such as cytolethal distending toxin operon, were upregulated in response to nutrient-limitation. The results suggest that accessory genes, including genomic islands, may be critical for bacterial adaptation under nutrient-limitation stress.

2. Results

2.1. Core Genes, Accessory Genes, and Genomic Islands

The 2041 protein-coding genes identified in the genome of *A. actinomycetemcomitans* strain D7S-1 were first categorized into core (N = 1608) and accessory (N = 433) genes. The latter included 191 non-island accessory genes, and 242 island genes organized into 26 genomic islands of 5 Kb or larger (see Supplementary Table S1 for details of the genomic islands). Fourteen islands were found in at least one other *A. actinomycetemcomitans* strain, while the remaining 12 islands were unique to strain D7S-1 (details of the distribution of genomic islands among all sequenced *A. actinomycetemcomitans* strains will be published elsewhere). Cumulatively these 26 islands had a footprint of 275,927 bps or 12% of the D7S-1 genome.

2.2. Differences in the Patterns of Gene Expression among Core, Accessory, and Island Genes

For each gene, the transcript level was the average of 3 biological replicates in each growth condition. To validate the expression levels obtained by RNA-Seq, quantitative real-time PCR (qRT-PCR) was also performed on selected genes (D7S_02294 *cdtA*, D7S_02295 *cdtB*, D7S_00244 *metF*, D7S_00604 *ltxA*). The correlations between the results obtained by qRT-PCR and RNA-Seq were shown in Supplementary Figure S1. Three of the four genes demonstrated excellent correlations between results obtained by qRT-PCR and RNA-Seq (R = 0.81–0.91). The expression levels of *ltxA* did not show good correlations between the two quantification methods probably due to experimental variables that were difficult to replicate between experiments, and this phenomenon had been observed previously [16].

The phenotypes of *A. actinomycetemcomitans* biofilms were first examined by assessing the optical density of the biofilm cultures. *A. actinomycetemcomitans* D7S-1 grew in the enriched mTSB, but did not show evidence of growth in the nutrient-limited media. We then determined the viability of *A. actinomycetemcomitans* D7S-1 by enumerating the CFU of the bacteria in the biofilms over time.

The results showed that *A. actinomycetemcomitans* D7S-1 grew in the enriched mTSB (as expected), maintained its viability in RPMI without apparent growth, and showed a reduced viability in keratinocyte medium (see Supplementary Materials Figure S2 for details). Therefore, RPMI and keratinocyte medium exerted two distinct types of nutrient-limitation stress to *A. actinomycetemcomitans*.

The combined expression levels of 4 experimental conditions for core, non-island accessory genes, and island genes are shown in Figure 1. The expression levels were statistically significantly different between core and non-island accessory genes or island genes in each of the tested conditions or in all conditions (the range of the p-values was 10^{-8} to 10^{-148} by Student's *t*-test. See Supplementary Table S2 for detailed information). The mode of the expression of non-island accessory or island genes was 2^7 transcripts, while the mode of expression of the core genes was 2^8 transcripts. The patterns of gene expressions were similar between non-island accessory and island genes (Supplementary Table S2). Henceforth, as appropriate, some results focused on the comparison between core and island genes.

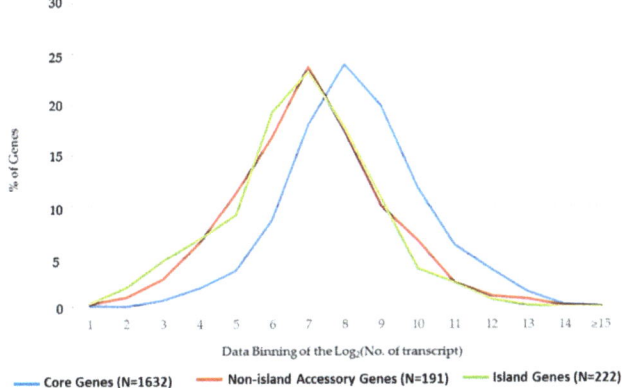

Figure 1. Distribution patterns of gene expression among core, non-island accessory and island genes. The expression signals were $\log_2$-transformed and binned 1 to ≥ 15 on the x-axis. 1 represents up to 2 copies of the transcript, and 2 represents up to 4 copies of transcripts et cetera.

The differences in the expression levels of core and island genes were examined in each of the four growth conditions. The mean and median expression levels of core and island genes were listed in Supplementary Table S3. We noted that island genes were expressed at higher levels in nutrient-limited media than in the enriched mTSB. Figure 2 showed that the activation of island genes was particularly pronounced when bacteria were cultured in RPMI. The results suggested that island genes were activated by stress associated with nutrient deprivation. Individual genes up- or down-regulated in these two nutrient-limited media were distinct (see Section 2.3 below).

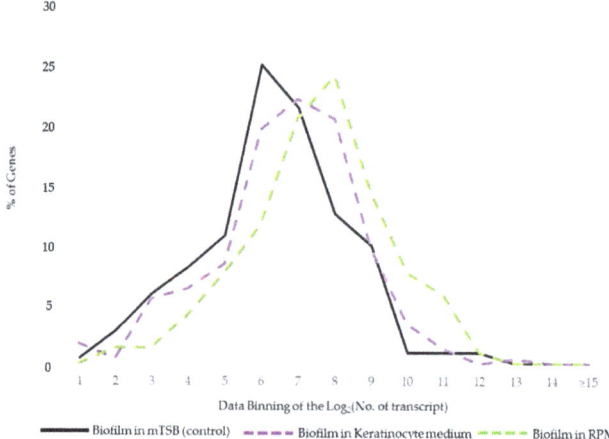

Figure 2. Differential expression of island genes in distinct growth conditions. The expression signals were $\log_2$-transformed and binned 1 to ≥15 on the x-axis.

2.3. Differentially Expressed Genes of A. actinomycetemcomitans

The numbers of differentially expressed genes in different growth conditions were listed in Table 1. Annotations of these genes were provided in Supplementary Table S4.

Table 1. Differentially expressed A. actinomycetemcomitans genes in different growth conditions.

	Up 1.5-Fold **			Down 1.5-Fold **		
Growth Condition *	Core	Non-Island Accessory Genes	Island Genes	Core	Non-Island Accessory Genes	Island Genes
Planktonic in mTSB	66	4	9	143	10	10
Biofilm in Keratinocyte Medium	454	53	72	145	13	13
Biofilm in RPMI	515	115	158	352	22	17

* As compared to biofilm in modified Trypticase Soy Broth (mTSB) control. ** Statistically significant at $p < 0.05$ by Student's t-test.

As expected, the greatest differences in gene expression levels between planktonic cells and biofilms were found in the fimbrial gene operon, which was down-regulated in planktonic cells (Supplementary Table S4). Other notable differentially expressed genes between planktonic and biofilms of *A. actinomycetemcomitans* included the genes PTS mannose transporter subunit IIAB (D7S_01753) (down-regulated), thiamine ABC transporter substrate-binding protein (D7S_02132) (upregulated), superoxide dismutase (D7S_01907) (upregulated), and peptide methionine sulfoxide reductase (D7S_00462) (upregulated). Relatively high numbers of differentially expressed genes were detected when *A. actinomycetemcomitans* strain D7S-1 was cultured in keratinocyte medium and more so in RPMI. More than 70% of island genes (as well as non-island accessory genes) of *A. actinomycetemcomitans* strain D7S-1 were differentially expressed in response to RPMI, with more than three-quarter of the genes upregulated.

Figure 3 showed differentially expressed genes (both accessory and core genes) in keratinocytes medium and RPMI grouped according to the Cluster of Orthologous Group (COG) categories. There were more upregulated genes compared to those that were downregulated in both media. Keratinocytes medium had about 35% of the upregulated genes belong to COG S whose functions were still unknown. About 46% of the genes in COG V (defense mechanism) were upregulated, and about 31% of genes in

COG Q (secondary metabolites biosynthesis, transport, and catabolism) were downregulated genes in RPMI. These might make good targets to determine genes and pathways involved in cellular responses to the stress of nutrient limitation.

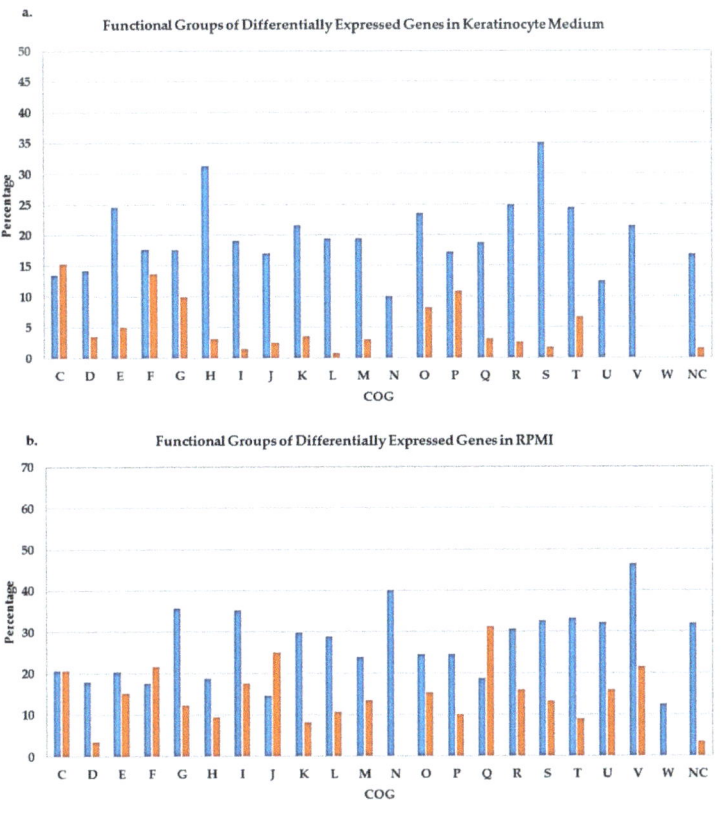

Figure 3. Cluster of Orthologous Groups (COG) functional categories of differentially expressed genes in keratinocyte medium (**a**) and RPMI (**b**). The y-axis is the percentage of differentially expressed genes. (**C**) Energy production and conversion, (**D**) cell cycle control, cell division, chromosome partitioning, (**E**) amino acid transport and metabolism, (**F**) nucleotide transport and metabolism, (**G**) carbohydrate transport and metabolism, (**H**) coenzyme transport and metabolism, (**I**) lipid transport and metabolism, (**J**) translation, ribosomal structure and biogenesis, (**K**) transcription, (**L**) replication, recombination and repair, (**M**) cell wall/membrane/envelope biogenesis, (**N**) cell motility, (**O**) posttranslational modification, protein turnover, chaperones, (**P**) inorganic ion transport and metabolism, (**Q**) secondary metabolites biosynthesis, transport and catabolism, (**R**) general function prediction only, (**S**) function unknown, (**T**) signal transduction mechanisms, (**U**) intracellular trafficking, secretion, and vesicular transport, (**V**) defense mechanism, (**W**) extracellular structure, (**NC**) not categorized.

KEGG-style metabolic networks were used to analyze biological pathways that might be affected by these differentially expressed genes. In keratinocyte medium, pathways affected included those involved in ribosomal biosynthesis, carbon metabolism, quorum sensing, microbial metabolism in diverse environments, and aminoacyl-tRNA biosynthesis. On the other hand, only ribosomal biosynthesis pathway was found to be affected significantly by the differentially expressed genes in RPMI medium.

These affected biological pathways seemed to have functions that might contribute to increasing the survival likelihood of *A. actinomycetemcomitans* under the stress of nutrient limitation.

Most of the genomic islands and a few selected *A. actinomycetemcomitans* virulence genes were upregulated in nutrient-limited media. These included the lipopolysaccharides biosynthesis genes in RPMI (2.3-fold) and keratinocyte medium (2.2-fold), the metal-binding heat shock protein upregulated in keratinocyte medium (1.5-fold) and RPMI (4-fold). Notably, a 24 Kb genomic island (here designated as *cdt*-island) that carried *cdtABC* was highly active and upregulated in *A. actinomycetemcomitans* exposed to RPMI, and also in keratinocyte medium to a lesser extent (Figure 4). The *cdtABC* was upregulated in both RPMI (2.5- to 3-fold) and keratinocyte medium (1.6- to 2-fold). Twenty of the 27 *cdt*-island genes, including *cdtABC* were upregulated in response to RPMI.

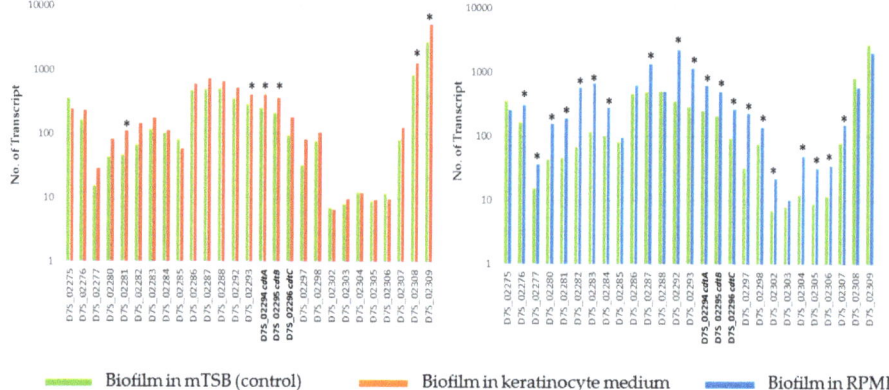

Figure 4. Expression levels of the 24 Kb cdt-island of D7S-1 biofilm in keratinocyte medium (**left** panel) or RPMI (**right** panel) in comparison to control in mTSB. The cdtABC are marked with bold font. See Supplementary Table S3 for annotation of other island genes. * Statistically significant at $p < 0.05$ by Student's t-test between biofilm in keratinocyte medium and control.

3. Discussion

Bacterial species are constantly evolving, and a prime example of this is the increasing occurrence of superbugs that are resistant to multiple antibiotics. Genomic islands are speculated to have contributed significantly to this phenomenon as they are involved in the dissemination of accessory genes, including antibiotic resistance and virulence genes. Genomic islands and the horizontal gene transfer process has been hypothesized to be a major force driving genome evolution [17–21]. Bioinformatics studies have also shown that genomic islands tend to carry genes that are considered novel, those with no orthologues in other species [22]. This suggests that genomic islands have been selected for adaptive and auxiliary functions [23].

The phenotypic variations observed in *A. actinomycetemcomitans* [5–9] are probably best explained by strain-to-strain variations in genome content. Core genes of *A. actinomycetemcomitans* presumably played significant housekeeping functions for the basic survival of the bacteria. In this study, the higher levels of expression of core genes and their relatively stable levels of expression in different conditions might, therefore, correlate with core genes' functions for basic functions of *A. actinomycetemcomitans*. In this study, the core genes were identified by comparative genomics and may or may not be the same as essential genes that require experimental confirmation. A previous study utilizing rapid transposon mutant sequencing (Tn-Seq) had established the presence of essential genomes in two divergent *A. actinomycetemcomitans* strains, VT1169 and 624 strains [24]. Notably, 307 of the 319 essential genes matched to our core gene pool. Other core genes of strain D7S-1 may also be essential for growth conditions not tested in the previous study.

The activation of *cdtABC* observed in this study may be a survival mechanism for *A. actinomycetemcomitans* in response to limited nutrients. The cytolethal distending toxin produced by *A. actinomycetemcomitans* is a trimeric holotoxin. *cdt*B is the toxin, while *cdt*A and *cdt*C facilitate the binding and entry of the toxin into the cells. The *cdt*B toxin enters the cells and traffics to the nucleus, where its DNase and lipid phosphatase activities lead to DNA damage and induce apoptosis and subsequently cell death in a variety of cell types [25–31]. *cdt*B may also elevate the expression level of receptor activator of nuclear factor kappa-B ligand with potential for osteoclastogenesis and bone loss [32,33]. The tissue damages and inflammatory responses triggered by *cdtABC* toxin could be a mechanism for nutrient acquisition by *A. actinomycetemcomitans*.

There is a paucity of information regarding the regulation of *cdtABC* in *A. actinomycetemcomitans*. Shenker et al. showed evidence for the expression of a 5-gene operon comprised of *orf1*, *orf2*, *cdtA*, *cdtB*, and *cdtC* [25]. The functions of the upstream *orf1*, *orf2* (homologous to D7S_02292 and D7S_02293 on the *cdt*-island in this study) were unknown. The environmental signals that activated the *cdtABC* operon remained to be determined. Here we showed evidence that, in addition to *cdtABC* and the homologs of *orf1* and *orf2*, several other genes on the D7S-1 *cdt*-island were similarly upregulated in response to RPMI. It is unclear whether D7S-1 *cdt*-island is regulated by a single promoter to generate a long polycistronic transcript for more than five genes defined by Shenker et al. [25]. We have noted the structural dis-similarities in the *cdtABC* loci among genetically distinct *A. actinomycetemcomitans* strains. There are at least three distinct *cdtABC* variants [13]. The first was represented by the 24 Kb *cdt*-island of strain D7S-1 in this study. The second is 5 Kb in size and found in serotype b and c strains [13]. The third is represented by a 22 Kb genomic island designated as GIY4-1 described by Doungudomdacha et al. [34]. It is likely that there are multiple regulation mechanisms for *cdtABC* in genetically distinct *A. actinomycetemcomitans* strains. More details of the structure and gene compositions of the distinct *cdtABC* loci among *A. actinomycetemcomitans* strains will be published elsewhere. Moreover, *A. actinomycetemcomitans* leukotoxin expression has been shown to be regulated by growth conditions such as iron availability and anaerobiosis [35,36]. The specific environmental signals that regulate the expression of *cdtABC* in D7S-1 remain to be elucidated.

Kawamoto et al. [37] examined the toxic activity of forty-one strains of *A. actinomycetemcomitans* on Chinese hamster ovary cells. The results demonstrated differences in cytotoxicity among strains. Serotype b and c strains appeared to be more cytotoxic than serotype a strains. Our study is limited to a single strain of serotype a and therefore the results are not comparable. It will be interesting to examine whether the differences in cytotoxicity attributed to cytolethal distending toxin could be explained by different genetic regulatory elements of *cdtABC* among *A. actinomycetemcomitans* strains.

Several genes involved in LPS biosynthesis were found to be upregulated in poor nutrient RPMI and keratinocyte media in this study. The transcription of LPS genes is upregulated under limited nutrient availability [38]. Changing the bacterial membrane structures and their fluidity have been proposed to be a stress response that allows bacteria to limit exchanges, save energy, and survive, which may also promote biofilm formation [39–43]. Therefore, the observed changes in LPS gene expression may be a stress response of A. actinomycetemcomitans to starvation. Whether nutrient-limitation of A. actinomycetemcomitans leads to greater amounts of biofilm formation requires further studies.

Differential gene expressions between *A. actinomycetemcomitans* in its planktonic and biofilm states had been observed previously [44], and our study confirmed their observations on several genes. The gene PTS mannose transporter subunit IIAB (D7S_01753) was found to be upregulated by both studies. On the other hand, the genes thiamine ABC transporter substrate-binding protein (D7S_02132), superoxide dismutase (D7S_01907), and peptide methionine sulfoxide reductase (D7S_00462) were found to be downregulated by both studies. The results may suggest different metabolic characteristics between planktonic and sessile *A. actinomycetemcomitans*.

During infection, bacteria cells are constantly exposed to various stresses of the environment, including drastic changes in temperature, pH, osmolarity, and nutritional availability. In order to survive, bacteria must cope with these stresses by regulating various gene expressions, and they are equipped with multiple mechanisms of stress responses. In the oral cavity, *A. actinomycetemcomitans* is subjected to the stress of different pH, heat, and nutrient availability [45]. In response to these environmental challenges, *A. actinomycetemcomitans* induces the expression of heat shock proteins (HSPs) that offered protection to them [46,47]. Our data provide additional evidence of HSPs involvement in *A. actinomycetemcomitans* stress response. In both keratinocyte and RPMI media, the transcription of metal-binding heat shock protein (D7S_01459) was found to be significantly upregulated. Although the importance of HSPs are evident, neither the mechanisms of protection by HSPs nor the cellular responses to the stress of nutrient limitation in *A. actinomycetemcomitans* is fully understood. Given the fact that a high percentage of upregulated genes in both RPMI and keratinocytes are those whose functions are still unknown, these genes can be targeted to study genes and pathways involved in cellular starvation responses.

In conclusion, our study showed that patterns and levels of expression of accessory genes (island and non-island genes) are different from core genes in *A. actinomycetemcomitans*. Notably, the accessory genes were activated in nutrient-limited growth conditions. We hypothesize that accessory genes, including genomic islands, are essential for the survival of *A. actinomycetemcomitans* in the in vivo-like conditions.

4. Materials and Methods

4.1. Bacterial Strains and Growth Conditions

A. actinomycetemcomitans strain D7S-1 and its isogenic nonfimbriated mutant D7SS were routinely grown in modified Trypticase Soy Broth (mTSB) containing 3% trypticase soy broth and 0.6% yeast extract, or on mTSB agar (mTSB with 1.5% agar (Becton Dickinson and Company)), and incubated in atmosphere supplemented with 5% CO_2 at 37 °C in a humidified incubator. The antibiotics rifampicin (100 µg/mL), nalidixic acid (50 µg/mL), and spectinomycin (50 µg/mL) were added when appropriate. In some experiments the bacteria were cultured in RPMI (Sigma, St. Louis, Missouri, USA, Catalog #: R0883), or in a keratinocyte medium (Green's medium) [48] consisted of 63% Dulbecco's modified Eagle's medium (DMEM, Life Technologies, Paisley, UK) supplemented with 0.14% $NAHCO_3$ and 13mM Hepes, 25% Ham-F-12-medium (Life Technologies), 10% Fetal bovine serum (Life Technologies), 4 mM L-glutamine (Life Technologies), 5 µg/mL Insulin (Sigma), 0.4 µg/mL Hydrocortisone (Sigma), 5 ng/mL Epidermal growth factor, EGF (Sigma), 0.1 nM Cholera toxin (Sigma), 1.8 µg/mL Adenine (Sigma) and 100 µg/mL freshly added Ascorbic acid (Sigma).

4.2. Transcriptomic Analysis via RNA-Seq

Transcriptomic analysis of log-phase bacteria was performed in 4 experimental conditions, each with three biological replicates. These included the growth of planktonic strain D7SS in mTSB, the growth of biofilm-forming strain D7S-1 in mTSB, RPMI and Green's medium. The starter bacterial cultures were prepared by transferring 10–15 colonies of bacteria from agar into 5 ml of mTSB and incubated overnight in atmosphere supplemented with 5% CO_2 at 37 °C in a humidified incubator. The colony forming unit/ml was estimated based on optical density (OD_{600} = 1 is equivalent to 10^9/mL).

An aliquot (0.2–0.4 mL) of the bacterial culture containing 10^8 CFU was transferred into each well of a polystyrene 6-well tissue culture plate (Multiwell™, Becton Dickinson, New Jersey, USA), and 3 mL of fresh mTSB was added to each well. The plate was then incubated for 20 h. For biofilm-forming D7S-1, the culture supernatant was removed and the biofilm attached to the bottom of the well was gently rinsed with warm fresh medium once, and then 2 mL of fresh mTSB, RPMI or keratinocyte medium was added, and incubated for 6 h. Afterward, the supernatant was removed, and 0.7 mL of RNAlater® (ThermoFisher Scientific, Waltham, Massachusetts, USA) was added to each well. The bacterial cells were then collected with the aid of a cell scraper (Greiner Bio-One, Monroe, North Carolina, USA), pelleted by centrifugation at 10,000 rpm for 2 min, kept at 4 °C for one hour, and then stored at −80 °C until used.

For the non-biofilm forming planktonic D7SS, after the same 20-hour incubation, 2 mL of the culture was removed (leaving 1 mL of the overnight culture), replaced with 2 mL of pre-warmed fresh mTSB, and incubated for 6 h. At the end of the 6-hour incubation, OD_{600} was measured again to assure that the bacteria were still in the log phase. Next, 1 mL of RNA*later*® was added into each well, and bacterial cells were harvested as above. After the supernatant was discarded, 0.7 mL of RNAlater® was added to the cells, incubated at 4 °C for 1 h, and then stored at −80 °C until use.

Total RNA was extracted using the Ribo-Pure Bacterial RNA isolation kit following the manufacturer's instructions (Life Technology, Grand Island, NY, USA). Briefly, 1.0×10^9 cells were lysed using zirconia beads, and the lysate was mixed with chloroform. The RNA was extracted in the top aqueous phase, cleaned, and treated with DNase to prepare for RNA sequencing. The purified mRNA was fragmented using divalent cations at elevated temperature. Cleaved RNA fragments were copied into first-strand cDNA using reverse transcriptase and random primers, followed by second-strand cDNA synthesis using DNA polymerase I and RNase H. cDNA products were purified and enriched by PCR to create a final cDNA library using the TruSeq Stranded Total RNA sample preparation kit (Illumina, San Diego, CA, USA). After sequencing, the reads for each sample were mapped to the corresponding genomes for each strain using the Geneious software (Biomatters LTD, Auckland, New Zealand). After mapping, the average coverage (number of sequences/nucleotide) was calculated for each predicted gene. Coverage was normalized by averaging across all genes for each sample and scaled up by multiplying by a factor of 1000. These RNA-Seq data are available via BioProject accession number PRJNA575215.

The replication and the viability of *A. actinomycetemcomitans* biofilms in tested media were evaluated. The replication of *A. actinomycetemcomitans* was examined by the measuring the optical density of the cell cultures at 600 nm. Briefly, the bacteria were collected from agar plates, resuspended in the media and adjusted to approximately 10^8 CFU/mL. The optical density of the cultures was recorded for 48 h. The viability of *A. actinomycetemcomitans* in the tested media was determined by enumerating CFU of the cultures. Briefly, biofilms were prepared in tissue culture wells as described above and incubated in each of the tested media. At specific time points, the cells were collected, serially diluted in the media and plated on mTSB agar. The plates were incubated in atmosphere supplemented with 5% CO_2 at 37 °C in a humidified incubator for 3–4 days to enumerate CFU. All experiments were performed in biological triplicates.

4.3. Metabolic Network

To determine pathways affected by the differentially expressed genes, we used the KEGG Mapper Search and Color Pathway tool as previously described [24,49] using the locus tag of each differentially expressed genes obtained from each media. A comparison of the pathways affected were then attempted.

4.4. Quantitative Real-Time PCR (qRT-PCR)

The relative gene expression levels by RNA-Seq were confirmed by qRT-PCR using BioRad iCycler iQ®Real-Time PCR Detection System as described previously [16] for the following genes: *cdtA* (D7S_02294), *cdtB* (D7S_02295), *ltxA* (D7S_00604), and *metF* (D7S_00244). A constitutively expressed house-keeping gene *clpX* (D7S_01693) was used as a reference to compare the expression levels [50]. For each sample, 1 μg of RNA in a 20 μL reaction mixture was reverse transcribed into first strand cDNA using SuperScript VILO kit (ThermoFisher Scientific). Reactions without reverse transcriptase or RNA template were included as controls. The first strand cDNA synthesis was performed at 25 °C for 10 min, 42 °C for 60 min, and 85 °C for 5 min. The 20 μL volume containing the cDNA was then diluted to 200 μL using sterile water. For qRT-PCR, a volume of 2 μL of the diluted cDNA from each sample was used following the protocol described by the manufacturer. Briefly, the reaction mixture included 2.5 μL of each primer (3 μM), 12.5 μL of 2X iQ SYBR Green Supermix (BioRad, Hercules, California, USA), 2 μL of cDNA, and water to 25 μL. The thermocycling profile consisted of four cycles as follows: Cycle 1: (1X) Step 1: 95 °C for 3 min. Cycle 2: (40X) Step 1: 95 °C for 10 s. Step 2: 55 °C for 30 s. Cycle 3: (1X) Step 1: 95 °C for 1 min. Cycle 4: (1X) Step 1: 55 °C for 1 min. For the melting curves, the final DNA products were denatured at 95 °C for 1 min. and then incubated at 5 °C below the annealing temperature for 1 min. before the temperature was increased to 95 °C at a ramp rate of 0.5 °C/10 s. For each sample, both target gene and reference gene were done in triplicate. Additional controls included samples without cDNA for each target gene. Data analysis was performed based on the protocol provided by BioRad. The transcript levels of the genes of interest were normalized to the transcript level of the house-keeping gene, *clpX*.

4.5. Statistical Analysis

Student's *t*-test was performed to compare the levels of transcripts in different gene categories (core, accessory and island) at $p < 0.01$. Differentially expressed genes were identified by Student's *t*-test at $p < 0.05$ and 1.5 or greater fold changes. The correlation between the expression levels by RNA-seq and qRT-PCR was determined by linear regression. Statistical analysis to determine the significance of the pathways affected by the differentially expressed genes was performed using the computing environment R [51].

Supplementary Materials: The following are available online at http://www.mdpi.com/2076-0817/8/4/282/s1, Figure S1: Correlations of genes expression levels obtained by qRT-PCR and RNA-Seq, Figure S2: Changes in optical density and CFU comparisons between *A. actinomycetemcomitans* cultured in rich mTSB, RPMI, and keratinocyte medium, Table S1: *A. actinomycetemcomitans* Genomic Islands, Table S2: Student's *t*-test of Gene Expression Levels between Gene Categories in All Tested Conditions, Table S3: Mean and Median Values of Gene Expression Levels of Core and Island Genes in Different Growth Conditions, Table S4: Upregulated and Downregulated *A. actinomycetemcomitans* Gene Expressions in Different Growth Conditions.

Author Contributions: Conception and study design C.C., A.T., R.E.B., and R.I.; performing experiments and data analysis N.O.T., A.T.; bioinformatics and sequence analysis C.C., W.K., and R.E.B.; writing—original draft preparation, C.C. and N.O.T.; writing—review and editing, C.C., N.O.T., W.K., R.E.B., R.I. All authors have read and agreed to the published version of the manuscript.

Funding: This research was funded by NIH R01 DE012212 (C.C.), and the Academy of Finland grants 126557 (AT and RI) and 265609 (R.I.).

Acknowledgments: We are grateful to Yong-Hwee Eddie Loh of USC Libraries Bioinformatics Services for his assistance in statistical analysis using the computing environment R in the analysis of the differentially expressed genes and the related metabolic networks.

Conflicts of Interest: The authors declare no conflict of interest.

References

1. Asikainen, S.; Chen, C. Oral ecology and person-to-person transmission of Actinobacillus actinomycetemcomitans and Porphyromonas gingivalis. *Periodontol 2000* **1999**, *20*, 65–81. [CrossRef]
2. Slots, J. Actinobacillus actinomycetemcomitans and Porphyromonas gingivalis in periodontal disease: Introduction. *Periodontology 2000* **1999**, *20*, 7–13. [CrossRef]
3. Fine, D.H.; Markowitz, K.; Furgang, D.; Fairlie, K.; Ferrandiz, J.; Nasri, C.; McKiernan, M.; Gunsolley, J. Aggregatibacter actinomycetemcomitans and its relationship to initiation of localized aggressive periodontitis: Longitudinal cohort study of initially healthy adolescents. *J. Clin. Microbiol.* **2007**, *45*, 3859–3869. [CrossRef]
4. Zambon, J.J. Actinobacillus actinomycetemcomitans in human periodontal disease. *J. Clin. Periodontol.* **1985**, *12*, 1–20. [CrossRef]
5. Haubek, D.; Ennibi, O.K.; Poulsen, K.; Vaeth, M.; Poulsen, S.; Kilian, M. Risk of aggressive periodontitis in adolescent carriers of the JP2 clone of Aggregatibacter (Actinobacillus) actinomycetemcomitans in Morocco: A prospective longitudinal cohort study. *Lancet* **2008**, *371*, 237–242. [CrossRef]
6. Kilian, M.; Frandsen, E.V.; Haubek, D.; Poulsen, K. The etiology of periodontal disease revisited by population genetic analysis. *Periodontol 2000* **2006**, *42*, 158–179. [CrossRef]

7. Asikainen, S.; Chen, C.; Saarela, M.; Saxen, L.; Slots, J. Clonal specificity of *Actinobacillus actinomycetemcomitans* in destructive periodontal disease. *Clin. Infect. Dis.* **1997**, *25* (Suppl. 2), S227–S229. [CrossRef]
8. Asikainen, S.; Lai, C.H.; Alaluusua, S.; Slots, J. Distribution of *Actinobacillus actinomycetemcomitans* serotypes in periodontal health and disease. *Oral Microbiol. Immunol.* **1991**, *6*, 115–118. [CrossRef]
9. Chen, C.; Wang, T.; Chen, W. Occurrence of *Aggregatibacter actinomycetemcomitans* serotypes in subgingival plaque from United States subjects. *Mol. Oral Microbiol.* **2010**, *25*, 207–214. [CrossRef]
10. Socransky, S.S.; Haffajee, A.D. The bacterial etiology of destructive periodontal disease: Current concepts. *J. Periodontol.* **1992**, *63*, 322–331. [CrossRef]
11. Schenkein, H.A.; Barbour, S.E.; Berry, C.R.; Kipps, B.; Tew, J.G. Invasion of human vascular endothelial cells by Actinobacillus actinomycetemcomitans via the receptor for platelet-activating factor. *Infect. Immun.* **2000**, *68*, 5416–5419. [CrossRef]
12. Socransky, S.S.; Haffajee, A.D.; Cugini, M.A.; Smith, C.; Kent, R.L., Jr. Microbial complexes in subgingival plaque. *J. Clin. Periodontol.* **1998**, *25*, 134–144. [CrossRef]
13. Kittichotirat, W.; Bumgarner, R.E.; Asikainen, S.; Chen, C. Identification of the pangenome and its components in 14 distinct Aggregatibacter actinomycetemcomitans strains by comparative genomic analysis. *PLoS ONE* **2011**, *6*, e22420. [CrossRef]
14. Kittichotirat, W.; Bumgarner, R.E.; Chen, C. Evolutionary Divergence of Aggregatibacter actinomycetemcomitans. *J. Dent. Res.* **2016**, *95*, 94–101. [CrossRef]
15. Kittichotirat, W.; Bumgarner, R.; Chen, C. Markedly different genome arrangements between serotype a strains and serotypes b or c strains of Aggregatibacter actinomycetemcomitans. *BMC Genom.* **2010**, *11*, 489. [CrossRef]
16. Huang, Y.; Kittichotirat, W.; Mayer, M.P.; Hall, R.; Bumgarner, R.; Chen, C. Comparative genomic hybridization and transcriptome analysis with a pan-genome microarray reveal distinctions between JP2 and non-JP2 genotypes of Aggregatibacter actinomycetemcomitans. *Mol. Oral Microbiol.* **2013**, *28*, 1–17. [CrossRef]
17. Ochman, H.; Lawrence, J.G.; Groisman, E.A. Lateral gene transfer and the nature of bacterial innovation. *Nature* **2000**, *405*, 299–304. [CrossRef]
18. Gogarten, J.P.; Townsend, J.P. Horizontal gene transfer, genome innovation and evolution. *Nat. Rev. Microbiol.* **2005**, *3*, 679–687. [CrossRef]
19. Dagan, T.; Artzy-Randrup, Y.; Martin, W. Modular networks and cumulative impact of lateral transfer in prokaryote genome evolution. *Proc. Natl. Acad. Sci. USA* **2008**, *105*, 10039–10044. [CrossRef]
20. Skippington, E.; Ragan, M.A. Within-species lateral genetic transfer and the evolution of transcriptional regulation in Escherichia coli and Shigella. *BMC Genom.* **2011**, *12*, 532. [CrossRef]
21. Treangen, T.J.; Rocha, E.P. Horizontal transfer, not duplication, drives the expansion of protein families in prokaryotes. *PLoS Genet.* **2011**, *7*, e1001284. [CrossRef] [PubMed]
22. Hsiao, W.W.; Ung, K.; Aeschliman, D.; Bryan, J.; Finlay, B.B.; Brinkman, F.S. Evidence of a large novel gene pool associated with prokaryotic genomic islands. *PLoS Genet.* **2005**, *1*, e62. [CrossRef] [PubMed]
23. Juhas, M.; van der Meer, J.R.; Gaillard, M.; Harding, R.M.; Hood, D.W.; Crook, D.W. Genomic islands: Tools of bacterial horizontal gene transfer and evolution. *FEMS Microbiol. Rev.* **2009**, *33*, 376–393. [CrossRef] [PubMed]
24. Narayanan, A.M.; Ramsey, M.M.; Stacy, A.; Whiteley, M. Defining Genetic Fitness Determinants and Creating Genomic Resources for an Oral Pathogen. *Appl. Environ. Microbiol* **2017**, *83*, e00797-17. [CrossRef]
25. Shenker, B.J.; Hoffmaster, R.H.; McKay, T.L.; Demuth, D.R. Expression of the cytolethal distending toxin (Cdt) operon in *Actinobacillus actinomycetemcomitans*: Evidence that the CdtB protein is responsible for G2 arrest of the cell cycle in human T cells. *J. Immunol.* **2000**, *165*, 2612–2618. [CrossRef]
26. Shenker, B.J.; McKay, T.; Datar, S.; Miller, M.; Chowhan, R.; Demuth, D. *Actinobacillus actinomycetemcomitans* immunosuppressive protein is a member of the family of cytolethal distending toxins capable of causing a G2 arrest in human T cells. *J. Immunol.* **1999**, *162*, 4773–4780.
27. Sato, T.; Koseki, T.; Yamato, K.; Saiki, K.; Konishi, K.; Yoshikawa, M.; Ishikawa, I.; Nishihara, T. p53-independent expression of p21(CIP1/WAF1) in plasmacytic cells during G(2) cell cycle arrest induced by *Actinobacillus actinomycetemcomitans* cytolethal distending toxin. *Infect. Immun.* **2002**, *70*, 528–534. [CrossRef]

28. Shenker, B.J.; Hoffmaster, R.H.; Zekavat, A.; Yamaguchi, N.; Lally, E.T.; Demuth, D.R. Induction of apoptosis in human T cells by *Actinobacillus actinomycetemcomitans* cytolethal distending toxin is a consequence of G2 arrest of the cell cycle. *J. Immunol.* **2001**, *167*, 435–441. [CrossRef]
29. Belibasakis, G.; Johansson, A.; Wang, Y.; Claesson, R.; Chen, C.; Asikainen, S.; Kalfas, S. Inhibited proliferation of human periodontal ligament cells and gingival fibroblasts by Actinobacillus actinomycetemcomitans: Involvement of the cytolethal distending toxin. *Eur. J. Oral Sci.* **2002**, *110*, 366–373. [CrossRef]
30. DiRienzo, J.M. Uptake and processing of the cytolethal distending toxin by mammalian cells. *Toxins (Basel)* **2014**, *6*, 3098–3116. [CrossRef]
31. Boesze-Battaglia, K.; Alexander, D.; Dlakic, M.; Shenker, B.J. A Journey of Cytolethal Distending Toxins through Cell Membranes. *Front. Cell Infect. Microbiol.* **2016**, *6*, 81. [CrossRef]
32. Belibasakis, G.N.; Johansson, A.; Wang, Y.; Chen, C.; Lagergard, T.; Kalfas, S.; Lerner, U.H. Cytokine responses of human gingival fibroblasts to Actinobacillus actinomycetemcomitans cytolethal distending toxin. *Cytokine* **2005**, *30*, 56–63. [CrossRef]
33. Belibasakis, G.N.; Johansson, A.; Wang, Y.; Chen, C.; Kalfas, S.; Lerner, U.H. The cytolethal distending toxin induces receptor activator of NF-kappaB ligand expression in human gingival fibroblasts and periodontal ligament cells. *Infect. Immun.* **2005**, *73*, 342–351. [CrossRef]
34. Doungudomdacha, S.; Volgina, A.; DiRienzo, J.M. Evidence that the cytolethal distending toxin locus was once part of a genomic island in the periodontal pathogen Aggregatibacter (Actinobacillus) actinomycetemcomitans strain Y4. *J. Med. Microbiol.* **2007**, *56*, 1519–1527. [CrossRef]
35. Balashova, N.V.; Diaz, R.; Balashov, S.V.; Crosby, J.A.; Kachlany, S.C. Regulation of Aggregatibacter (Actinobacillus) actinomycetemcomitans leukotoxin secretion by iron. *J. Bacteriol.* **2006**, *188*, 8658–8661. [CrossRef]
36. Kolodrubetz, D.; Phillips, L.; Jacobs, C.; Burgum, A.; Kraig, E. Anaerobic regulation of Actinobacillus actinomycetemcomitans leukotoxin transcription is ArcA/FnrA-independent and requires a novel promoter element. *Res. Microbiol.* **2003**, *154*, 645–653. [CrossRef]
37. Kawamoto, D.; Ando, E.S.; Longo, P.L.; Nunes, A.C.; Wikstrom, M.; Mayer, M.P. Genetic diversity and toxic activity of Aggregatibacter actinomycetemcomitans isolates. *Oral Microbiol. Immunol.* **2009**, *24*, 493–501. [CrossRef]
38. Amarasinghe, J.J.; Scannapieco, F.A.; Haase, E.M. Transcriptional and translational analysis of biofilm determinants of Aggregatibacter actinomycetemcomitans in response to environmental perturbation. *Infect. Immun.* **2009**, *77*, 2896–2907. [CrossRef]
39. Alexander, C.; Rietschel, E.T. Bacterial lipopolysaccharides and innate immunity. *J. Endotoxin Res.* **2001**, *7*, 167–202. [CrossRef]
40. Dubois-Brissonnet, F.; Trotier, E.; Briandet, R. The Biofilm Lifestyle Involves an Increase in Bacterial Membrane Saturated Fatty Acids. *Front. Microbiol.* **2016**, *7*, 1673. [CrossRef]
41. Costerton, J.W.; Lewandowski, Z.; Caldwell, D.E.; Korber, D.R.; Lappin-Scott, H.M. Microbial biofilms. *Annu. Rev. Microbiol.* **1995**, *49*, 711–745. [CrossRef]
42. Loo, C.Y.; Corliss, D.A.; Ganeshkumar, N. Streptococcus gordonii biofilm formation: Identification of genes that code for biofilm phenotypes. *J. Bacteriol.* **2000**, *182*, 1374–1382. [CrossRef]
43. Yoshida, A.; Kuramitsu, H.K. Multiple Streptococcus mutans Genes Are Involved in Biofilm Formation. *Appl. Env. Microbiol.* **2002**, *68*, 6283–6291. [CrossRef]
44. Llama-Palacios, A.; Potupa, O.; Sanchez, M.C.; Figuero, E.; Herrera, D.; Sanz, M. Aggregatibacter actinomycetemcomitans Growth in Biofilm versus Planktonic State: Differential Expression of Proteins. *J. Proteome Res.* **2017**, *16*, 3158–3167. [CrossRef]
45. Bowden, G.H.; Hamilton, I.R. Survival of oral bacteria. *Crit. Rev. Oral Biol. Med.* **1998**, *9*, 54–85. [CrossRef]
46. Lindquist, S.; Craig, E.A. The heat-shock proteins. *Annu. Rev. Genet.* **1988**, *22*, 631–677. [CrossRef]
47. Watson, K. Microbial stress proteins. *Adv. Microb. Physiol.* **1990**, *31*, 183–223.
48. Green, H.; Fuchs, E.; Watt, F. Differentiated structural components of the keratinocyte. *Cold Spring Harb. Symp. Quant. Biol.* **1982**, *46*, 293–301. [CrossRef]

49. Kanehisa, M.; Furumichi, M.; Tanabe, M.; Sato, Y.; Morishima, K. KEGG: New perspectives on genomes, pathways, diseases and drugs. *Nucleic Acids Res.* **2017**, *45*, D353–D361. [CrossRef]
50. Ramsey, M.M.; Whiteley, M. Polymicrobial interactions stimulate resistance to host innate immunity through metabolite perception. *Proc. Natl. Acad. Sci. USA* **2009**, *106*, 1578–1583. [CrossRef]
51. R Development Core Team. *R: A Language and Environment for Statistical Computing*; R Foundation for Statistical Computing: Vienna, Austria, 2018.

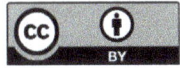

© 2019 by the authors. Licensee MDPI, Basel, Switzerland. This article is an open access article distributed under the terms and conditions of the Creative Commons Attribution (CC BY) license (http://creativecommons.org/licenses/by/4.0/).

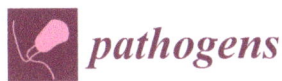

Article

Aggregatibacter actinomycetemcomitans Biofilm Reduces Gingival Epithelial Cell Keratin Expression in an Organotypic Gingival Tissue Culture Model

Arzu Beklen [1], Annamari Torittu [1], Riikka Ihalin [1] and Marja Pöllänen [2,*]

[1] Department of Biochemistry, University of Turku, 20014 Turku, Finland; arzu.beklen@gmail.com (A.B.); atorittu@abo.fi (A.T.); riikka.ihalin@utu.fi (R.I.)
[2] Institute of Dentistry, University of Turku, 20014 Turku, Finland
* Correspondence: marja.pollanen@duodecim.fi; Tel.: +358-40-723-5818

Received: 11 November 2019; Accepted: 29 November 2019; Published: 1 December 2019

Abstract: Epithelial cells express keratins, which are essential for the structural integrity and mechanical strength of the cells. In the junctional epithelium (JE) of the tooth, keratins such as K16, K18, and K19, are expressed, which is typical for non-differentiated and rapidly dividing cells. The expression of K17, K4, and K13 keratins can be induced by injury, bacterial irritation, smoking, and inflammation. In addition, these keratins can be found in the sulcular epithelium and in the JE. Our aim was to estimate the changes in K4, K13, K17, and K19 expression in gingival epithelial cells exposed to *Aggregatibacter actinomycetemcomitans*. An organotypic gingival mucosa and biofilm co-culture was used as a model system. The effect of the biofilm after 24 h was assessed using immunohistochemistry. The structure of the epithelium was also studied with transmission electron microscopy (TEM). The expression of K17 and K19, as well as total keratin expression, decreased in the suprabasal layers of epithelium, which were in close contact with the *A. actinomycetemcomitans* biofilm. The effect on keratin expression was biofilm specific. The expression of K4 and K13 was low in all of the tested conditions. When stimulated with the *A. actinomycetemcomitans* biofilm, the epithelial contact site displayed a thick necrotic layer on the top of the epithelium. The *A. actinomycetemcomitans* biofilm released vesicles, which were found in close contact with the epithelium. After *A. actinomycetemcomitans* irritation, gingival epithelial cells may lose their resistance and become more vulnerable to bacterial infection.

Keywords: *Aggregatibacter actinomycetemcomitans*; keratins; organotypic gingival mucosa

---

1. Introduction

Periodontal disease is an inflammatory disease caused by growing biofilm, which gradually develops to a bacterial community rich in inflammophilic Gram-negative species [1]. The formation of such biofilm and the subsequent inflammation affects the supporting tissues of the tooth, including the epithelium and the connective tissue. Cytoskeletal intermediate filaments are essential for the structural integrity and function of the epithelial cells. Intermediate filaments constitute the acidic (Type I) and basic (Type II) keratins. The molecular weight of Type I keratin ranges from 40 to 57 kDa and encompasses keratins K9–K20. The molecular weight of Type II keratin ranges from 50 to 70 kDa and encompasses keratins K1–K8.

Keratins play an important functional role in the integrity and mechanical stability of both individual epithelial cells and cell–cell contacts in tissues. Thus, they contribute not only to the stability of the epithelium itself but also to the basement membrane attachment to the connective tissue underlying the epithelium. In the epithelia of internal organs, which are under little mechanical stress, there are only a few loosely-distributed keratin filaments in the cytoplasm. Conversely, keratins are abundant and are densely bound in the lining of outer surfaces. The composition of keratins varies depending on the epithelial cell type and the differentiation status of the epithelial cells. The keratin composition may also be affected by external stimuli, inflammation, or other types of disease development (e.g., cancer). The oral epithelium is a keratinizing form of epithelium and provides an effective physical barrier to microbial invasion. In the oral epithelium, basal dividing cells express simple epithelial cell keratins (K5, K14, and K19), whereas suprabasal cells express keratins typical of differentiated cells (K1, K10, K6, and K16). The keratin profile of the junctional epithelium (JE) differs from the oral epithelium, as only keratins typical for non-differentiated and rapidly dividing cells are expressed both basally (K5, K14, and K19) and suprabasally (K19). In addition, keratins such as K4, K13, and K17 have been found in the sulcular area of the dentogingival junction and may be induced by acute injury, bacterial irritation, smoking, and inflammation [2,3].

In contrast, in patients with severe and rapidly progressive periodontitis (previous term aggressive periodontitis), K17 gene expression was found to be repressed in disease site gingival samples compared to healthy site samples [4]. An open issue of significant interest is whether the expression of those keratins is altered by irritation from biofilm bacteria, such as *Aggregatibacter actinomycetemcomitans*, in periodontal diseases. The Gram-negative bacterium *A. actinomycetemcomitans* is an aggressive pathogen that is frequently associated with subgingival biofilms and has been strongly implicated in the development of rapidly progressive periodontal disease involving the invasion of *A. actinomycetemcomitans* into epithelial layers. Although *A. actinomycetemcomitans* represents only one species in multispecies periodontal biofilm, it most likely is able to suppress the host defense with its virulence factors. To gain insight into this question, we examined keratin K4, K13, K17, and K19 expression and distribution in an organotypic gingival tissue culture model co-cultured with a periodontopathogenic *A. actinomycetemcomitans* biofilm. Keratin K19 was chosen since it is typical and most dominant keratin in the JE [5,6] and we wanted to investigate how well the tissue culture model mimics the JE. We found that the expression of K17 and K19, as well as total keratin expression, decreased in the suprabasal layers of epithelium, which were in close contact with the *A. actinomycetemcomitans* biofilm. The decreased keratin expression may lead to decreased resistance of gingival epithelial cells to bacterial infection.

2. Results

2.1. Control Cultures Showed Strong Expression of K17 and K19 and Only Weak or No Expression of K4 and K13

Both control cultures grown without anything on the top of the epithelium or with an empty sterile filter disc showed similar immunohistochemical staining. Pancytokeratin staining was strong and was evenly distributed throughout the epithelium (Figure 1a,b). Similarly, the specific cytokeratins K17 and K19 were found to be expressed from the basal layer throughout the epithelium to the surface (Figure 1a,b). Keratin 4 was not found in the control cultures (Figure 2a,b), and K13 expression was only observed occasionally in single cells (Figure 2a,b).

2.2. A. actinomycetemcomitans Biofilm Decreased the Expression of Keratin 17 and 19, Which Was in Accordance with the Decreased Expression of Total Keratin

When exposed to pre-grown *A. actinomycetemcomitans* biofilm for 24 h, the human gingival keratinocytes showed no or very weak expression of K17 and K19 throughout the epithelium and especially in areas in close contact to the biofilm (Figure 1c). Some expression of K17 was evident further away from the biofilm-epithelium contact site (Figure 1c) as well as in the basal layer adjacent to the connective tissue. K19 expression was almost totally absent (Figure 1c). No expression of K4 or K13 was observed in the co-cultures with the biofilm (Figure 2c). The decrease in the expression levels of total keratins (pan-cytokeratin staining, Figure 1c) in the co-cultures with the *A. actinomycetemcomitans* biofilm was in accordance with the decrease in specific keratin expression.

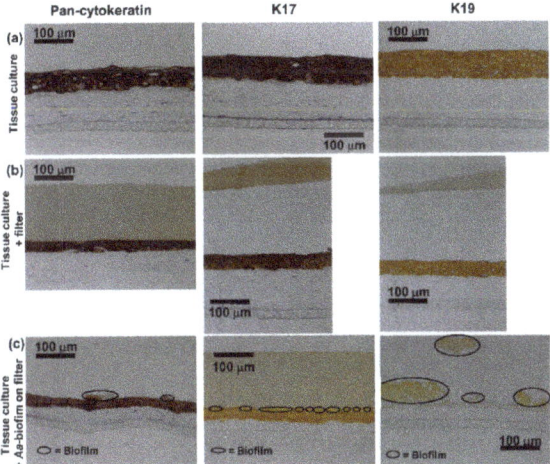

Figure 1. *A. actinomycetemcomitans* biofilm decreased the total keratin as well as K17 and K19 expression in the suprabasal layers of the epithelium. (**a,b**) Immunohistochemical staining (peroxidase-3,3′-diaminobenzidine (DAB)) with anti-pan-cytokeratin/anti-cytokeratin 17/anti-cytokeratin 19 shows strong staining in the control cultures. (**c**) Pan-cytokeratin/K17/K19 expression is decreased in the co-cultures with the *A. actinomycetemcomitans* biofilm.

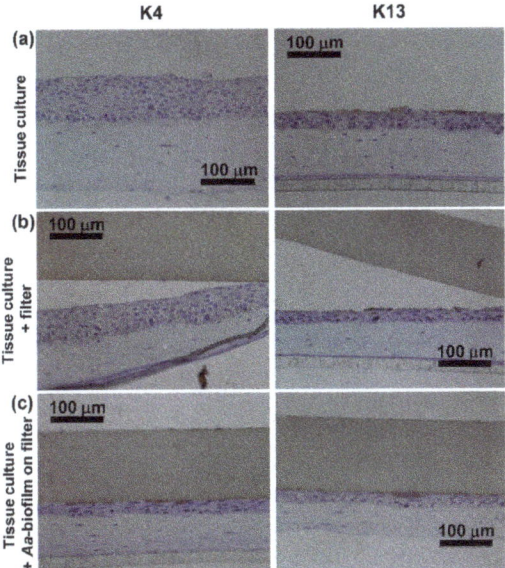

Figure 2. The expression of K4 and K13 was low in all of the tested conditions. (**a,b**) Immunohistochemical staining (DAB) with anti-cytokeratin 4 in the control cultures or (**c**) in the co-cultures with the *A. actinomycetemcomitans* biofilm shows no expression of K4. (**a,b**) Immunohistochemical staining (DAB) with anti-cytokeratin 13 shows only a few stained cells in the control cultures. (**c**) In the co-cultures with *A. actinomycetemcomitans* biofilm, no expression of K13 is observed.

2.3. A. actinomycetemcomitans Biofilm Caused Necrosis of the Epithelial Surface

Using TEM analysis, the control culture surface showed a thin layer of exfoliating, necrotic cells (Figure 3a,b). The cell structures and cell–cell contacts appeared normal. When exposed to the *A. actinomycetemcomitans* biofilm, the necrotic area of the epithelial surface was thick (Figure 4a,b), and the thickness of the necrotic area increased in areas in close contact to the biofilm and with an increasing amount of biofilm (Figure 4b). Necrosis of the epithelium in contact with the biofilm was consistently seen in EM, as visualized in Figure 4b, where right beneath the increasing mass of *A actinonmycetemcomitans* (on the left side of the picture) the necrotic epithelial layer increases clearly in thickness. This is a descriptive result, but was consistently seen in EM. In the co-cultures, nuclear breakdown was observed in areas in close contact to the biofilm (Figure 4a,c). When in close contact with the epithelium, the biofilm bacteria released vesicles, and similar structures could be observed intraepithelially (Figure 5a,b). The necrotic area appeared to act as a barrier to the biofilm bacteria; however, a few structures which resembled bacteria were observed inside the epithelium after the 24 h co-culture (Figure 5c).

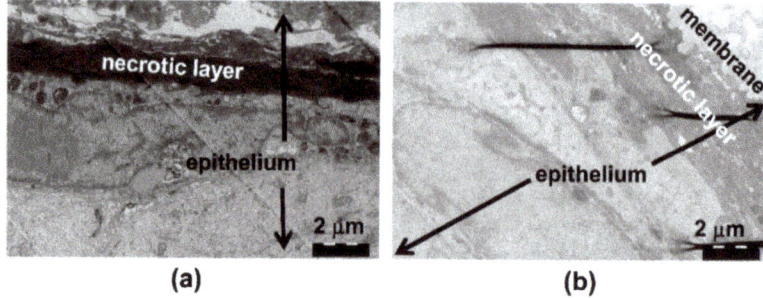

Figure 3. Normal structure of the epithelial cells and the epithelial cell nuclei. (**a**) Transmission electron microscopy (TEM) of the control cultures grown with nothing on the surface and (**b**) with the sterile membrane on the epithelium shows the normal structure of the cells and nuclei. On the top of the epithelium, a thin area of exfoliating and necrotic cells is observed (dark area).

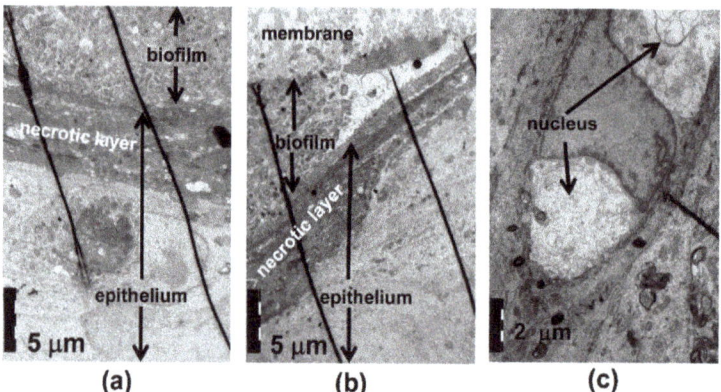

Figure 4. *A. actinomycetemcomitans* biofilm caused necrosis of the epithelial cells. (**a,b**) TEM of the co-cultures with *A. actinomycetemcomitans* shows the thickening of the necrotic layer in areas in close contact to the biofilm and (**a,c**) disruption of the nuclei beneath the biofilm.

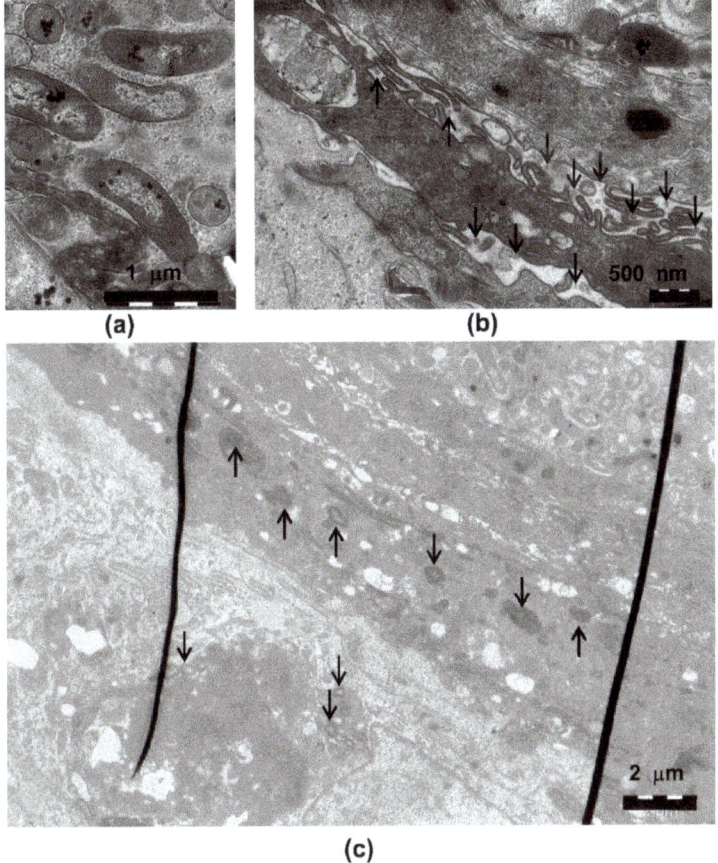

Figure 5. Vesicle-like structures are released by *A. actinomycetemcomitans* biofilm. (**a**) *A. actinomycetemcomitans* cells in the biofilm release vesicles, and (**b**) similar structures can be observed inside the epithelium. (**c**) (arrows) A few particles resembling single *A. actinomycetemcomitans* cells are observed inside the necrotic epithelium and inside the epithelial cells beneath the necrotic layer.

3. Discussion

Our major findings were that the *A. actinomycetemcomitans* biofilm caused decreased expression of cytokeratins, which is typical for the dentogingival junction and necrosis of the epithelial surface layers in close contact to the biofilm. Our tissue culture model appeared to mimic JE well, as K19, the typical keratin for JE, was highly expressed in the control cultures [6]. Our finding of decreased K19 expression adjacent to the *A. actinomycetemcomitans* biofilm is in disagreement with earlier reports showing that the inflammation in the periodontal pocket increases K19 expression [3,7]. However, our result may reflect the specific nature of the *A actinomycetemcomitans* biofilm–host tissue interaction. Previous work has shown that *A. actinomycetemcomitans* can invade buccal epithelial cells [8] and gingival tissue [9]. By decreasing the expression of one major structural protein, K19, in JE cells, *A. actinomycetemcomitans* could disturb the epithelial integrity, ease the invasion of the bacteria into deeper tissues, and lead to subsequent periodontal connective tissue destruction. In fact, structures resembling single *A. actinomycetemcomitans* cells were observed in the TEM analysis of epitheliums of co-cultures. Tissue destruction may even be further accelerated by decreased epithelial cell proliferation, which we showed in a previous study of tissue cultures exposed to an *A. actinomycetemcomitans* biofilm [10].

K17 was also strongly expressed in our control cultures. In vivo, K17 has been found in the sulcular epithelium of the dentogingival junction [2]. In addition, JE seems to express the genes encoding K17 [11]. Furthermore, it has been previously suggested that short chain fatty acids produced by some Gram-negative periodontal pathogens increase the expression of K17 [2] and that the inflammatory mediators would play a role in the regulation of the K17 expression [12]. Our finding that an *A. actinomycetemcomitans* biofilm decreased the expression of K17 seems to conflict with the earlier studies showing increased K17 expression after treatment with short chain fatty acids [2]. However, *A. actinomycetemcomitans*, although resistant to the antimicrobial activity of short chain fatty acids [13], produces only long chain fatty acids [14], which may at least partly explain these contradictory findings. Furthermore, K17 gene expression has been found depressed in clinical specimens from patients with severe and rapidly progressive periodontitis, which is in agreement with our results [4].

The model showed no evidence of K4 or K13 expression, which have been shown to be expressed in healthy oral sulcular epithelium [15]. Although K4 is typically absent in JE, its expression can be observed in JE of smoking periodontitis patients [15]. In our model, the *A. actinomycetemcomitans* biofilm did not increase or decrease K4 or K13 expression, of which the latter has been shown increasingly expressed in inflamed tissues [3]. However, the increase in K13 expression in inflammation may require the presence of host immune cells, such as macrophages, which were not included to our tissue co-culture model.

A closer investigation of the epithelial surface structure by TEM revealed that *A. actinomycetemcomitans* biofilm exposure caused necrosis of the epithelial surface in the co-culture models. The thick necrotic layer most likely inhibited the invasion of *A. actinomycetemcomitans* cells into the deeper layers of epithelium, as we could only detect a few structures resembling *A. actinomycetemcomitans* cells in the surface layers of the epithelium. However, the *A. actinomycetemcomitans* biofilm secreted high amounts of vesicles, which could have greater invasive potential than whole bacterial cells. For instance, *A. actinomycetemcomitans* vesicles have been shown to invade human HeLa and gingival fibroblast cells and release cytolethal distending toxin to the host cell nucleus [16,17]. *A. actinomycetemcomitans* vesicle-like structures could be observed in the epithelium. However, these vesicles may also originate from the host epithelial cells, and thus their origin needs to be confirmed in further studies.

In conclusion, *A. actinomycetemcomitans* biofilm decreases the expression of K17 and K19 and the total expression levels of keratins in an organotypic gingival mucosa model. However, the epithelium appears to utilize additional measures to withstand attack by the *A. actinomycetemcomitans* biofilm, which is suggested by the thicker necrotic layer between the epithelial cells and biofilm. Whether host immune cells and macrophages, in particular, change the keratin expression pattern during biofilm attack requires further investigation in a more complex environment.

4. Materials and Methods

4.1. A. actinomycetemcomitans Biofilm Culture

The *A. actinomycetemcomitans* biofilm cultures were generated as described previously [10]. Briefly, *A. actinomycetemcomitans* strain D7S was first cultured from trypticase soy agar blood plates. From the plates, an even bacterial suspension was made [18], and 5×10^7 cells/well were added to a 48-well plate containing porous filter discs. The biofilms were first grown in a rich trypticase soy broth medium for 24 h on a filter disc, and after which they were washed with a 0.85% NaCl solution. The cultivation was continued for an additional 24 h in glutamine supplemented RPMI-1640 medium. The 48-well plate also contained wells with sterile filter discs in the appropriate media for use as controls.

4.2. Gingival Mucosa Co-Culture Models

The *A. actinomycetemcomitans* biofilm/gingival mucosa co-culture models were constructed as described previously [10]. Briefly, human gingival fibroblasts [19] were grown in a collagen suspension with a cell culture insert (ThinCert™, Greiner Bio-One GmbH, Germany) for one day before 4×10^5

spontaneously immortalized human gingival keratinocyte cells [20] were seeded on top of the fibroblast-collagen matrix. The epithelial cells were cultured for one day submerged in the growth medium before the tissue model was lifted to the air–liquid interface. The model was air exposed for five days before a separately cultured *A. actinomycetemcomitans* D7S [21] biofilm (see above) was added on top of the tissue culture. The co-cultures were incubated without antibiotics in the cell culture medium. The gingival mucosa was co-cultured with the biofilm/control disc/no added components for 24 h, and the co-cultures were the fixed with a 10% formalin solution overnight. After the fixation step, the samples were embedded in paraffin and were sectioned.

4.3. Immunohistochemical Staining of Keratins K4, K13, K17, and K19

Before staining, the specimens were deparaffinized and heat-mediated antigen retrieval in 10 mM citrate buffer (pH 6.0) with microwaving was performed, which was followed by proteinase K treatment [22]. The staining was performed with a Dako TechMate™ 500 Plus Autostainer (Dako, Glostrup; Denmark) using the primary antibodies listed in Table 1 and the Dako REAL™ Detection System, Peroxidase/DAB+, Rabbit/Mouse (Code K5001; Dako) according to manufacturer's instructions.

Table 1. Primary anti-keratin antibodies used in the study.

Keratin	Dilution	Host	Type	Code	Manufacturer
Keratin 4	1/10	mouse	monoclonal	MON3015-1	Sanbio, Holland
Keratin 13	1/50	mouse	monoclonal	MUB0340S	Nordic MUbio, Holland
Keratin 17	1/20	mouse	monoclonal	M704601-2	Dako, Denmark
Keratin 19	1/100	mouse	monoclonal	M088801-2	Dako, Denmark
Pan-cytokeratin 5,6,8,17,(19)	1/50	mouse	monoclonal	M0821	Dako, Denmark

4.4. Transmission Electron Microscopic (TEM) Studies of the Biofilm-Epithelium Contact Site

The *A. actinomycetemcomitans* biofilm gingival mucosa co-culture models were assembled as described above. The samples were prefixed for TEM with a freshly prepared 5% glutaraldehyde solution (5% glutaraldehyde, 0.16 M s-collidin-HCl buffer, pH 7.4) for at least 3 h at room temperature. After prefixation, the samples were washed with s-collidin-HCl buffer three times for 3 min each. Then, the samples were postfixed (1% OsO4, 1.5% K-ferrocyanide) for 2 h [23], washed with s-collidin buffer three times for 5 min each, and were dehydrated with ethanol (70% ethanol, 1 min at 4 °C; 96% ethanol, 1 min, at 4 °C; 100% ethanol, 30 min, at 4 °C; 100% ethanol, three times, 30 min each, at 20 °C). The dehydrated samples were embedded in epoxy using the following series: propylene oxide, two times, 15 min each; propylene oxide + epoxy resin + DMP (10:10:0.15), 2 h; epoxy resin + DMP (10:0.15), 12 h; epoxy resin + DMP (10:0.15), at 60 °C, 36 h. The sectioning of the samples was accomplished with an ultramicrotome to a thickness of approximately 70 nm. After sectioning, the samples were stained with uranyl acetate (1% uranyl acetate in pure water for 30 min) and were rinsed three times with pure water for 30 s. Finally, the samples were stained with lead citrate (0.3% lead citrate in pure water for 3 min) and were rinsed with water as in the previous step. The samples were examined with a JEM-1400 Plus Transmission Electron Microscope (JEOL USA, Inc., Peabody, MA, USA).

Author Contributions: Conceptualization, R.I. and M.P.; formal analysis, A.B., R.I., and M.P.; investigation, A.B. and A.T.; methodology, A.T. and M.P.; visualization, R.I. and M.P., project administration, R.I.; resources, R.I. and M.P.; supervision, R.I. and M.P.; writing—original draft, A.B., A.T., R.I., and M.P.; and writing—review and editing, R.I. and M.P., funding acquisition, R.I.

Funding: This work was supported by the Academy of Finland grant numbers 126557, 265609, 272960, and 322817 to R.I. A.B. was funded by The Scientific and Technological Research Council of Turkey (TUBITAK).

Acknowledgments: We thank Katja Sampalahti, Marja-Riitta Uola, and Essi Hautamäki for their skillful technical assistance in the organotypic tissue cultures and histological staining. The transmission electron microscopic studies were performed in the EM core facility, and the light microscopic imaging was performed at the Cell Imaging Core (Turku Centre for Biotechnology, University of Turku and Åbo Akademi University).

Conflicts of Interest: The authors declare no conflict of interest.

References

1. Lamont, R.J.; Koo, H.; Hajishengallis, G. The oral microbiota: Dynamic communities and host interactions. *Nat. Rev. Microbiol.* **2018**, *16*, 745–759. [CrossRef] [PubMed]
2. Pöllänen, M.T.; Salonen, J.I. Effect of short chain fatty acids on human gingival epithelial cell keratins in vitro. *Eur. J. Oral Sci.* **2000**, *108*, 523–529. [CrossRef] [PubMed]
3. Mackenzie, I.C.; Gao, Z. Patterns of cytokeratin expression in the epithelia of inflamed human gingiva and periodontal pockets. *J. Periodontal Res.* **1993**, *28*, 49–59. [CrossRef] [PubMed]
4. Kebschull, M.; Guarnieri, P.; Demmer, R.T.; Boulesteix, A.L.; Pavlidis, P.; Papapanou, P.N. Molecular differences between chronic and aggressive periodontitis. *J. Dent. Res.* **2013**, *92*, 1081–1088. [CrossRef] [PubMed]
5. Pöllänen, M.T.; Salonen, J.I.; Uitto, V.J. Structure and function of the tooth-epithelial interface in health and disease. *Periodontol 2000* **2003**, *31*, 12–31. [CrossRef] [PubMed]
6. Jiang, Q.; Yu, Y.; Ruan, H.; Luo, Y.; Guo, X. Morphological and functional characteristics of human gingival junctional epithelium. *BMC Oral Health* **2014**, *14*, 30. [CrossRef] [PubMed]
7. Nagarakanti, S.; Ramya, S.; Babu, P.; Arun, K.V.; Sudarsan, S. Differential expression of E-cadherin and cytokeratin 19 and net proliferative rate of gingival keratinocytes in oral epithelium in periodontal health and disease. *J. Periodontol.* **2007**, *78*, 2197–2202. [CrossRef]
8. Johnson, J.D.; Chen, R.; Lenton, P.A.; Zhang, G.; Hinrichs, J.E.; Rudney, J.D. Persistence of extracrevicular bacterial reservoirs after treatment of aggressive periodontitis. *J. Periodontol.* **2008**, *79*, 2305–2312. [CrossRef]
9. Christersson, L.A.; Albini, B.; Zambon, J.J.; Wikesjo, U.M.; Genco, R.J. Tissue localization of Actinobacillus actinomycetemcomitans in human periodontitis. I. Light, immunofluorescence and electron microscopic studies. *J. Periodontol.* **1987**, *58*, 529–539. [CrossRef]
10. Paino, A.; Lohermaa, E.; Sormunen, R.; Tuominen, H.; Korhonen, J.; Pöllänen, M.T.; Ihalin, R. Interleukin-1beta is internalised by viable Aggregatibacter actinomycetemcomitans biofilm and locates to the outer edges of nucleoids. *Cytokine* **2012**, *60*, 565–574. [CrossRef]
11. Hayashi, Y.; Matsunaga, T.; Yamamoto, G.; Nishii, K.; Usui, M.; Yamamoto, M.; Tachikawa, T. Comprehensive analysis of gene expression in the junctional epithelium by laser microdissection and microarray analysis. *J. Periodontal Res.* **2010**, *45*, 618–625. [CrossRef] [PubMed]
12. Zhang, W.; Dang, E.; Shi, X.; Jin, L.; Feng, Z.; Hu, L.; Wu, Y.; Wang, G. The pro-inflammatory cytokine IL-22 up-regulates keratin 17 expression in keratinocytes via STAT3 and ERK1/2. *PLoS ONE* **2012**, *7*, e40797. [CrossRef] [PubMed]
13. Huang, C.B.; Alimova, Y.; Myers, T.M.; Ebersole, J.L. Short- and medium-chain fatty acids exhibit antimicrobial activity for oral microorganisms. *Arch. Oral Biol.* **2011**, *56*, 650–654. [CrossRef] [PubMed]
14. Braunthal, S.D.; Holt, S.C.; Tanner, A.C.; Socransky, S.S. Cellular fatty acid composition of Actinobacillus actinomycetemcomitans and Haemophilus aphrophilus. *J. Clin. Microbiol.* **1980**, *11*, 625–630.
15. Pritlove-Carson, S.; Charlesworth, S.; Morgan, P.R.; Palmer, R.M. Cytokeratin phenotypes at the dento-gingival junction in relative health and inflammation, in smokers and nonsmokers. *Oral Dis.* **1997**, *3*, 19–24. [CrossRef]
16. Rompikuntal, P.K.; Thay, B.; Khan, M.K.; Alanko, J.; Penttinen, A.M.; Asikainen, S.; Wai, S.N.; Oscarsson, J. Perinuclear localization of internalized outer membrane vesicles carrying active cytolethal distending toxin from Aggregatibacter actinomycetemcomitans. *Infect. Immun.* **2012**, *80*, 31–42. [CrossRef]
17. Thay, B.; Damm, A.; Kufer, T.A.; Wai, S.N.; Oscarsson, J. Aggregatibacter actinomycetemcomitans outer membrane vesicles are internalized in human host cells and trigger NOD1- and NOD2-dependent NF-kappaB activation. *Infect. Immun.* **2014**, *82*, 4034–4046. [CrossRef]
18. Karched, M.; Paul-Satyaseela, M.; Asikainen, S. A simple viability-maintaining method produces homogenic cell suspensions of autoaggregating wild-type Actinobacillus actinomycetemcomitans. *J. Microbiol. Methods* **2007**, *68*, 46–51. [CrossRef]

19. Oksanen, J.; Hormia, M. An organotypic in vitro model that mimics the dento-epithelial junction. *J. Periodontol.* **2002**, *73*, 86–93. [CrossRef]
20. Mäkelä, M.; Salo, T.; Larjava, H. MMP-9 from TNF alpha-stimulated keratinocytes binds to cell membranes and type I collagen: A cause for extended matrix degradation in inflammation? *Biochem. Biophys. Res. Commun.* **1998**, *253*, 325–335. [CrossRef]
21. Wang, Y.; Shi, W.; Chen, W.; Chen, C. Type IV pilus gene homologs pilABCD are required for natural transformation in Actinobacillus actinomycetemcomitans. *Gene* **2003**, *312*, 249–255. [CrossRef]
22. Paino, A.; Tuominen, H.; Jaaskelainen, M.; Alanko, J.; Nuutila, J.; Asikainen, S.E.; Pelliniemi, L.J.; Pöllönen, M.T.; Chen, C.; Ihalin, R. Trimeric form of intracellular ATP synthase subunit beta of Aggregatibacter actinomycetemcomitans binds human interleukin-1beta. *PLoS ONE* **2011**, *6*, e18929. [CrossRef]
23. Karnovsky, M.J. Use of ferrocyanide-reduced osmium tetroxide in electron microscopy. In Proceedings of the 11th Annual Meeting of American Society for Cell Biology, New Orleans, LA, USA, 17–20 November 1971; p. 146.

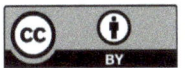

© 2019 by the authors. Licensee MDPI, Basel, Switzerland. This article is an open access article distributed under the terms and conditions of the Creative Commons Attribution (CC BY) license (http://creativecommons.org/licenses/by/4.0/).

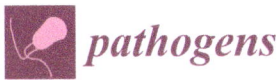

Article

Whole Genome Sequencing of *Aggregatibacter actinomycetemcomitans* Cultured from Blood Stream Infections Reveals Three Major Phylogenetic Groups Including a Novel Lineage Expressing Serotype a Membrane O Polysaccharide

Signe Nedergaard [1], Carl M. Kobel [1,2], Marie B. Nielsen [1,3], Rikke T. Møller [1], Anne B. Jensen [1,4] and Niels Nørskov-Lauritsen [1,*]

[1] Department of Clinical Microbiology, Aarhus University Hospital, DK-8200 Aarhus N, Denmark; nedergaardsigne@gmail.com (S.N.); kobel@pm.me (C.M.K.); mabanielsen@health.sdu.dk (M.B.N.); torsbjerg-92@hotmail.com (R.T.M.); abj@dent.au.dk (A.B.J.)
[2] Bioinformatics Research Centre, Aarhus University, DK-8000 Aarhus C, Denmark
[3] Department of Clinical Biochemistry and Pharmacology, Odense University hospital, DK-5000 Odense C, Denmark
[4] Department of Dentistry, Aarhus University, DK-8000 Aarhus C, Denmark
* Correspondence: nielnoer@rm.dk

Received: 1 October 2019; Accepted: 19 November 2019; Published: 22 November 2019

Abstract: Twenty-nine strains of *Aggregatibacter actinomycetemcomitans* cultured from blood stream infections in Denmark were characterised. Serotyping was unremarkable, with almost equal proportions of the three major types plus a single serotype e strain. Whole genome sequencing positioned the serotype e strain outside the species boundary; moreover, one of the serotype a strains was unrelated to other strains of the major serotypes and to deposited sequences in the public databases. We identified five additional strains of this type in our collections. The particularity of the group was corroborated by phylogenetic analysis of concatenated core genes present in all strains of the species, and by uneven distribution of accessory genes only present in a subset of strains. Currently, the most accurate depiction of *A. actinomycetemcomitans* is a division into three lineages that differ in genomic content and competence for transformation. The clinical relevance of the different lineages is not known, and even strains excluded from the species sensu stricto can cause serious human infections. Serotyping is insufficient for characterisation, and serotypes a and e are not confined to specific lineages.

Keywords: taxonomy; core and accessory genes; average nucleotide identity; principal component analysis

1. Introduction

Aggregatibacter actinomycetemcomitans is a fastidious Gram-negative bacterium that inhabits the mucosal surfaces of humans and certain primates [1,2]. The species has attracted attention due to its association with periodontitis [3]. Particularly, a single serotype b clonal lineage is associated with a silent but aggressive orphan disease of adolescents that results in periodontitis and tooth loss [4]. Rather than being the causative agent of aggressive periodontitis, *A. actinomycetemcomitans* may be necessary for the action of a consortium of bacterial partners by suppressing host defences [5].

A. actinomycetemcomitans is a member of the HACEK group of fastidious Gram-negative bacteria (*Haemophilus*, *Aggregatibacter*, *Cardiobacterium*, *Eikenella* and *Kingella*), a recognized but unusual cause of infective endocarditis responsible for 1.4% to 3% of cases [2]. A recent population-based study of the incidence of HACEK bacteraemia in Denmark identified 147 cases corresponding to an annual incidence of 0.44 per 100,000 population [6]. A retrospective study from New Zealand with 87 cases of HACEK bacteraemia confirmed a strong association with infective endocarditis, although the association with endocarditis ranged from 0 of 11 cases (*Eikenella corrodens*) to 18 of 18 cases (*A. actinomycetemcomitans*) [7].

Traditional classification of *A. actinomycetemcomitans* into serotypes is based on the chemical structures of the outer membrane O polysaccharide. Other studies have addressed the species' population structure by subjecting selected strains to multilocus enzyme electrophoresis [8], 16S rRNA gene sequencing [9], or multilocus sequence typing [10]. All methods identified an outgroup consisting of a subset of serotype e strains, but the grouping of serotypes was not consistent between methods. Finally, whole genome sequences (WGSs) of *A. actinomycetemcomitans* have become available. The first comparison of 14 strains found two major groups composed of serotypes a, d, e, plus f, and b plus c, respectively, while a serotype e strain outgroup showed a conspicuous lack of the cytolethal distending toxin gene cluster [11]. Jorth and Whiteley added three additional WGSs and calculated average nucleotide identity (ANI); strains within the two major groups were ~99% identical, while comparisons of strains belonging to separate groups disclosed significant differences (ANI of ~97%), and the outgroup strain was positioned outside the recommended species boundary [12]. The most recent comparison of WGSs included non-*actinomycetemcomitans Aggregatibacter* strains and was restricted to 397 concatenated core genes. The analysis suggested a division of the species into five clades: clade b (serotype b), clade c (serotype c), clade e/f (serotypes e and f), clade a/d (serotypes a and d), and clade e' (outgroup serotype e strains) [13].

The few studies that have characterised *A. actinomycetemcomitans* from cases of bacteraemia were limited to serotyping [14], or serotyping supplemented with arbitrarily primed PCR [15]. Here, we present WGSs of 29 Danish bacteraemia isolates. We include five additional oral strains to characterise a novel group within the species designated lineage III.

2. Results

Twenty-nine blood stream isolates of *A. actinomycetemcomitans* were identified as part of an investigation of Danish HACEK bacteraemia cases [6]. Serotyping by PCR identified seven serotype a, 11 serotype b, 10 serotype c, and one serotype e strain—this distribution is similar to the observed prevalence among oral strains in Scandinavia ([16] and references therein). Comparison of WGSs did, however, show that the single serotype e strain (PN_561) was unrelated to common isolates of this serotype, but clustered with the clade e' outgroup [13]. Moreover, one serotype a strain (PN_696) was unrelated to the other six isolates of this serotype and did not cluster with any *A. actinomycetemcomitans* WGSs present in the public databases. We tried to identify further isolates of this peculiar genotype. An early characterisation by multilocus enzyme electrophoresis of 97 strains isolated over a period of 45 years identified four minor groups that deviated from the two major divisions [8]. By WGSs, the three strains of division V (HK_907, HK_973, and HK_974) clustered with the aberrant serotype a blood stream isolate. An investigation of stored serotype a strains revealed two additional members of this lineage (K51, HK_1710), and these five oral isolates are included in the comparison.

The neighbour-joining comparison of core gene sequences of 35 study strains (including the type strain NCTC 9710 of serotype c) plus seven selected reference sequences downloaded from the public databases is shown in Figure 1. One blood stream isolate (PN_561) plus a reference sequence comprise the clade e' outgroup that is used to root the tree. Although serotype b and serotype c strains are distributed in two separate branches, the overall population structure of the species consists of three separate lineages.

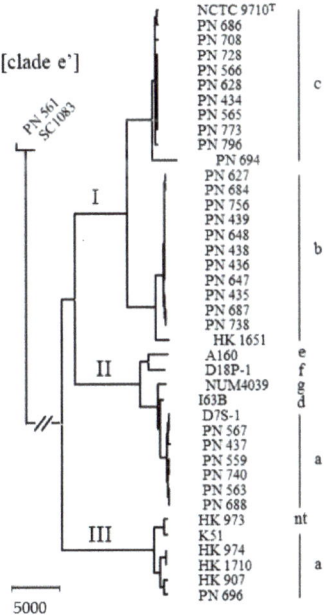

Figure 1. Neighbour-joining dendrogram of *Aggregatibacter actinomycetemcomitans* based on 1146 concatenated core genes (1,104,001 nucleotides) of 42 whole genome-sequenced strains. The type strain is designated with a superscript T. Twenty-nine strains were from cases of bacteraemia (designated PN), five oral strains were included to describe lineage III, and seven WGSs were downloaded from Genbank; see Supplementary Table S1 for further description and origin of strains. The outgroup (strains PN_561 and SC1083) reduces the number of core genes and should probably be excluded from the species. Serotypes and phylogenetic lineages are shown; nt, non-typeable by immunodiffusion with antisera [8]. The bar represents 5000 residue substitutions.

2.1. Delineation of the Species

Serotype e strain PN_561 was cultured from a case of bacteraemia in 2005. The patient underwent aortic valve replacement for infective endocarditis, and the bacterium was also cultured from the removed valve. The strain was identified as *Actinobacillus (Aggregatibacter) actinomycetemcomitans* based on selected phenotypic tests; re-examination using matrix-assisted laser desorption/ionization time-of-flight (MALDI-TOF) mass spectrometry confirmed the identification with a log-score value above 2. The clinical case demonstrates the aggregative potential of the clade e' outgroup, and the WGSs reveal the presence of a *tad* cluster and leukotoxin operon, but a lack of the cytolethal distending toxin gene cluster (GenBank accession number VSEC00000000). We performed in silico DNA–DNA hybridisation (DDH) by use of the Genome-to-Genome Distance Calculator 2.1, which estimates the DDH values that would have resulted from classic hybridisation experiments [17]. The in silico DDH value for strain PN_561 versus the type strain NCTC 9710 was 54.7%, which is below the phylogenetic species boundary of 70% suggested by classic hybridisation [18]. Similar in silico DDH values were obtained for PN_561 versus selected reference strains from other serotypes (range: 54.2% (D18P-1, serotype f) to 55.4% (HK_1651, serotype b)).

Average nucleotide identity (ANI) is a powerful method to estimate overall genome relatedness and is widely used as a substitute of the classic DDH methods. ANI is calculated for two genome sequences by breaking the genome sequence of the query strain into 1020-bp-long fragments. Then, nucleotide identity values for individual fragments of the query strain and the genome of the subject strain are calculated using the NCBI BLASTn program. Using OrthoANI [19], where both genomes are fragmented and only reciprocal BLASTn hits are included, strain PN_561 was 93.89% identical with the type strain of *A. actinomycetemcomitans*; restricting ANI calculation to 1146 concatenated core gene sequences gave an ANI value of 94.72%. An ANI threshold value of 95% is considered the species boundary [20,21], and the two clade e' outgroup strains are excluded from further analysis.

2.2. Natural Competence and Genomic Characteristics of Lineages

Twenty-eight invasive strains plus five oral strains of *A. actinomycetemcomitans* were tested for natural competence by plating on kanamycin-containing agar in the presence of donor DNA. All strains belonged to the three dominant serotypes a–c. In accordance with previous findings [22], only a subset of serotype a strains were competent for transformation, while serotype b and c were invariably noncompetent. Specifically, competence was associated with lineage II (strains PN_437, PN_559, PN_563, PN_567, and PN_688), while all strains of lineage III were noncompetent. Competence is a primary mechanism of horizontal gene transfer and DNA acquisition in bacteria, and it has previously been shown that competent strains of *A. actinomycetemcomitans* are, on average, 200,000 bp larger than noncompetent strains [12]. In accordance with this, the mean genome size of strains of lineage II was 2.26 Mb, while the mean genome size of invariably noncompetent strains of lineage I was 2.07 Mb. With an average genome size of 2.22 Mb, lineage III was closely related to the mean size of competent lineage II, but the range (2113–2316 Kb) did overlap the size of the largest genome in lineage I (strain PN_738; 2134 Kb).

Analysis of competence genes in the six strains of lineage III revealed major disruptions within the essential repository (Figure 2). All strains carried large (11–28 Kb) mobile elements impeding *comM*, but no genome contained all 16 genes, and 31 of 84 identified competence genes were inactivated. It is possible that future analysis will reveal some competent strains of lineage III, but the investigated genomes indicate an ancestral noncompetent lineage, which questions the relationship between competence and genome size.

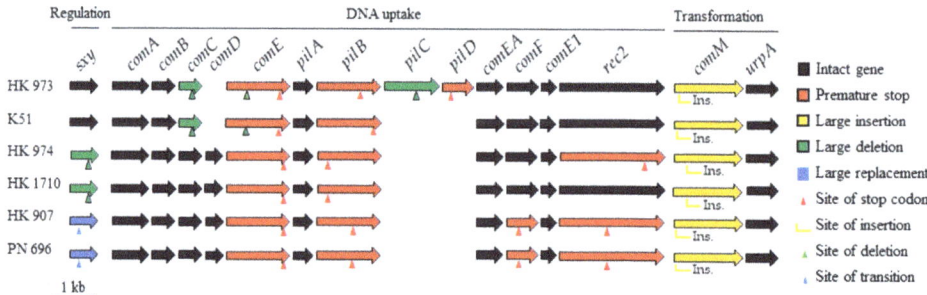

Figure 2. Intact and inactivated competence genes from lineage III strains using strain HK_1651 as reference. Red genes have premature stop codons caused by single base substitutions, single base deletions, or double nucleotide insertions. Yellow genes are disrupted by large insertions (11–28 Kb). Green genes have deletions (150–722 bp) of either the first (*sxy*, *pilC*, *comE*) or the last part (*comC*) of a gene. The first 73 amino acids of gene *sxy* in strains HK_907 and PN_696 are replaced with an unrelated coding sequence (blue genes). Green and blue arrows mark the transition from competence gene to unrelated sequence, or vice versa.

Excluding the two clade e' outgroup strains from Figure 1 increased the number of core gene sequences from 1146 to 1357 but did not distort the dendrogram (not shown). The total number of genes identified by Prokka was 4631, and the distribution of accessory genes is of interest. We used principal component analysis (PCA) of the dichotomous presence/absence of orthologs, analysing 3274 genes present in 1–39 of 40 strains. Figure 3A shows a scatterplot of this accessory genome of 40 *A. actinomycetemcomitans* strains, represented by the two principal components that account for a major part of the variance in the gene presence/absence matrix (Figure 3B). Analysis of the accessory genome supports the division of the species into three distinct lineages. The first principal component (PC) primarily serves to separate lineage I from lineages II and III, while PC2 dissociates all three lineages (Figure 3A). Indeed, nine of the 10 annotated genes (excluding hypothetical genes) with the highest loadings in PC1 were only present in 23 strains of lineage I, while nine of the 10 annotated genes with the highest negative loadings were predominantly associated with 17 strains of lineage II plus III (range 15–18). For PC2, the highest loadings were associated either with 34 strains of lineage I plus II, or with six strains of lineage III, while the highest negative loadings were more unevenly distributed among lineages (not shown).

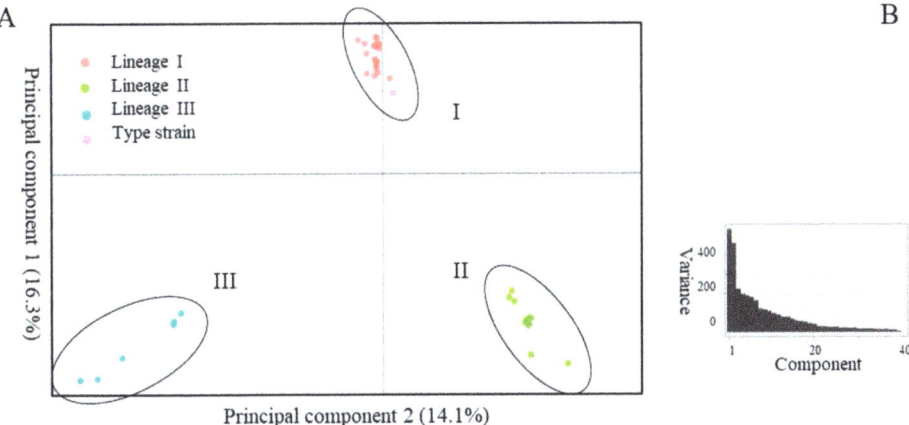

Figure 3. (**A**), principal component analysis of presence/absence of accessory homologs in 40 strains of *A. actinomycetemcomitans*. (**B**), line plot of the eigenvalues of factors or principal components in the analysis. The two principal components depicted in 3A comprise 30% of the sum of variances of all individual principal components (3B).

By scatterplot of PC1 vs. PC2, strains of lineage III appear more diverse than those of lineage II, which are more diverse than those of lineage I (Figure 3A); this may, in part, be caused by the decreasing number of strains included in the lineages. The accessory gene content of serotype g strain NUM4039 was the most divergent in lineage II, followed by serotype a strain D7S-1 (Figure 3A); this segregation is not apparent from single-nucleotide polymorphism (SNP) analysis of core gene sequences (Figure 1). Three strains of lineage III clustered closely by PCA, while HK_907, HK_973 and PN_696 were more individually positioned (Figure 3A). Again, this pattern of accessory gene content is not reflected in the SNP analysis of core gene sequences (Figure 1).

Lineage-specific gene homologs were abstracted from the Roary output, and the annotated genes (excluding hypotheticals) are listed in Supplementary Table S2. Thirty-seven gene homologs (14 annotated, 23 hypothetical) were detected in 23 lineage I strains and not in strains of other lineages; the corresponding numbers are 16 annotated genes only present in 11 lineage II strains, and 20 annotated genes only present in six lineage III strains. Several unexpected associations are observed, such as homologs of the multidrug exporter MdtA restricted to lineage II, and several CRISPR-associated nucleases confined to lineage II or III. Clearly, phenotypic and pathobiological significance must be addressed in biologic experiments, and the true relationship between marker genes and lineages awaits analysis of a larger number of strains. Nevertheless, the existence of lineage-specific marker genes encourages the development of lineage-specific PCRs that will be simpler and more informative than the currently employed serotype-specific PCRs.

3. Discussion

A. actinomycetemcomitans was linked to aggressive periodontitis in 1976, and this association was supported by elevated serum antibodies in patients [5]. Three distinct bacterial surface antigens were identified by 1983, and this typing has remained the cornerstone of the initial characterisation of cultured strains. More advanced methods for dissection of the population structure [8–10] have not gained acceptance, although multilocus sequence typing (MLST) holds promise as a general, versatile typing method. WGSs have unequivocally shown that serotyping is inadequate for assessment of the phylogenetic positioning of a clinical strain.

We performed whole genome sequencing of *A. actinomycetemcomitans* cultured from blood stream infections. By serotype, the population resembled oral strains from our region with almost equal proportions of the three dominant serotypes. However, comparison of WGSs revealed some interesting observations. First, the serotype e strain PN_561 was not related to common serotype e strains within the species but belonged to an outgroup that has been designated clade e' [13]. Aberrant strains of serotype e also deviate by 16S rRNA [9] and MLST [10,23], but distinctive phenotypic markers have not yet been described. Assessment of overall genome relatedness by ANI and in silico DDH positioned PN_561 and the reference clade e' outgroup strain outside the species boundary. These strains are negative for the cytolethal distending toxin genes but encode the *tad* cluster that is decisive for autoaggregation and adherence to a wide range of solid surfaces. Strain HK_921 of the clade e' outgroup was included in the investigation of *Aggragatibacter* strains that resulted in the description of the new species *Aggregatibacter kilianii*, and the difference between HK_921 and the other strains of *A. actinomycetemcomitans* was similar to or exceeded the difference between *Aggregatibacter kilianii* and *Aggregatibacter aphrophilus* [24]. Valid publication of bacterial names generally requires key phenotypic tests for discriminatory purposes, while identification by matrix-assisted laser desorption/ionisation time-of-flight (MALDI-TOF) mass spectrometry is only dependent on the composition of mass spectre in the database. The frequent detection of these outgroup strains in clinical samples may give impetus to taxonomic rearrangements in genus *Aggregatibacter*; the clinical significance of the clade e' outgroup is emphasised by strain PN_561 being the cause of infective endocarditis.

Second, strain PN_696 of serotype a was neither related to other strains of this serotype nor to any previously deposited WGSs of *A. actinomycetemcomitans*. We were able to identify five additional strains cultured from the oral cavity with high genotypic resemblance to PN_696. In contrast to the clade e' outgroup, aberrant serotype a strains were positioned inside the *A. actinomycetemcomitans* species boundary. Accepted and used designations are helpful, and clade a' would be in line with a recent description of the population structure of *A. actinomycetemcomitans* by WGSs [13]. We suggest a different term. The population structure of *A. actinomycetemcomitans* is more accurately described by a division of the species into three phylogenetic lineages I–III. Although clearly separate entities, this designation would bundle serotype b and c strains into a common lineage. Strains of five separate serotypes are present in lineage II, while a subset of serotype a strains constitute lineage III.

4. Materials and Methods

4.1. Bacterial Strains and DNA Accession Numbers

Twenty-nine strains of *A actinomycetemcomitans* were collected from blood stream infections from seven Danish departments of clinical microbiology. Initial analysis of WGSs revealed a peculiar sequence from a serotype a strain, and we were able to identify five additional oral strains with high resemblance to the invasive strain; these five strains were included in the study, as was the type strain NCTC 9710 of serotype c. Representative WGSs of serotypes other than c were downloaded from the public databases, including an additional serotype e strain allocated to the outgroup tentatively designated clade e' [13]. Supplementary Table S1 lists the origin, host characteristics, and accession numbers of all investigated strains and sequences.

4.2. Identification and Phenotyping

All clinical strains were subjected to renewed identification by matrix-assisted, laser desorption/ionization time-of-flight mass spectrometry (MALDI-TOF) as described [24]. Serotyping by PCR was performed as previously described [25]. Natural competence was investigated by transformation assays [22] using donor DNA from the D7S *hns* mutant that carries the kanamycin resistance gene cluster from pUC4K in the *H-NS* gene [26]. In brief, 20 µl of a dense bacterial suspension (OD_{600nm} = 0.3) was spread in a small area (diameter of ~10 mm) on a brain-heart infusion (BHI) agar plate. After incubation for 2 h, 10 µl of donor DNA (~1 µg) was added, gently mixed by using a loop, and further incubated for an additional 6 h. The bacteria were collected with a cotton swab, suspended in 400 µl of BHI broth, and plated on selective media containing kanamycin 50 (µg/mL); in parallel, diluted samples were plated on chocolate agar plates. Colonies were counted after two and seven days, and the transformation frequency was the ratio of the number of transformants to the number of cells plated.

4.3. DNA Sequencing, Genome Assembly, and Analysis

DNA libraries were prepared from 200 ng of genomic DNA with a Sciclone NGS robot (PerkinElmer), using the QIAseq FX DNA Library Kit (QIAGEN), according to the manufacturer's protocol. Quality control of the libraries was conducted by on-chip electrophoresis (TapeStation, Agilent) and by Qubit (Thermofisher) concentration measurements. Dual-indexed paired-end sequencing (2 by 150 bp) was performed with an Illumina NextSeq 500 system (Illumina) aiming at 200 x coverage. Paired demultiplexed FASTQ files were generated using CASAVA software (Illumina), and initial quality control was performed using FastQC. Reads were assembled using Unicycler (version 0.4.7), an optimiser for SPAdes (version 3.13.9). Contigs with a length below 500 nt were disregarded. Draft assemblies of study strains plus FASTA files from reference strains downloaded from GenBank were annotated with Prokka [27]. Roary [28], a rapid, large-scale, prokaryote pan-genome analysis tool, was used with default settings for identification of core genes to create clusters of genes that share amino acid sequence similarity and coverage above a given threshold and orders strains by the presence or absence of orthologs. Core genes (present in all strains) were aligned with ClustalW and concatenated, before SNPs were called and evolutionary analyses conducted in MEGA X [29].

In silico DNA hybridisation between selected strains was performed with the Genome-to-Genome Distance Calculator (version 2.1), using standard settings and the recommended identity/high-scoring segment pair length calculation [17]. Average nucleotide identity (ANI) values of draft genomes were calculated using online tools (http://www.ezbiocloud.net/sw/oat) [19]; additionally, ANI values of concatenated *A. actinomycetemcomitans* core genes were calculated with Panito (version 0.0.2b1) (https://github.com/sanger-pathogens/panito). Principal component analysis (PCA) of binary absence/presence gene matrix from Prokka was computed in R with built-in packages.

Supplementary Materials: The following are available online at http://www.mdpi.com/2076-0817/8/4/256/s1, Table S1: List of strains and sequence accession number; Table S2: Lineage-specific, annotated genes.

Author Contributions: All authors made a substantial, direct, and intellectual contribution to the work. N.N.-L. conceived and planned the study and made the first draft of the manuscript. A.B.J., M.B.N., R.T.M., and S.N. performed molecular and phenotypic experiments. C.M.K. completed the bioinformatics. All authors approved the manuscript for publication.

Funding: This research did not receive any specific grant from funding agencies in the public, commercial, or not-for-profit sectors.

Acknowledgments: Members of the Danish HACEK Study Group Jens J. Christensen, Slagelse Hospital; Gitte Hartmeyer, Odense University Hospital; Kristian Schønning, Hvidovre Hospital; Lisbeth Lützen, Aarhus University Hospital; Claus Moser, Rigshospitalet; Bente Olesen, Herlev and Gentofte Hospital; and Henrik C. Schønheyder, Aalborg University Hospital provided strains and clinical information on patient cases.

Ethical Statement: The study is an extension the incidence of HACEK bacteraemia in Denmark [6] and was conducted in accordance with the regional guidelines for the use of clinical and laboratory data and was approved by the Danish Data Protection Agency (record number 2012-58-0004) and the National Board of Health (record number 3-3013-1170/1).

Conflicts of Interest: The authors declare no conflict of interest.

Abbreviations

ANI, average nucleotide identity; BHI, brain-heart infusion; DDH, DNA–DNA hybridization; HACEK, *Haemophilus*, *Aggregatibacter*, *Cardiobacterium*, *Eikenella* and *Kingella*; MALDI-TOF, matrix-assisted laser desorption/ionisation time-of-flight; MLST, multilocus sequence typing; PCA, principal component analysis; SNP, single-nucleotide polymorphism; WGSs, whole genome sequences.

References

1. Karched, M.; Furgang, D.; Planet, P.J.; DeSalle, R.; Fine, D.H. Genome Sequence of *Aggregatibacter actinomycetemcomitans* RHAA1, Isolated from a Rhesus Macaque, an Old World Primate. *J. Bacteriol.* **2012**, *194*, 1275–1276. [CrossRef] [PubMed]
2. Nørskov-Lauritsen, N. Classification, identification, and clinical significance of *Haemophilus* and *Aggregatibacter* species with host specificity for humans. *Clin. Microbiol. Rev.* **2014**, *27*, 214–240. [CrossRef] [PubMed]
3. Henderson, B.; Ward, J.M.; Ready, D. *Aggregatibacter (Actinobacillus) actinomycetemcomitans*: A triple A* periodontopathogen? *Periodontology 2000* **2010**, *54*, 78–105. [CrossRef] [PubMed]
4. Haubek, D.; Ennibi, O.K.; Poulsen, K.; Vaeth, M.; Poulsen, S.; Kilian, M. Risk of aggressive periodontitis in adolescent carriers of the JP2 clone of *Aggregatibacter (Actinobacillus) actinomycetemcomitans* in Morocco: A prospective longitudinal cohort study. *Lancet* **2008**, *371*, 237–242. [CrossRef]
5. Fine, D.H.; Patil, A.G.; Velusamy, S.K. *Aggregatibacter actinomycetemcomitans* (Aa) Under the Radar: Myths and Misunderstandings of Aa and Its Role in Aggressive Periodontitis. *Front. Immunol.* **2019**, *10*, 728. [CrossRef]
6. Lützen, L.; Olesen, B.; Voldstedlund, M.; Christensen, J.J.; Moser, C.; Knudsen, J.D.; Fuursted, K.; Hartmeyer, G.N.; Chen, M.; Søndergaard, T.S.; et al. Incidence of HACEK bacteraemia in Denmark: A 6-year population-based study. *Int. J. Infect. Dis.* **2018**, *68*, 83–87. [CrossRef]
7. Yew, H.S.; Chambers, S.T.; Roberts, S.A.; Holland, D.J.; Julian, K.A.; Raymond Beardsley, J.; Read, K.M.; Murdoch, D.R. Association between HACEK bacteraemia and endocarditis. *J. Med. Microbiol.* **2014**, *63*, 892–895. [CrossRef]
8. Poulsen, K.; Theilade, E.; Lally, E.T.; Demuth, D.R.; Kilian, M. Population structure of *Actinobacillus actinomycetemcomitans*: A framework for studies of disease-associated properties. *Microbiology* **1994**, *140*, 2049–2060. [CrossRef]
9. Kaplan, J.B.; Schreiner, H.C.; Furgang, D.; Fine, D.H. Population Structure and Genetic Diversity of *Actinobacillus actinomycetemcomitans* Strains Isolated from Localized Juvenile Periodontitis Patients. *J. Clin. Microbiol.* **2002**, *40*, 1181–1187. [CrossRef]
10. Haubek, D.; Poulsen, K.; Kilian, M. Microevolution and patterns of dissemination of the JP2 clone of *Aggregatibacter (Actinobacillus) Actinomycetemcomitans*. *Infect. Immun.* **2007**, *75*, 3080–3088. [CrossRef]
11. Kittichotirat, W.; Bumgarner, R.E.; Asikainen, S.; Chen, C. Identification of the Pangenome and Its Components in 14 Distinct *Aggregatibacter actinomycetemcomitans* Strains by Comparative Genomic Analysis. *PLoS ONE* **2011**, *6*, e22420. [CrossRef] [PubMed]
12. Jorth, P.; Whiteley, M. An Evolutionary Link between Natural Transformation and CRISPR Adaptive Immunity. *MBio* **2012**, *3*, e00309-12. [CrossRef] [PubMed]
13. Kittichotirat, W.; Bumgarner, R.E.; Chen, C. Evolutionary Divergence of Aggregatibacter actinomycetemcomitans. *J. Dent. Res.* **2016**, *95*, 94–101. [CrossRef] [PubMed]
14. Zambon, J.J.; Umemoto, T.; De Nardin, E.; Nakazawa, F.; Christersson, L.A.; Genco, R.J. *Actinobacillus actinomycetemcomitans* in the pathogenesis of human periodontal disease. *Adv. Dent. Res.* **1988**, *2*, 269–274. [CrossRef]

15. Paju, S.; Carlson, P.; Jousimies-Somer, H.; Asikainen, S. Heterogeneity of *Actinobacillus actinomycetemcomitans* Strains in Various Human Infections and Relationships between Serotype, Genotype, and Antimicrobial Susceptibility. *J. Clin. Microbiol.* **2000**, *38*, 79–84.
16. Rylev, M.; Kilian, M. Prevalence and distribution of principal periodontal pathogens worldwide. *J. Clin. Periodontol.* **2011**, *3*, 346–361. [CrossRef]
17. Meier-Kolthoff, J.P.; Auch, A.F.; Klenk, H.P.; Göker, M. Genome sequencebased species delimitation with confidence intervals and improved distance functions. *BMC Bioinform.* **2013**, *14*, 60. [CrossRef]
18. Wayne, L.; Brenner, D.J.; Colwell, R.R.; Grimont, P.A.D.; Kandler, O.; Krichevsky, M.I.; Moore, L.H.; Moore, W.E.C.; Murray, R.G.E.; Stackebrandt, E.; et al. Report of the Ad Hoc Committee on Reconciliation of Approaches to Bacterial Systematics. *Int. J. Syst. Bacteriol.* **1987**, *37*, 463–464. [CrossRef]
19. Lee, I.; Ouk Kim, Y.; Park, S.C.; Chun, J. OrthoANI: An improved algorithm and software for calculating average nucleotide identity. *Int. J. Syst. Evol. Microbiol.* **2016**, *66*, 1100–1103. [CrossRef]
20. Gevers, D.; Cohan, F.M.; Lawrence, J.G.; Spratt, B.G.; Coenye, T.; Feil, E.J.; Stackebrandt, E.; Van de Peer, Y.; Vandamme, P.; Thompson, F.L.; et al. Opinion: Re-evaluating prokaryotic species. *Nat. Rev. Microbiol.* **2005**, *3*, 733–739. [CrossRef]
21. Richter, M.; Rosselló-Móra, R. Shifting the genomic gold standard for the prokaryotic species definition. *Proc. Natl. Acad. Sci. USA* **2009**, *106*, 19126–19131. [CrossRef] [PubMed]
22. Wang, Y.; Goodman, S.D.; Redfield, R.J.; Chen, C. Natural transformation and DNA uptake signal sequences in *Actinobacillus actinomycetemcomitans*. *J. Bacteriol.* **2002**, *184*, 3442–3449. [CrossRef] [PubMed]
23. Nørskov-Lauritsen, N.; Kilian, M. Reclassification of *Actinobacillus actinomycetemcomitans*, *Haemophilus aphrophilus*, *Haemophilus paraphrophilus* and *Haemophilus segnis* as *Aggregatibacter actinomycetemcomitans* gen. nov., comb. nov., *Aggregatibacter aphrophilus* comb. nov. and *Aggregatibacter segnis* comb. nov., and emended description of *Aggregatibacter aphrophilus* to include V factor-dependent and V factor-independent isolates. *Int. J. Syst. Evol. Microbiol.* **2006**, *56*, 2135–2146.
24. Murra, M.; Lützen, L.; Barut, A.; Zbinden, R.; Lund, M.; Villesen, P.; Nørskov-Lauritsen, N. Whole-Genome Sequencing of *Aggregatibacter* Species Isolated from Human Clinical Specimens and Description of *Aggregatibacter kilianii* sp. nov. *J. Clin. Microbiol.* **2018**, *56*, e00053-18. [CrossRef] [PubMed]
25. Jensen, A.B.; Haubek, D.; Claesson, R.; Johansson, A.; Nørskov-Lauritsen, N. Comprehensive antimicrobial susceptibility testing of a large collection of clinical strains of *Aggregatibacter actinomycetemcomitans* does not identify resistance to amoxicillin. *J. Clin. Periodontol.* **2019**, *46*, 846–854. [CrossRef]
26. Bao, K.; Bostanci, N.; Thurnheer, T.; Grossmann, J.; Wolski, W.E.; Thay, B.; Belibasakis, G.N.; Oscarsson, J. *Aggregatibacter actinomycetemcomitans* H-NS promotes biofilm formation and alters protein dynamics of other species within a polymicrobial oral biofilm. *NPJ Biofilms Microbiomes* **2018**, *4*, 12. [CrossRef] [PubMed]
27. Seemann, T. Prokka: Rapid prokaryotic genome annotation. *Bioinformatics* **2014**, *30*, 2068–2069. [CrossRef]
28. Page, A.J.; Cummins, C.A.; Hunt, M.; Wong, V.K.; Reuter, S.; Holden, M.T.; Fookes, M.; Falush, D.; Keane, J.A.; Parkhill, J. Roary: Rapid large-scale prokaryote pan genome analysis. *Bioinformatics* **2015**, *31*, 3691–3693. [CrossRef]
29. Kumar, S.; Stecher, G.; Li, M.; Knyaz, C.; Tamura, K. MEGA X: Molecular Evolutionary Genetics Analysis across computing platforms. *Mol. Biol. Evol.* **2018**, *35*, 1547–1549. [CrossRef]

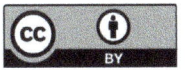

© 2019 by the authors. Licensee MDPI, Basel, Switzerland. This article is an open access article distributed under the terms and conditions of the Creative Commons Attribution (CC BY) license (http://creativecommons.org/licenses/by/4.0/).

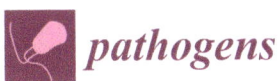

Article

Differential Cell Lysis Among Periodontal Strains of JP2 and Non-JP2 Genotype of *Aggregatibacter actinomycetemcomitans* Serotype B Is Not Reflected in Dissimilar Expression and Production of Leukotoxin

Anne Birkeholm Jensen [1,2], Marianne Lund [2], Niels Nørskov-Lauritsen [2], Anders Johansson [3], Rolf Claesson [4], Jesper Reinholdt [5] and Dorte Haubek [1,*]

[1] Section for Pediatric Dentistry, Department of Dentistry and Oral Health, Health, Aarhus University, 8000 Aarhus, Denmark; abj@dent.au.dk
[2] Department of Clinical Microbiology, Aarhus University Hospital Skejby, 8200 Aarhus, Denmark; marialun@rm.dk (M.L.); nielnoer@rm.dk (N.N.-L.)
[3] Section of Molecular Periodontology, Department of Odontology, Faculty of Medicine, Umeå University, 901 87 Umeå, Sweden; anders.p.johansson@umu.se
[4] Division of Oral Microbiology, Department of Odontology, Faculty of Medicine, Umeå University, 901 87 Umeå, Sweden; rolf.claesson@umu.se
[5] Department of Biomedicine, Aarhus University, 8000 Aarhus, Denmark; reinholdt8240@gmail.com
* Correspondence: dorte.haubek@dent.au.dk; Tel.: +45-87168092

Received: 11 October 2019; Accepted: 26 October 2019; Published: 30 October 2019

Abstract: Leukotoxic potential of *Aggregatibacter actinomycetemcomitans* strains has been studied by the use of several methods, and results differ depending on the methods used. The aim of the present study was to perform a comprehensive examination of the leukotoxic potential of a collection of *A. actinomycetemcomitans* strains by use of three quantitative methods, Western blotting, ELISA, and mRNA expression assay and compare these results with previous data obtained by a cell lysis assay. A higher leukotoxic potential among JP2 genotype strains compared to non-JP2 genotype strains of *A. actinomycetemcomitans* was found by Western blotting, ELISA and mRNA expression assay. Leukotoxicity as determined by cell lysis assay showed a variation among strains examined, not only depending on being part of JP2 genotype *vs.* non-JP2 genotype group of *A. actinomycetemcomitans*. The leukotoxicity of *A. actinomycetemcomitans* strains as determined by cell lysis assay did not correspond to the leukotoxic potential of *A. actinomycetemcomitans* strains as determined by three quantitative methods. A comparison of the results obtained by ELISA and mRNA expression assay showed a reasonable correlation between these two methods. It seems important to use more than one method to assess the LtxA-related virulence capacity of *A. actinomycetemcomitans* in order to obtain comprehensive understanding of the leukotoxic potential of *A. actinomycetemcomitans* strains.

Keywords: mRNA assay; quantitative ELISA; cell lysis assay; leukotoxin; JP2 genotype

1. Introduction

Aggregatibacter actinomycetemcomitans is a Gram-negative member of the human oral microbiota [1] and is involved in human infections and diseases [2–5]. One of these diseases is periodontitis, characterized by destruction of tooth-supporting periodontal tissues due to an inflammatory response [6]. *A. actinomycetemcomitans* possesses several virulence factors [3], of which the production of the RTX (repeats-in-toxin) leukotoxin (LtxA) has received much attention [7–12]. LtxA induces cell lysis, degranulation and an inflammatory response in human leukocytes by interaction with the β2-integrins in the cell membrane of human immune cells [8,13,14]. A 530-bp deletion in the promoter region of the

LtxA gene operon was identified in the original JP2 strain, cultured from a young individual diagnosed with juvenile periodontitis [15]. This discovery marked the beginning of an era, where the detection of the 530-bp deletion categorized highly leukotoxic *A. actinomycetemcomitans* strains as a member of the JP2 clone of *A. actinomycetemcomitans*, possessing enhanced virulence. Based on in vitro studies, it was reported that the JP2 genotype of *A. actinomycetemcomitans* has a 10–20 fold higher lytic activity than the non-JP2 genotypes of *A. actinomycetemcomitans* [15]. Furthermore, longitudinal clinical studies reported a clear correlation between being carrier of the JP2 genotype of *A. actinomycetemcomitans* and having an increased risk of developing periodontitis at a young age [16,17].

Often the leukotoxic potential of *A. actinomycetemcomitans* is characterized by the leukotoxicity in in vitro studies [11,15,18–21]. This leukotoxicity is determined by use of cell lysis assays, where human immune cells are exposed either to the bacteria or to purified LtxA, and most often the leukotoxicity is correlated with the JP2 or non-JP2 genotype of the *A. actinomycetemcomitans* strain. Therefore, it has been the common believe that the leukotoxicity of an *A. actinomycetemcomitans* strain could be explained by the 530-bp deletion, an explanation supported by recent results presented by Sampathkumar and co-workers [21]. However, *A. actinomycetemcomitans* strains without the 530-bp deletion with high leukotoxicity according to results obtained by cell lysis assay have been reported on [20]. Furthermore, the leukotoxic potential of *A. actinomycetemcomitans* strains has been explained by different mechanisms [15,18,19]. A higher expression of the mRNA, encoding the *ltxA*, has been reported to correspond with a higher leukotoxic potential [15,18], but also a variation in the activity of LtxA in some *A. actinomycetemcomitans* has been reported [19]. Only a few studies have compared the leukotoxicity of *A. actinomycetemcomitans* with the LtxA expression and production defined as a quantification of the LtxA, e.g., by enzyme-linked immunosorbent assay (ELISA), or mRNA coding for LtxA [15,18,21], but it seems reasonable to assume that the two factors are related.

In the present study, we aimed to investigate if the leukotoxicity of a collection of Ghanaian *A. actinomycetemcomitans*, serotype b, is related to the LtxA production of the strains determined by Western blotting and ELISA, and LtxA expression as determined in a mRNA expression assay. Furthermore, we wanted to compare the results obtained by ELISA and mRNA expression assay to elucidate the relationship between the two quantification methods used to determine leukotoxic potential as the LtxA production and expression of *A. actinomycetemcomitans*, respectively.

2. Results

2.1. LtxA Expression and Production of the 20 Ghanaian Strains by Western Blotting, ELISA and mRNA Expression Assay

Western blotting clearly showed that the JP2 genotype strains of *A. actinomycetemcomitans* had a higher LtxA production than the non-JP2 genotype strains (Figure S1).

The non-JP2 genotype strains 575G, 605G, 638G, 443G, and 486G were previously characterized as having high leukotoxicity by cell lysis assay (Table 1) [20].

Strains 443G and 486G might have a tendency towards a higher LtxA production than the other non-JP2 genotype strains, but not at comparable levels as to the JP2 genotype strains. Furthermore, the Western blotting demonstrated that the strains with high LtxA production had a higher amount of LtxA in the growth supernatant than in the cell pellet extract (Figure S1).

By visual inspection of Figure 1, the ELISA showed the same division of JP2 and non-JP2 genotype strains of *A. actinomycetemcomitans* as demonstrated by the Western blotting (Figure S1). In Figures 1 and 2, the cell lysis assay (LDH) characterizes the leukotoxicity of the strains, and the results are from the publication by Höglund Åberg and coworkers (2014) [20]. The results are given as a percentage of total lysis of THP-1 cells by Triton X. The ELISA determines the leukotoxic production of the *A. actinomycetemcomitans* strains as a percentage of the reference *A. actinomycetemcomitans* strain HK921, and results are the mean of two separate runs. The mRNA expression assay determines the leukotoxin expression of *A. actinomycetemcomitans* strains as a ratio to *adk* and *pgi*, and the results are the mean of three separate runs.

Table 1. Characterization of the collection of *A. actinomycetemcomitans* strains, serotype b.

Bacterial Strains	Genotype	Origin	Leukotoxicity *
1 G	non-JP2	Ghana	Average
153 G	non-JP2	Ghana	Average
212 G	non-JP2	Ghana	Average
217 G	non-JP2	Ghana	Average
640 G	non-JP2	Ghana	Average
443 G	non-JP2	Ghana	High
486 G	non-JP2	Ghana	High
575 G	non-JP2	Ghana	High
605 G	non-JP2	Ghana	High
638 G	non-JP2	Ghana	High
369 G	non-JP2	Ghana	Low
467 G	non-JP2	Ghana	Low
493 G	non-JP2	Ghana	Low
708 G	non-JP2	Ghana	Low
744 G	non-JP2	Ghana	Low
331 M	non-JP2	Morocco	
394 M	non-JP2	Morocco	
416 M	non-JP2	Morocco	
HK1605	non-JP2	USA	
HK908	non-JP2	Porto-Brazil [1]	
HK911	non-JP2	Holland	
HK912	non-JP2	Holland	
HK975 (Y4)	non-JP2	USA	
437 G	JP2	Ghana	High
488 G	JP2	Ghana	High
524 G	JP2	Ghana	High
654 G	JP2	Ghana	High
666 G	JP2	Ghana	High
HK1199	JP2	USA	
HK1507	JP2	Cape Verde Isands-Sweden [2]	
HK1519	JP2	Cape Verde Islands-Sweden [2]	
HK1547	JP2	USA	
HK1609	JP2	USA	
HK1615	JP2	USA	
HK1626	JP2	Tel Aviv-Switzerland [3]	
HK1630	JP2	Algeria-Denmark [4]	
HK1631	JP2	Morocco-Denmark [5]	
HK1651	JP2	Ghana-Denmark [6]	
HK1659	JP2	Morocco-Denmark [5]	
HK1702	JP2	Brazil	
HK1707	JP2	Brazil	
HK1990	JP2	Portugal-Holland	
HK2000	JP2	Morocco	
HK2017	JP2	Tel Aviv	
HK921 (JP2)	JP2	USA	

* As defined by Höglund Åberg and coworkers (2014): 0–30% LDH release = low leukotoxicity, 31–60% = average leukotoxicity and 60% ≤ = high leukotoxicity. [1] Originating from Portugal, [2] Originating from Cape Verde Islands, [3] Originating from Tel Aviv, [4] Originating from Algeria, [5] Originating from Morocco, [6] Originating from Ghana.

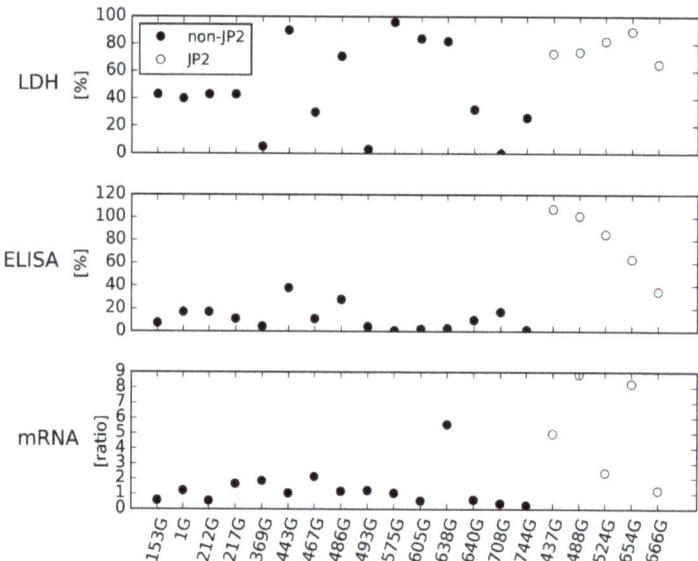

Figure 1. Leukotoxicity, leukotoxin production and leukotoxin expression of 20 Ghanaian *A. actinomycetemcomitans*, serotype b, JP2 and non-JP2 genotype strains determined by a cell lysis assay (LDH), an ELISA, and a mRNA expression assay.

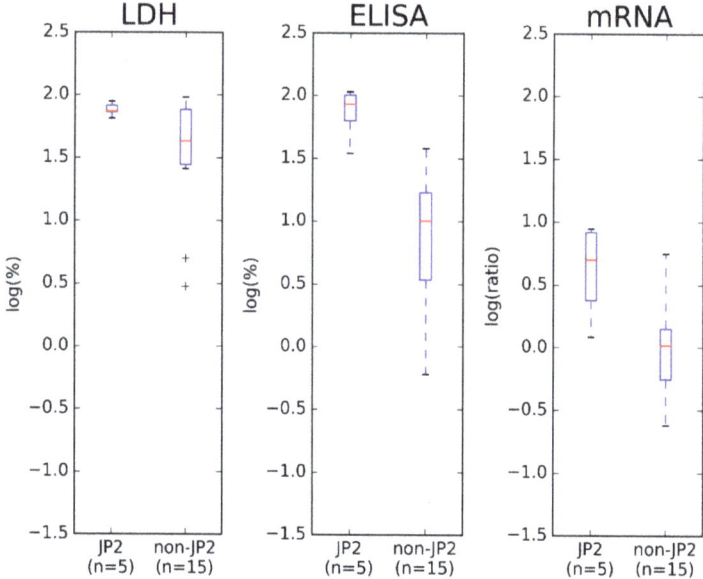

Figure 2. Box plot of the distribution of the 20 Ghanaian *A. actinomycetemcomitans* strains according to JP2 genotype and non-JP2 genotype strains.

Two non-JP2 genotype strains of *A. actinomycetemcomitans* (443G and 486G) showed almost the same LtxA production as one of the JP2 genotype strains of *A. actinomycetemcomitans*. However, in general the JP2 genotype strains of *A. actinomycetemcomitans* showed a higher LtxA production than the non-JP2 genotype strains of *A. actinomycetemcomitans*. Furthermore, this finding was supported by comparing the group of JP2 genotype strains of *A. actinomycetemcomitans* to the group of non-JP2 genotype strains of *A. actinomycetemcomitans* (Figure 2). The group of JP2 genotype of *A. actinomycetemcomitans* had a statistically significant higher LtxA production than the group of non-JP2 strains of *A. actinomycetemcomitans* ($p < 0.05$) (Figure 2).

Expression of mRNA encoding LtxA did not correlate with the leukotoxicity either (Figure 1). By visual inspection, the mRNA expression assay showed a greater variation in the LtxA expression of the *A. actinomycetemcomitans* strains and found one non-JP2 genotype strain (638G) with a LtxA expression at comparable levels to the JP2 genotype strains. The average mRNA expression of JP2 genotype strains of *A. actinomycetemcomitans* was higher than observed for non-JP2 genotype strains, and the difference did attain statistical significance (Figure 2) ($p < 0.05$).

Conclusively, the high leukotoxicity of some of the non-JP2 strains of *A. actinomycetemcomitans* found by Höglund Åberg and coworkers (2014) could not be reproduced according to the LtxA expression and production found by neither the Western blotting, the ELISA, nor the mRNA expression assay.

2.2. Comparison of Results Obtained by ELISA and mRNA Expression Assay

For further comparison of the two quantitative methods, ELISA and mRNA expression assay, 45 strains of *A. actinomycetemcomitans*, serotype b, were analyzed (Figure 3). The ELISA determines the leukotoxin production of the *A. actinomycetemcomitans* strains as a percentage of the reference strain HK921, and the results are the mean of two separate runs. The mRNA expression assay determines the leukotoxin expression of the *A. actinomycetemcomitans* strains as a ratio to *adk* and *pgi*, and the results are the mean of three separate runs.

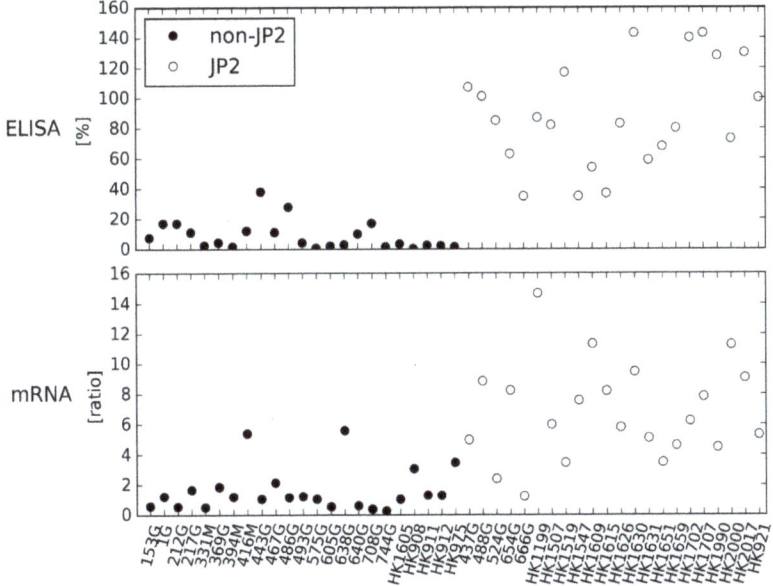

Figure 3. The distribution of the expanded bacterial collection of 45 *A. actinomycetemcomitans* strains for comparison of the results obtained by ELISA and in mRNA expression assay.

By visual inspection of Figure 3, both methods divided the *A. actinomycetemcomitans* strains, serotype b, according to their genotype, although the division was most clearly demonstrated by ELISA. A comparison of the group of JP2 genotype strains of *A. actinomycetemcomitans* and the group of non-JP2 genotype strains of *A. actinomycetemcomitans* is illustrated in Figure 4.

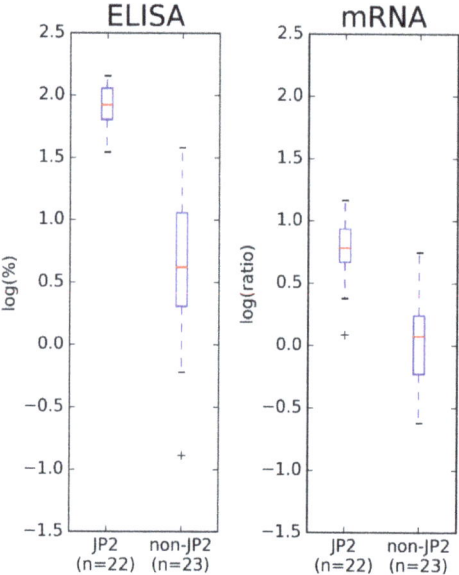

Figure 4. A comparison of the group of JP2 genotype strains and the group of non-JP2 genotype strains of *A. actinomycetemcomitans* based on the expanded bacterial collection of 45 strains for comparison of results obtained by ELISA and in mRNA expression assays by use of log-transformed data.

As for the analysis of the 20 Ghanaian *A. actinomycetemcomitans* strains, the group of JP2 genotype strains had a higher LtxA production and expression than the group of non-JP2 genotype strains of *A. actinomycetemcomitans* ($p < 0.05$) by both ELISA and mRNA expression assay.

By visual inspection of the scatter plot (Figure 5), where the points correspond to a particular strain, a reasonable fit between the results obtained by the ELISA and in the mRNA expression assay was seen.

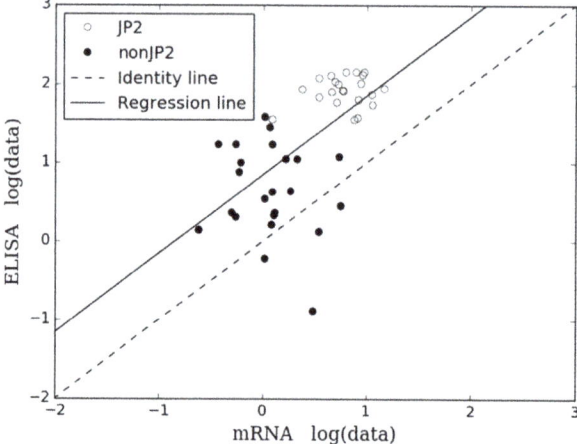

Figure 5. A comparison of ELISA and mRNA expression assay by an ordinary least square regression model based on the expanded bacterial collection consisting of 23 non-JP2 genotype strains of *A. actinomycetemcomitans* (black dots) and 22 JP2 genotype strains of *A. actinomycetemcomitans* (white dots) by use of log-transformed data.

However, the points tended to fall above the identity line indicating bias in the data. An ordinary least squares regression model was used to compare the ELISA and the mRNA expression assay based on the results of the collection of 45 *A. actinomycetemcomitans*, serotype b, strains. The regression fit of the two methods is given by the R^2 at 0.37 indicating a reasonable relationship between the methods. The intercept differed from 0.0 (0.85) indicating that the regression model possesses consistent bias. A slope > 0.00 (1.00) ($p < 0.05$) illustrated a proportional (log-log linear) relationship between the two methods. Furthermore, the scatter plot (Figure 5) illustrated a greater variation in the data among the non-JP2 genotype of *A. actinomycetemcomitans*, whereas the data for the JP2 genotype strains of *A. actinomycetemcomitans* was more equal.

3. Discussion

In the present study, we aimed to investigate if the leukotoxic potential determined by a leukotoxicity assay of 20 Ghanaian *A. actinomycetemcomitans*, serotype b, is related to the LtxA production and expression of the strains determined by three different quantitative methods. Quantification of the LtxA production and expression using Western blotting, ELISA and mRNA expression assay could not reproduce the high leukotoxicity found among some of the Ghanaian non-JP2 genotype strains by use of cell lysis assay previously reported on by Höglund Åberg and coworkers (2014) [20]. All JP2 genotype strains of *A. actinomycetemcomitans* showed high LtxA expression and production. Furthermore, the non-JP2 genotype strains of *A. actinomycetemcomitans*, serotype b, previously characterized as having a high leukotoxicity, were all below the JP2 genotype strains when using LtxA expression and production assays. Furthermore, supplementary analysis of the expanded bacterial collection of *A. actinomycetemcomitans* strains, serotype b, revealed a reasonable relationship between the results obtained by ELISA and mRNA expression assay.

To our knowledge, this is the first study relating the leukotoxicity of a large collection of *A. actinomycetemcomitans* strains, serotype b, to the LtxA expression and production determined by three different quantitative methods. Studies have previously related the leukotoxicity of *A. actinomycetemcomitans* strains to the LtxA expression and production, often determined by quantification of mRNA or by Western blotting [15,18,21]. In addition, many studies have related a high leukotoxicity and a high LtxA expression to the presence of the 530-bp deletion in the strains [14,15,18,21,22]. The results from the present study do agree with such previous findings (Figure S1, Figures 1–5). Both ELISA and Western blotting characterize the JP2 genotype of *A. actinomycetemcomitans* as having a higher LtxA production than the non-JP2 genotype strains (Figure S1 and Figure 1). Furthermore, the comparison of the group of JP2 genotype strains and the group of non-JP2 genotype strains did classify the JP2 genotype strains with a higher LtxA expression and production than the non-JP2 genotype strains regardless of using mRNA expression assay or ELISA (Figures 2 and 4). The difference between JP2 and non-JP2 genotype strains of *A. actinomycetemcomitans* applied to both the collection of the 20 Ghanaian *A. actinomycetemcomitans* and to the expanded collection consisting of 45 *A. actinomycetemcomitans*, serotype b. Surprisingly, a poor relation between the leukotoxicity and the LtxA expression and production of the Ghanaian *A. actinomycetemcomitans* strains, serotype b, was found (Figure S1 and Figure 1).

Since other researchers have reported on correlating data concerning the leukotoxicity and the LtxA expression, e.g., the mRNA expression, of *A. actinomycetemcomitans*, one has to speculate if methodological complexities may explain the lack of correlation between the results obtained by cell lysis assay compared to the three quantitative assays in the present study. It has been proposed that other factors than the *ltxA* expression, LtxA production, and LtxA secretion may influence the leukotoxic potential of a strain; Diaz and co-workers did describe a higher activity of the LtxA in a fresh clinical strain compared to the original JP2 strain [19]. Still, this higher activity of the protein did correlate to a higher amount of LtxA detected on the cell pellet of the clinical strain analyzed by Western blotting [19]. Diaz and co-workers also reported that the LtxA from the fresh clinical *A. actinomycetemcomitans* strain of JP2 genotype was located on the cell pellet in larger amounts than in the supernatant [19]. However, the clinical strain was described with features comparable to a rough strain phenotype. Kachlany and co-workers studied the difference between rough and smooth strains of *A. actinomycetemcomitans*, and they found that the smooth strains secreted more LtxA into the growth supernatant than the rough strains [23]. In order to accommodate the risk of differences between the strains due to rough-smooth phenotype in the present study, all strains were converted to smooth phenotypes, and the procedures of each method were adjusted according to this. Also in the study by Åberg and coworkers, analyzing the leukotoxicity of the Ghanaian *A. actinomycetemcomitans*, serotype b, smooth strain variants were used [20]. Still, the LtxA was purified from the cell pellet and not from the growth supernatant. However, when using the Peptone-Yeast-Glucose (PYG) medium (as done in the study by Åberg and co-workers) LtxA stays attached to the cell membrane and is not secreted into the growth medium [10]. The LtxA was extracted by NaCl in the study by Åberg et al. 2014; a protocol that has been criticized by others [19]. In addition, the use of different culture broth could also interfere with the LtxA production. However, whether or not these methodological aspects may explain the lack of correlation between the leukotoxicity and the LtxA expression and production among the Ghanaian *A. actinomycetemcomitans*, serotype b, found in this study, has to be a matter of further investigation in the future.

Environmental factors are of great importance and have been reported to influence on both the production and the secretion of the LtxA [18,22–25]. Previous studies have reported that the secretion of LtxA occurs into the environment both as a water-soluble protein and as an attached protein to membrane vesicles [26–28]. The LtxA attached to the vesicle is expected to be found in the supernatant used in the ELISA and the Western blot; however, this is not the case for the cell lysis assay used by Åberg and coworkers [20]. Although, the amount of cell membrane-attached LtxA and the vesicle membrane-attached LtxA should be relative [29], Kato et al. showed a 5-fold greater leukotoxic activity in the LtxA purified from the vesicles compared to the cell membrane-attached LtxA [29]. Therefore, the aspect of membrane vesicles may contribute to the surprising results in the present study as well.

The results from the present study show that the leukotoxicity of the Ghanaian *A. actinomycetemcomitans* strains is not explained by a greater leukotoxin expression and production. Johansson and coworkers have described different genetic similarities among the highly leukotoxic strains in the Ghanaian collection of *A. actinomycetemcomitans* [30]. The genetic similarity among the strains characterized by the *cagE* may be an indicator of a higher toxicity of the strains, but perhaps not an indicator of a higher leukotoxicity. The protocol used for purification of the LtxA in the study by Åberg and coworkers [20] may lead to presence of other protein and membrane components in the supernatant added to the THP-1 cells used in the cell lysis assay to measure the leukotoxicity of the *A. actinomycetemcomitans* strains [31]. Therefore, it is possible that the activity of the Ghanaian *A. actinomycetemcomitans* strains towards THP-1 cells is influenced by other components, either by interference directly with the THP-1 cells or by interference with the activity of the LtxA. It would be interesting to reproduce the leukotoxicity of the Ghanaian *A. actinomycetemcomitans* strains with other LtxA-purification protocols, where the LtxA is more strictly purified [11,19,32].

The leukotoxicity reported by Åberg and co-workers is given as a percentage of total lysis of the THP-1 cells by Triton X [20]. The results of the three LtxA-quantitative methods (Western blotting, ELISA and mRNA expression assay) used in the present study do not have a maximum value in the same way, and therefore it is possible for a strain to be characterized with a value above, e.g., 100%. If a certain amount of LtxA is needed for the total lysis of THP-1 cells [18], it is possible for strains with different amounts of produced and secreted LtxA to be classified with the same level of high leukotoxicity. However, they may still be very different according to LtxA expression and production. Therefore, some of the Ghanaian non-JP2 genotype strains of *A. actinomycetemcomitans*, serotype b, might produce enough LtxA to lead to a high percentage of cell lysis, but still not produce comparable amounts of LtxA to the JP2 genotype strains of *A. actinomycetemcomitans*. Of course, such presumptions depend on the fact that there is no difference in the activity of the LtxA. This is a notion that is unanswered for the bacterial collections used in the present study.

The results obtained by use of the ELISA and the mRNA expression assay did not correlate completely. Still, there is a reasonable relationship between the methods by visual inspection of Figures 3 and 5. Furthermore, both methods did determine the group of JP2 genotype of *A. actinomycetemcomitans*, serotype b, with a statistical significant higher leukotoxin expression and production than the group of non-JP2 genotype strains (Figure 4). The ELISA and the mRNA expression assay are both quantitative assays, and comparison of the results by a regression model seems reasonable [33,34]. Therefore, we performed a Bland-Altman plot for detection of difference between methods (not shown) [34], but this analysis showed no bias in our data; a result refuted by our scatter plot analysis. However, Ludbrook (2002) does discuss that the Bland-Altman analysis is not always safe to use when comparing methods that do not measure the exact same quantity and have a proportional relationship [33]. The results in the present study did show a reasonable relationship (Figure 5) when studying the scatter plot and the regression model, but with a higher agreement between the two methods among the JP2 genotype strains of *A. actinomycetemcomitans* than for the non-JP2 genotype strains. Generally, the data based on analysis of JP2 genotype strains seems more equal than for the non-JP2 genotype strains. This is probably reasonable considering that the group of JP2 genotype strains of *A. actinomycetemcomitans* is a very genetically homogeneous group of isolates, whereas the non-JP2 genotype strains, although all being of serotype b, is a more genetically diverse group of isolates. Still, based on the visual inspection of the Figures 3 and 5, it seems reasonable to assume that one can predict the LtxA production based on an analysis by use of a mRNA expression assay.

Some limitations of the present study should be addressed. Our mRNA analysis consists of quite high standard deviations, but our results from the mRNA expression assay are still consistent with previous findings by others [18,24,25]. In addition, the method is very similar to the one used by Longo et al. [25], but they reported no standard deviations, and, therefore, comparison is impossible. Whether or not the high standard deviation is caused by a biological phenomenon or by technical difficulties is unknown and needs to be investigated further. We are currently preparing for analysis of the *ltxA* gene expression by Nanostrings technologies; Nanostrings technologies are based on hybridization probes and require no amplification of RNA, thus, the inherent variabilities in the PCR technique will be avoided.

In the present study, we characterized 20 Ghanaian *A. actinomycetemcomitans*, serotype b, according to the LtxA expression and production by three different quantitative methods. The LtxA expression and production of the Ghanaian *A. actinomycetemcomitans*, serotype b, was not fully related with previously published results on leukotoxicity of the strains [20]. Therefore, these findings indicate that the non-JP2 genotype strains of *A. actinomycetemcomitans*, serotype b, originating from Ghana and previously reported on as highly leukotoxic, may have enhanced leukotoxicity, but probably not at comparable levels to JP2 genotype strains. Furthermore, the results from the present study showed a reasonable relationship between the expression of *ltxA* and the amount of produced and secreted LtxA. Conclusively, it is possible that only using one method to describe the LtxA-related virulence potential of *A. actinomycetemcomitans* could result in incomplete or misleading conclusions. Therefore, it is recommendable to use more than one method, combining analysis of both the leukotoxicity and the LtxA expression and/or production, when characterizing the leukotoxic potential of *A. actinomycetemcomitans*.

4. Materials and Methods

4.1. Bacterial Strains and Cell Lysis Assay

Table 1 shows the characteristics of 45 *A. actinomycetemcomitans* strains of serotype b, originally collected as subgingival plaque samples. The highly leukotoxic JP2 genotype of *A. actinomycetemcomitans*, characterized by a 530-bp deletion in the LtxA gene operon, belongs to serotype b, and is in particular linked to individuals of African descent [20,35,36]. Out of the 45 strains studied, 20 isolates from Ghanaian adolescents were previously analysed in a cell lysis assay based on the determination of lactate dehydrogenase (LDH) release from the monocytic leukemia cell line, THP-1 [20] as an expression of the leukotoxicity. Of these 20 *A. actinomycetemcomitans* strains of serotype b, 15 were non-JP2 genotype strains, and, among these strains, five were characterized as low leukotoxic, five as intermediate leukotoxic, and five as highly leukotoxic (0–30% LDH release = low leukotoxicity, 31–60% = average leukotoxicity, and 60% ≤ = high leukotoxicity, respectively) according to the study by Åberg and coworkers [20] (Table 1). The remaining five Ghanaian strains from that study belonged to the JP2 genotype of *A. actinomycetemcomitans* and were all highly leukotoxic towards THP-1 cells (Table 1).

The results obtained by the three quantitative assays being Western blotting, ELISA, and mRNA expression assay in the present study were compared with cell lysis assay results obtained in a previous study reported by Åberg and coworkers [20]. In addition to the 20 strains from Ghana, the bacterial collection in the present study was expanded with another 25 strains collected mainly from individuals originating from Africa or with African origin for comparison reasons. These 25 *A. actinomycetemcomitans* strains were 17 JP2 and five non-JP2 genotypes of *A. actinomycetemcomitans*, serotype b, previously characterized by Haubek et al. [36], and three non-JP2 genotype of *A. actinomycetemcomitans*, serotype b, from a collection of Moroccan isolates not previously reported on. The complete collection of 45 *A. actinomycetemcomitans* strains, serotype b, was analysed by ELISA and in an mRNA expression assay for comparison of the two different methods determining leukotoxic production and expression of *A. actinomycetemcomitans*, respectively (Table 1).

All strains were transformed into smooth variants by repeated subculture before being analysed by three different biochemical methods.

4.2. LtxA Isolation from the Cell Pellet and the Growth Supernatant

For isolation of LtxA, 50 ml volumes of pre-warmed TY×2 (Tryptone-yeast) medium were inoculated with a few colonies from a chocolate agar plate and incubated for 24 h in an atmosphere of 5% CO_2 in air to an $OD_{600, 1\,cm}$ at approximately 0.3. Tubes were centrifuged at 3000× g for 20 min, and 1 mL of the supernatant was transferred to Eppendorf tubes, supplied with sodium azide to 3 mM, and stored at −20 °C for later quantification of LtxA by ELISA and Western blotting. The cell pellet was isolated and five ml of 10 mM phosphate-buffered saline (PBS, 0.3 M NaCl) pH 7.2, containing 3 mM sodium azide, was added to the bacterial pellet with the purpose of releasing the cell membrane-attached LtxA as described by Johansson and co-workers [10]. The tube was vortexed and rotated end-over-end for 30 min at room temperature. One ml of the suspension of the cell pellet in buffer was transferred to an Eppendorf tube and prepared for quantification of LtxA by Western blotting.

4.3. Western Blotting

Western blotting was performed on the 20 Ghanaian *A. actinomycetemcomitans* (Table 1) for semi-quantitative comparison of the level of LtxA between the different strains and for semi-quantitative comparison of the level of LtxA in the cell pellet extract and the growth supernatant. Cell pellet extracts for SDS-page were prepared from suspensions of the bacteria in five ml 0.3 M NaCl (as described above) and subsequently diluted 10-fold with SDS-containing sample buffer in order to reflect bacteria-bound LtxA in the 50 mL culture volume. Supernatant samples were prepared as described above. The Western blotting was performed as described by Reinholdt and co-workers [14] using a polyclonal rabbit anti-LtxA antibody (Ab-LtxA) (unlabelled for coating, labelled for detection) raised against the C-terminal half (recombinant) of the LtxA molecule in collaboration with the DAKO laboratories (Glostrup, Denmark). Briefly, samples of supernatant and cell pellet extract were applied to a 7% Tris-acetat buffered gel (Nu-PAGE™, Invitrogen) in identical volumes in neighbouring lanes, providing visual semi-quantitative comparison of LtxA.

4.4. ELISA for Quantification of LtxA in Growth Supernatants

Quantification of the production of LtxA was performed by an ELISA as described by Reinholdt and co-workers [14]. Briefly, the LtxA isolated in the growth supernatant treated with sodium azide to

3 mM was used to quantify the LtxA production of the different strains. To detect LtxA by ELISA, polystyrene microplates (Nunc, Roskilde, Denmark) were coated overnight with Ab-LtxA in 10 mM phosphate-buffered saline, pH 7.4 (PBS). After washing and blocking the plate with washing solution (PBS containing 0.25 M NaCl and 0.15%Tween 20), test samples appropriately diluted in washing solution were incubated in wells for 2 h. Bound LtxA was detected by sequential incubations with biotinylated Ab-LtxA and alkaline phosphatase-conjugated streptavidine (DAKO). The assay was developed with a chromogenic substrate of p-nitrophenylenephosphate in diethanolamine buffer, pH 9.0, and plates were read at 405 nm by a Multiscan RC reader (Labsystems). The analysis was performed in duplicates, and the original strain HK921 (JP2) served as a reference. The results are the mean of the two runs and are given as a percentage of the results when testing *A. actinomycetemcomitans* strain HK921 (JP2).

4.5. mRNA Analysis

The purification of RNA, the synthesis of cDNA, and the performing of the real-time PCR for the determination of the expression of mRNA, coding for the production of LtxA in each strain, were performed as described by Søndergaard and co-workers with a few modifications [37]. Briefly, bacterial suspensions were made with smooth colonies in 1.5 ml Brain Heart Infusion (BHI) broth to an OD_{600} at approximately 0.4. The suspensions were centrifuged, and the cell pellets were isolated. The cell pellets were re-suspended in one ml of RNAprotect (Qiagen, by GmbH, Hilden, Germany), and the RNA was purified with Magna Pure Compact instrument using a MagnaPure Compact Nucleic Acid Isolation kit (large volume) (Roche Diagnostics GmbH, Mannheim, Germany). Residual DNA was degraded from the RNA sample using a Turbo DNA free kit (Ambion by ThermoFischer Scientific, Waltham, Massachusetts, USA) and 50% more DNase than recommended by the manufacturer in a Veriti 96-well Thermal Cycler (Applied Biosystems by ThermoFischer Scientific, Waltham, Massachusetts, USA) for 30 min at 37 °C, and 5 min at 95 °C. cDNA was prepared with TaqMan Reverse Transcription reagents (Life Technologies) in a Veriti 96-well Thermo Cycler for 10 min at 25 °C, 30 min at 48 °C and 5 min at 95 °C. The complete digestion of the genomic DNA in each RNA sample was confirmed by running a cDNA reaction without reverse transcriptase in the cDNA reaction mix, followed by PCR. The cDNA was mixed with primers, probes, and TaqMan Fast Advanced Master Mix (Life Technologies by ThermoFischer Scientific, Waltham, Massachusetts, USA) and quantitative PCR was run in triplicates in a LightCycler 480 (Roche, Germany). Relative gene expression of *ltxA* was quantified with LightCycler Relative Quantification software (Roche Applied Science) and normalized to the single-copy housekeeping genes *adk* and *pgi*. The assay was performed in triplicates, and the results are given as the mean of the three runs. Primers and probes are listed in Table 2.

Table 2. Primers and probes used in the mRNA expression analysis of *A. actinomycetemcomitans*.

Gene	Primer F (5′ → 3′)	Primer R (3′ → 5′)	Probe (5′ → 3′)
pgi	TAACCATGCACTTCGTGTCTAAC	CACAAGGGTGGTTTCCGGATT	TGGACGGCACGCACATTGCGGAAAC
adk	GATATGTTACGTTCCGCGATCA	GCACTAATTGACCGGCATCCA	AGCTGGCACCGAGTTAGGCAAACAAGC
ltxA	CTGTCGCAGGGTTAATTGCCT	GATCAAATTGTTTCGCAATACCTAG	TGTGGTCAGCTTGGCAATCAGCCCTTTG

4.6. Statistical Analysis

All the statistics were analyzed by the use of SciPy [38] that is an open source scientific tool for Python® (Beaverton, USA). The statistical analysis were performed on log-transformed data in order to attain normal distributed data.

The difference between the group of JP2 and the group of non-JP2 genotype strains of *A. actinomycetemcomitans*, serotype b, determined for each method separately was analyzed by an unpaired sample t-test for parametric data.

A scatter plot for comparison of ELISA and the mRNA expression assay was performed as described by Ludbrook [33] with a few modifications. The relationship between the two methods was tested by use of a regression analysis. Because the ELISA quantifies the protein and the mRNA expression assay measures the mRNA coding for the protein, the two methods do not measure the exactly same quantity of the *A. actinomycetemcomitans* strains. Therefore, an ordinary least squares regression model was used, since the relationship between the two methods can be viewed as a calibration problem [33].

Supplementary Materials: The following are available online at http://www.mdpi.com/2076-0817/8/4/211/s1, Figure S1. A semi-quantitative determination of the leukotoxin expression by Western blotting of 20 Ghanaian *A. actinomycetemcomitans*, serotype b, both JP2 and non-JP2 genotypes. The cell membrane-attached LtxA isolated from the cell pellet (C), and the released LtxA into the growth supernatant (S). HK921 (JP2) is illustrated as a reference. The LtxA is given as the band with a size of 116 kDa.

Author Contributions: Conceptualization, D.H., N.N.-L., A.J., and A.B.J.; methodology, J.R., M.L., N.N.-L., A.J., R.C. and A.B.J.; software, N.K.C. and A.B.J.; validation, D.H., N.N.-L., A.J. and A.B.J.; formal analysis, A.B.J. and N.K.C.; investigation, J.R., M.L., N.N.-L., D.H., A.J., R.C. and A.B.J.; resources, D.H., N.N.-L. and A.J.; data curation, D.H., A.J., N.N.-L., M.L. and A.B.J.; writing—original draft preparation, A.B.J.; writing—review and editing, A.B.J., D.H., N.N.-L., M.L., A.J., and R.C.; visualization, A.B.J.; supervision, D.H., A.J. and N.N.-L.; project administration, A.B.J., N.N.-L. and D.H.; funding acquisition, D.H. and A.J.

Funding: This research was funded by the University Strategic Fundings (USM-fundings) of Aarhus University, Danish Dental Association, the Ingeborg and Leo Danin Foundation, and by the Västerbotten County Foundation (TUA), Sweden.

Acknowledgments: We thank laboratory technician, Mette Nikolajsen for the preparation of bacterial isolates and growth media for the use in the ELISA and Western Blot analysis. We thank laboratory technician Mette Jensen for laboratory work carried out while performing the mRNA analysis. We thank Nikolaj Kruse Christensen (N.K.C) for a great contribution in the statistical analysis performance.

Conflicts of Interest: The authors declare to have no conflict of interest.

References

1. Slots, J.; Ting, M. *Actinobacillus actinomycetemcomitans* and Porphyromonas Gingivalis in Human Periodontal Disease: Occurrence and Treatment. *Periodontology 2000* **1999**, *20*, 82–121. [CrossRef] [PubMed]
2. Zambon, J.J. Actinobacillus actinomycetemcomitans in Human Periodontal Disease. *J. Clin. Periodontol.* **1985**, *12*, 1–20. [CrossRef] [PubMed]
3. Fives-Taylor, P.M.; Meyer, D.H.; Mintz, K.P.; Brissette, C. Virulence Factors of *Actinobacillus actinomycetemcomitans*. *Periodontology 2000* **1999**, *20*, 136–167. [CrossRef] [PubMed]
4. Henderson, B.; Ward, J.M.; Ready, D. *Aggregatibacter* (*Actinobacillus*) *actinomycetemcomitans*: A Triple A* Periodontopathogen? *Periodontology 2000* **2010**, *54*, 78–105. [CrossRef]
5. Norskov-Lauritsen, N. Classification, Identification, and Clinical Significance of *Haemophilus* and *Aggregatibacter* Species with Host Specificity for Humans. *Clin. Microbiol. Rev.* **2014**, *27*, 214–240. [CrossRef]
6. Pihlstrom, B.L.; Michalowicz, B.S.; Johnson, N.W. Periodontal Diseases. *Lancet* **2005**, *366*, 1809–1820. [CrossRef]
7. Lally, E.T.; Kieba, I.R.; Demuth, D.R.; Rosenbloom, J.; Golub, E.E.; Taichman, N.S.; Gibson, C.W. Identification and Expression of the *Actinobacillus actinomycetemcomitans* Leukotoxin Gene. *Biochem. Biophys. Res. Commun.* **1989**, *159*, 256–262. [CrossRef]
8. Korostoff, J.; Wang, J.F.; Kieba, I.; Miller, M.; Shenker, B.J.; Lally, E.T. Actinobacillus actinomycetemcomitans Leukotoxin Induces Apoptosis in HL-60 Cells. *Infect. Immun.* **1998**, *66*, 4474–4483.
9. Kachlany, S.C.; Fine, D.H.; Figurski, D.H. Purification of Secreted Leukotoxin (LtxA) from *Actinobacillus actinomycetemcomitans*. *Protein Expr. Purif.* **2002**, *25*, 465–471. [CrossRef]
10. Johansson, A.; Claesson, R.; Hänström, L.; Kalfas, S. Serum-Mediated Release of Leukotoxin from the Cell Surface of the Periodontal Pathogen *Actinobacillus actinomycetemcomitans*. *Eur. J. Oral Sci.* **2003**, *111*, 209–215. [CrossRef]
11. Balashova, N.V.; Shah, C.; Patel, J.K.; Megalla, S.; Kachlany, S.C. *Aggregatibacter actinomycetemcomitans* LtxC Is Required for Leukotoxin Activity and Initial Interaction between Toxin and Host Cells. *Gene* **2009**, *443*, 42–47. [CrossRef] [PubMed]

12. Balashova, N.; Dhingra, A.; Boesze-Battaglia, K.; Lally, E.T. *Aggregatibacter actinomycetemcomitans* Leukotoxin Induces Cytosol Acidification in LFA-1 Expressing Immune Cells. *Mol. Oral Microbiol.* **2016**, *31*, 106–114. [CrossRef] [PubMed]
13. Johansson, A. *Aggregatibacter actinomycetemcomitans* Leukotoxin: A Powerful Tool with Capacity to Cause Imbalance in the Host Inflammatory Response. *Toxins* **2011**, *3*, 242–259. [CrossRef] [PubMed]
14. Reinholdt, J.; Poulsen, K.; Brinkmann, C.R.; Hoffmann, S.V.; Stapulionis, R.; Enghild, J.J.; Jensen, U.B.; Boesen, T.; Vorup-Jensen, T. Monodisperse and LPS-Free *Aggregatibacter actinomycetemcomitans* Leukotoxin: Interactions with Human B2 Integrins and Erythrocytes. *Biochim. Biophys. Acta Proteins Proteom.* **2013**, *1834*, 546–558. [CrossRef]
15. Brogan, J.M.; Lally, E.T.; Poulsen, K.; Kilian, M.; Demuth, D.R. Regulation of *Actinobacillus actinomycetemcomitans* Leukotoxin Expression: Analysis of the Promoter Regions of Leukotoxic and Minimally Leukotoxic Strains. *Infect. Immun.* **1994**, *62*, 501–508.
16. Haubek, D.; Ennibi, O.-K.; Poulsen, K.; Væth, M.; Poulsen, S.; Kilian, M. Risk of Aggressive Periodontitis in Adolescent Carriers of the JP2 Clone of *Aggregatibacter* (*Actinobacillus*) *actinomycetemcomitans* in Morocco: A Prospective Longitudinal Cohort Study. *Lancet* **2008**, *371*, 237–242. [CrossRef]
17. Åberg, C.H.; Kwamin, F.; Claesson, R.; Johansson, A.; Haubek, D. Presence of JP2 and Non-JP2 Genotypes of *Aggregatibacter actinomycetemcomitans* and Attachment Loss in Adolescents in Ghana. *J. Periodontol.* **2012**, *83*, 1520–1528. [CrossRef]
18. Spitznagel, J.; Kraig, E.; Kolodrubetz, D. Regulation of Leukotoxin in Leukotoxic and Nonleukotoxic Strains of *Actinobacillus actinomycetemcomitans*. *Infect. Immun.* **1991**, *59*, 1394–1401.
19. Diaz, R.; Al Ghofaily, L.; Patel, J.; Balashova, N.V.; Freitas, A.C.; Labib, I.; Kachlany, S.C. Characterization of Leukotoxin from a Clinical Strain of *Actinobacillus actinomycetemcomitans*. *Microb. Pathog.* **2006**, *40*, 48–55. [CrossRef]
20. Höglund Åberg, C.; Haubek, D.; Kwamin, F.; Johansson, A.; Claesson, R. Leukotoxic Activity of *Aggregatibacter actinomycetemcomitans* and Periodontal Attachment Loss. *PLoS ONE* **2014**, *9*, e104095. [CrossRef]
21. Sampathkumar, V.; Velusamy, S.K.; Godboley, D.; Fine, D.H. Increased Leukotoxin Production: Characterization of 100 Base Pairs within the 530 Base Pair Leukotoxin Promoter Region of *Aggregatibacter actinomycetemcomitans*. *Sci. Rep.* **2017**, *7*, 1887. [CrossRef] [PubMed]
22. Balashova, N.V.; Diaz, R.; Balashov, S.V.; Crosby, J.A.; Kachlany, S.C. Regulation of Aggregatibacter (Actinobacillus) actinomycetemcomitans Leukotoxin Secretion by Iron. *J. Bacteriol.* **2006**, *188*, 8658–8661. [CrossRef] [PubMed]
23. Kachlany, S.C.; Fine, D.H.; Figurski, D.H. Secretion of RTX Leukotoxin by *Actinobacillus actinomycetemcomitans*. *Infect. Immun.* **2000**, *68*, 6094–6100. [CrossRef] [PubMed]
24. Fukui, K.; Tada, T.; Tanimoto, I.; Inoue, T.; Ohta, H.; Ohashi, T. Fermentable-Sugar-Level-Dependent Regulation of Leukotoxin Synthesis in a Variably Toxic Strain of *Actinobacillus actinomycetemcomitans*. *Microbiology* **2001**, *147*, 2749–2756. [CrossRef]
25. Longo, P.L.; Nunes, A.C.R.; Umeda, J.E.; Mayer, M.P.A. Gene Expression and Phenotypic Traits of *Aggregatibacter actinomycetemcomitans* in Response to Environmental Changes. *J. Periodontal Res.* **2013**, *48*, 766–772. [CrossRef] [PubMed]
26. Nowotny, A.; Behling, U.H.; Hammond, B.; Lai, C.H.; Listgarten, M.; Pham, P.H.; Sanavi, F. Release of Toxic Microvesicles by *Actinobacillus actinomycetemcomitans*. *Infect. Immun.* **1982**, *37*, 151–154. [PubMed]
27. Berthold, P.; Forti, D.; Kieba, I.R.; Rosenbloom, J.; Taichman, N.S.; Lally, E.T. Electron Immunocytochemical Localization of *Actinobacillus actinomycetemcomitans* Leukotoxin. *Oral Microbiol. Immunol.* **1992**, *7*, 24–27. [CrossRef]
28. Nice, J.; Balashova, N.; Kachlany, S.; Koufos, E.; Krueger, E.; Lally, E.; Brown, A. *Aggregatibacter actinomycetemcomitans* Leukotoxin Is Delivered to Host Cells in an LFA-1-Indeppendent Manner When Associated with Outer Membrane Vesicles. *Toxins* **2018**, *10*, 414. [CrossRef]
29. Kato, S.; Kowashi, Y.; Demuth, D.R. Outer Membrane-like Vesicles Secreted by *Actinobacillus actinomycetemcomitans* Are Enriched in Leukotoxin. *Microb. Pathog.* **2002**, *32*, 1–13. [CrossRef]
30. Johansson, A.; Claesson, R.; Höglund Åberg, C.; Haubek, D.; Oscarsson, J. The CagE Gene Sequence as a Diagnostic Marker to Identify JP2 and Non-JP2 Highly Leukotoxic *Aggregatibacter actinomycetemcomitans* Serotype b Strains. *J. Periodontal Res.* **2017**, *52*, 903–912. [CrossRef]

31. Johansson, A.; Hänström, L.; Kalfas, S. Inhibition of *Actinobacillus actinomycetemcomitans* Leukotoxicity by Bacteria from the Subgingival Flora. *Oral Microbiol. Immunol.* **2000**, *15*, 218–225. [CrossRef] [PubMed]
32. Velusamy, S.K.; Sampathkumar, V.; Godboley, D.; Fine, D.H. Survival of an *Aggregatibacter actinomycetemcomitans* Quorum Sensing *Lux* S Mutant in the Mouths of Rhesus Monkeys: Insights into Ecological Adaptation. *Mol. Oral Microbiol.* **2017**, *32*, 432–442. [CrossRef] [PubMed]
33. Ludbrook, J. Statistical Techniques for Comparing Measurers and Methods of Measurement: A Critical Review. *Clin. Exp. Pharmacol. Physiol.* **2002**, *29*, 527–536. [CrossRef] [PubMed]
34. Altman, D.G.; Bland, J.M. Measurement in Medicine: The Analysis of Method Comparison Studies. *J. R. Stat. Soc. Ser. D (Stat.)* **1983**, *32*, 307–317. [CrossRef]
35. Haubek, D.; Poulsen, K.; Westergaard, J.; Dahlèn, G.; Kilian, M. Highly Toxic Clone of *Actinobacillus actinomycetemcomitans* in Geographically Widespread Cases of Juvenile Periodontitis in Adolescents of African Origin. *J. Clin. Microbiol.* **1996**, *34*, 1576–1578. [PubMed]
36. Haubek, D.; Poulsen, K.; Kilian, M. Microevolution and Patterns of Dissemination of the JP2 Clone of *Aggregatibacter* (*Actinobacillus*) *actinomycetemcomitans*. *Infect. Immun.* **2007**, *75*, 3080–3088. [CrossRef]
37. Nørskov-Lauritsen, N.; Søndergaard, A.; Lund, M. TEM-1-Encoding Small Plasmids Impose Dissimilar Fitness Costs on *Haemophilus influenzae* and *Haemophilus parainfluenzae*. *Microbiology* **2015**, *161*, 2310–2315. [CrossRef]
38. SciPy—SciPy v1.3.0 Reference Guide. Available online: https://docs.scipy.org/doc/scipy-1.3.0/reference/ (accessed on 8 July 2019).

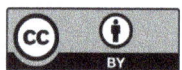

© 2019 by the authors. Licensee MDPI, Basel, Switzerland. This article is an open access article distributed under the terms and conditions of the Creative Commons Attribution (CC BY) license (http://creativecommons.org/licenses/by/4.0/).

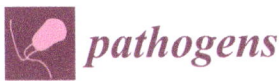

Article

Genetic Profiling of *Aggregatibacter actinomycetemcomitans* Serotype B Isolated from Periodontitis Patients Living in Sweden

Anders Johansson [1], Rolf Claesson [2], Carola Höglund Åberg [1], Dorte Haubek [3], Mark Lindholm [2], Sarah Jasim [2] and Jan Oscarsson [2,*]

1. Division of Molecular Periodontology, Department of Odontology, Umeå University, 907 00 Umeå, Sweden
2. Division of Oral Microbiology, Department of Odontology, Umeå University, 907 00 Umeå, Sweden
3. Section for Pediatric Dentistry, Department of Dentistry and Oral Health, Aarhus University, 8000 Aarhus, Denmark
* Correspondence: jan.oscarsson@umu.se

Received: 28 August 2019; Accepted: 15 September 2019; Published: 17 September 2019

Abstract: The bacterium *Aggregatibacter actinomycetemcomitans* is associated with aggressive forms of periodontitis and with systemic diseases, such as endocarditis. By assessing a Ghanaian longitudinal adolescent cohort, we earlier recognized the *cagE* gene as a possible diagnostic marker for a subgroup of JP2 and non-JP2 genotype serotype b *A. actinomycetemcomitans* strains, associated with high leukotoxicity as determined in a semi-quantitative cell assay. This group of *A. actinomycetemcomitans* is associated with the progression of attachment loss. In the present work, we used conventional polymerase chain reaction (PCR) and quantitative PCR to perform the *cagE* genotyping of our collection of 116 selected serotype b *A. actinomycetemcomitans* strains, collected over a period of 15 years from periodontitis patients living in Sweden. The *A. actinomycetemcomitans* strains carrying *cagE* (referred to as $cagE^+$; n = 49) were compared to the *cagE*-negative strains (n = 67), present at larger proportions in the subgingival plaque samples, and were also much more prevalent in the young (≤35 years) compared to in the old (>35 years) group of patients. Our present results underline the potential use of *cagE* genotyping in the risk assessment of the development of periodontal attachment loss in Swedish adolescents.

Keywords: *Aggregatibacter actinomycetemcomitans*; *cagE*; *virB1*; *virB4*; genotype; virulence

1. Introduction

Aggregatibacter actinomycetemcomitans is a Gram-negative opportunistic pathogen associated with rapidly progressing periodontitis and with extra-oral diseases, such as endocarditis [1–3]. Several longitudinal studies have demonstrated that adolescents colonized with *A. actinomycetemcomitans*, as compared to those that are not, have a significantly increased risk of the development of periodontal attachment loss (AL) [4–7]. *A. actinomycetemcomitans* produces an array of virulence factors that allow this bacterium to evade and suppress the host immune response, including two exotoxins, i.e., leukotoxin and cytolethal distending toxin (CDT) [8–10]. A large genetic diversity within the *A. actinomycetemcomitans* species has been found, and seven different serotypes (a–g) exist, representing genetically divergent lineages [11–13]. *A. actinomycetemcomitans* genotypes can have extensively different pathogenic potentials [5,14,15]. For example, carriers of the JP2 serotype b-specific genotype of *A. actinomycetemcomitans* are at higher risk of development of AL compared to carriers of a non-JP2 genotype of *A. actinomycetemcomitans*. Typical for JP2 genotype strains is the deletion of 530 base pairs (bp) in the promoter region of the *ltxCABD* gene operon, which encodes leukotoxin (LtxA), and an enhanced leukotoxicity [16,17]. LtxA is a virulence factor of *A. actinomycetemcomitans* with the capacity to cause imbalance in the host inflammatory response [9]. The *ltx* promoter deletion has been frequently used as genetic marker to identify *A. actinomycetemcomitans* carriers with an increased risk for periodontal disease onset and progression [17], and this genotype is easily detected using a DNA-based assay (PCR) [18]. In addition to the JP2 genotype, a subgroup of non-JP2 genotype serotype b strains exhibits a similar disease association and high leukotoxicity, as has been shown in a semi-quantitative cell assay [14]. Genetic characterization has revealed that this particular subgroup of non-JP2 genotype of *A. actinomycetemcomitans* strains of serotype b are genetically closely related to the JP2 genotype by sharing the same arbitrarily-primed (AP) PCR gel electrophoresis banding pattern, referred to as AP-PCR genotype 1 in the present work [14]. Another property shared between the JP2 genotype and highly leukotoxic non-JP2 genotype serotype b strains was recently recognized, i.e., the carriage of the *cagE* gene sequence [19]. The *cagE* gene in *A. actinomycetemcomitans* was initially characterized by Teng and Hu [20], presenting evidence that the encoded CagE protein could induce apoptosis on primary human epithelial cells. However, consistent with leukotoxicity being a major virulence property of *cagE*-positive *A. actinomycetemcomitans* serotype b strains, one JP2 genotype bacterial cell was enough to lyse the majority of macrophage cells in vitro [20], whereas, as in comparison, a ratio of 50,000 JP2 genotype bacterial cells per epithelial cell was used to detect the CagE-induced apoptotic effects in vitro [21]. This suggests that CagE may have limited overall contribution to the virulence at biologically-relevant bacterial levels. In the present study, we utilized the *cagE* gene sequence as a diagnostic risk marker for the PCR detection of highly leukotoxic JP2 and non-JP2 genotypes of *A. actinomycetemcomitans* serotype b [19].

Furthermore, a type IV secretion system (T4SS) is a large macromolecular complex in Gram-negative bacteria which mediates conjugation, DNA transport and the secretion of virulence factors. Experimental work on model organisms, such as *Agrobacterium tumefaciens* and *Helicobacter pylori*, has revealed an archetypal T4SS system composed of 12 proteins, referred to as VirB1–VirB11, and VirD4 [22,23]. *A. actinomycetemcomitans* T4SS gene clusters are found in approximately 50% of strains and can be encoded both on the chromosome and on plasmids [24–26]. Interestingly, CagE exhibits homology to two T4SS proteins. The CagE N-terminus is homologous to VirB1 (lytic transglycosylase; also known as MagB01), and the CagE C-terminus is homologous to VirB4 (ATP:ase; MagB03) [19]. As judged by in silico analysis of the serotype b genomes available in the National Center for Biotechnology (NCBI) database, the *cagE* gene locus is not present in any of the strains encoding VirB1 and VirB4 on the chromosome. Whether the *cagE* and *virB1/virB4* genes are consistently inversely carried in serotype b strains has not earlier been thoroughly assessed but would support the notion that CagE may represent the result of a recombination event in which parts of the *virB1* and *virB4* genes were fused together to encode a chimeric VirB1–VirB4 protein in *A. actinomycemcomitans* [19].

In our previous work, delineating the role of *cagE* as a potential diagnostic marker, we studied a collection of *A. actinomycetemcomitans* strains collected from a prospective cohort of Ghanaian adolescents [19]. To further evaluate the role of *cagE* and *virB1/virB4* as diagnostic tools, we assessed our collection of *A. actinomycetemcomitans* strains that were collected during 15 years from periodontitis patients living in Sweden [27]. Data from microbiological analyses of this collection revealed that the young individuals ($\leq$35 years) had a higher prevalence of *A. actinomycetemcomitans* and larger proportions of it in the samples compared to the older patients (>35 years). Moreover, serotype b was highly prevalent in the samples collected from young patients [27]. The aim of the present work was to determine the prevalence of the *cagE* genotype among the serotype b strains from this aforementioned collection (n = 116) and also to evaluate the potential use of *cagE* as a diagnostic marker for the carriage of highly leukotoxic serotype b strains among periodontitis patients living in Sweden.

2. Results

2.1. Validation of PCR Assays to Detect VirB1 and VirB4 Sequences in A. actinomycetemcomitans Serotype B Reference Strains

All *A. actinomycetemcomitans* serotype b strains assessed in the present study were grouped according to their AP-PCR genotype—1, 2 or "other" (i.e., AP-PCR types 3–11 as defined earlier [27]) (Figure 1A).

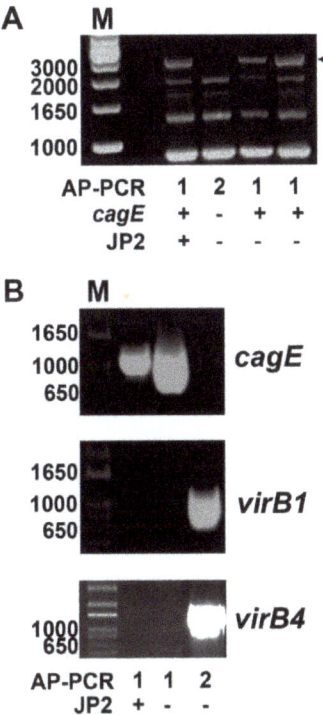

Figure 1. PCR genotyping of *Aggregatibacter actinomycetemcomitans* serotype b strains. (**A**) Distinct arbitrarily-primed (AP)-PCR banding patterns distinguish *cagE*-positive and *cagE*-negative serotype b strains of *A. actinomycetemcomitans*. The approximately 3000-bp DNA-band (arrowed) detected in AP-PCR type 1 is unique for this genotype and was earlier demonstrated to contain the *cagE* gene sequence [19]. Typically, this DNA band reflects the difference between AP-PCR types 1 and 2. The presence/absence of the *cagE* gene and *ltxA* JP2 promoter type in AP-PCR types 1 and 2 is indicated. (**B**) PCR detection of *cagE*, *virB1*, and *virB4*, respectively. An amplicon specific for *cagE* was revealed in both JP2 and non-JP2 AP-PCR genotype 1 strains. In AP-PCR genotype 2 strains, amplicons specific for *virB1* and *virB4* were detected, whereas *cagE* was not. Sizes (bp) of selected bands in the DNA molecular weight marker (M) are indicated. Figures illustrate representative experiments.

To test the hypothesis that the presence of chromosomal *virB1* and *virB4* genes can serve as genetic markers that are suitable for the detection of *cagE*-negative serotype b strains, PCR was employed as described in the Materials and Methods section. To evaluate the PCR approach, we initially assessed 25 *A. actinomycetemcomitans* strains of serotype b which have previously been subject to whole genome sequencing (Table 1) (Figure 1B). As expected, this revealed presence of both *virB1* and *virB4* in the *cagE*-negative strains only (n = 7; 4 type 2 AP-PCR and 3 "other" AP-PCR type), whereas neither *virB1* nor *virB4* were detected by PCR in the *cagE*-positive strains (n = 18; all AP-PCR type 1). This finding prompted us to further investigate this apparent inverse relationship between the carriage of *cagE* and *virB1/virB4* in the assessment of our local collection of serotype b *A. actinomycetemcomitans* strains. As *virB1* and *virB4* were carried simultaneously in the strains studied, we continued our analyses, mainly screening for the presence of *virB4*.

Table 1. Genotyping of *A. actinomycetemcomitans* serotype b strains (n = 25) that were earlier subjected to whole genome sequencing.

Strain	Origin [a]	*virB1* [b]	*virB4* [b]	JP2 [c]	*cagE* [d]	AP-PCR [e]
ANH9381	Finland/Caucasian	+	+	-	-	2
HK908	Denmark/USA	+	+	-	-	2
HK909	Denmark	-	-	+	+	1
HK912	Denmark/USA	-	-	-	+	1
HK921	Denmark/USA	-	-	+	+	1
HK1651	Denmark/Ghana	-	-	+	+	1
I23C	Finland/Caucasian	+	+	-	-	2
S23A	Finland/Caucasian	+	+	-	-	2
SCC1398	Finland/Caucasian	+	+	-	-	other
SCC4092	Finland/Caucasian	+	+	-	-	other
Y4	USA	+	+	-	-	other
133A1-08U	Sweden [f]	-	-	+	+	1
196A1-10U	Sweden	-	-	+	+	1
115A-11U	Sweden	-	-	+	+	1
245-12U	Sweden	-	-	+	+	1
338A1-13U	Sweden	-	-	+	+	1
304A1-14U	Sweden	-	-	+	+	1
299A1-15U	Sweden	-	-	+	+	1
456A1-13U	Sweden	-	-	+	+	1
520A-01U	Sweden	-	-	+	+	1
443G	Sweden/Ghana	-	-	-	+	1
486G	Sweden/Ghana	-	-	-	+	1
575G	Sweden/Ghana	-	-	-	+	1
605G	Sweden/Ghana	-	-	-	+	1
638G	Sweden/Ghana	-	-	-	+	1

[a] Geographic location of laboratories from where strains were obtained/origin of donor (where known); [b] determined by PCR as described in Materials and Methods; [c] previously determined by PCR [14,28,29]; [d] previously determined by PCR [19]; [e] previously determined by AP-PCR [19], or deduced in the present work; [f] Sweden residents unless specified otherwise.

2.2. Screening of CagE and VirB4 in Serotype B A. actinomycetemcomitans Strains Collected from Patients with Periodontitis Living in Sweden

We screened the 116 serotype b *A. actinomycetemcomitans* strains, collected from periodontitis patients living in Sweden, using qPCR to determine the prevalence of the *cagE* and *virB4* genes (Table 2) (Table S1) (Figure 2).

Table 2. Inverse relationship in the carriage of *cagE* and *virB4*. Presence of chromosomal *cagE* and *virB4* genes in serotype b strains of *A. actinomycetemcomitans* (n = 116) in different AP-PCR genotypes. The number of strains and percent (%) of all strains are indicated. The *cagE*-positive strains all (100%) belong to AP-PCR type 1 and lack the *virB4* gene.

	AP-PCR Type 1	AP-PCR Type 2	Other (Types 3–11)
cagE+/*virB4*-	49 (42.2)	0 (0)	0 (0)
cagE-/*virB4*+	0 (0)	11 (9.5)	15 (12.9)
cagE+/*virB4*+	0 (0)	0 (0)	0 (0)
cagE-/*virB4*-	0 (0)	14 (12.1)	27 (23.3)
All strains	49 (42.2)	25 (21.6)	42 (36.2)

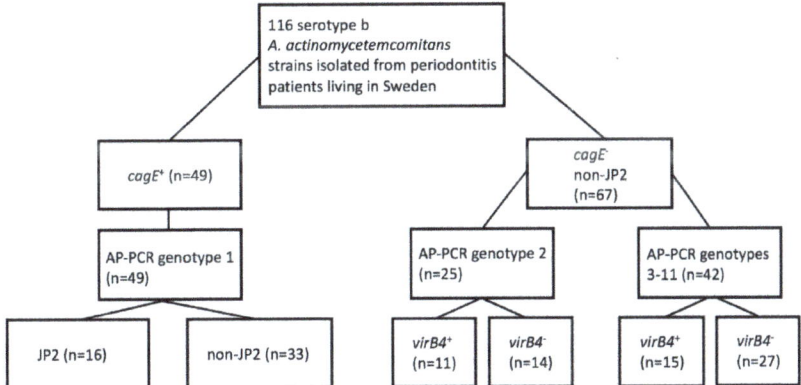

Figure 2. Genotype patterns of *A. actinomycetemcomitans* serotype b strains. Schematic overview of AP-PCR type, as well as the JP2- and *virB4*-genotype patterns of the *cagE*-positive and *cagE*-negative strains, respectively. The collection of 116 serotype b strains was earlier sampled from periodontitis patients living in Sweden [27].

According to our results, *cagE* was present in 49 (42.2%) strains, including all 16 JP2 genotype strains, and hence absent in 67 (57.8%) strains. Of the *cagE*-positive strains, all (100%) belonged to AP-PCR genotype 1. Interestingly, three *cagE*-positive strains (all non-JP2 genotypes) were found to carry the *virB4* gene. However, PCR analysis, using the primers *magB01*-F and *ssb*-R, supported that all three strains most likely carried *virB4* on a plasmid rather than on the chromosome (data not shown). Thus, we concluded that a property common among the *cagE*-positive strains is an apparent lack of a chromosomal *virB4* gene. Of the *cagE*-negative *A. actinomycetemcomitans* strains, 25 (37.3%) belonged to AP-PCR genotype 2, and 42 (62.7%) belonged to AP-PCR genotypes 3–11. The prevalence of *virB4* was somewhat higher among the AP-PCR genotype 2 *A. actinomycetemcomitans* strains (44%) compared to the strains belonging to AP-PCR genotypes 3–11 (35.7%), suggesting that *virB4* might be usable as a genetic marker for a subgroup of *cagE*-negative strains. Thus, taken together, as none of the 116 strains studied encoded both *cagE* and *virB4* on the chromosome, we concluded that there is an apparent inverse relationship in the carriage of these genes in the *A. actinomycetemcomitans* strains of serotype b.

2.3. Higher Proportions of CagE-Positive A. actinomycetemcomitans Serotype B in Subgingival Plaque Samples

Furthermore, we assessed whether the *cagE* genotype may correlate with the proportion of *A. actinomycetemcomitans* found in the subgingival plaque samples. For this, the serotype b *A. actinomycetemcomitans* strains (n = 116) were divided into two groups, i.e., *cagE*-positive (n = 49) and *cagE*-negative (n = 67), and then they were matched with the determined total viable counts (%) of *A. actinomycetemcomitans* in the respective samples [27]. This clearly revealed that *cagE*-positive strains were carried in patients at significantly higher ($p < 0.001$) proportions than *cagE*-negative *A. actinomycetemcomitans* (Figure 3A). However, among the *cagE*-positive, the proportion of *A. actinomycetemcomitans* in samples with a JP2 genotype strain (n = 16) was not significantly different from that with a non-JP2 genotype strain (n = 33) (Figure 3B).

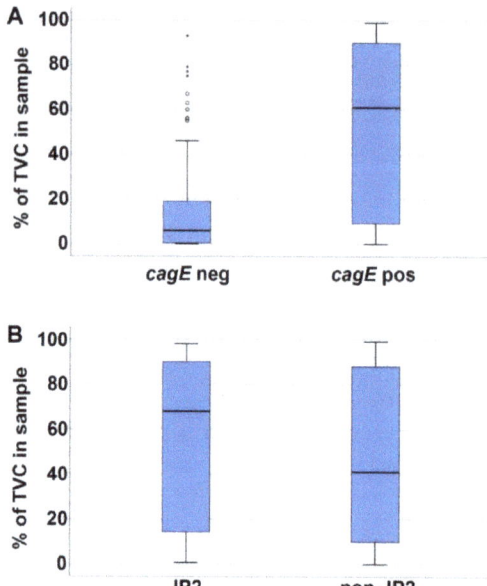

Figure 3. Higher proportions of *A. actinomycetemcomitans* in subgingival plaque samples containing a *cagE*-positive serotype b. The proportion of *A. actinomycetemcomitans* (total viable count—TVC; %) in the subgingival plaque samples was determined earlier for each of the serotype b strains (n = 116) [27]. (**A**) The *cagE*-positive strains (n = 49) were present in significantly higher ($p < 0.001$) proportions than the *cagE*-negative strains (n = 67). (**B**) The JP2 (n = 16) and non-JP2 (n = 33) strains were present at similar proportions. Median and quartiles from the samples are shown in each panel.

2.4. Higher Prevalence of CagE-Positive A. actinomycetemcomitans Serotype B in Young Patients

To further evaluate the virulence of the *cagE*-positive serotype b *A. actinomycetemcomitans* strains (n = 49) among periodontitis patients living in Sweden, we also assessed the age-associated prevalence of these strains. For this purpose, the patients (n = 116) were grouped into young (≤35 years; n = 62) and old (>35 years; n = 54) groups (Table 3). This revealed that among the young patients, $cagE^+$ *A. actinomycetemcomitans* strains (n = 40; 64.5%) were much more common than among the older patients (n = 9; 16.7%), i.e., these strains had a significantly higher ($p < 0.001$, odds ratio (OR) = 9.1, 95% CI: 3.8–22.0) prevalence among the young patients.

Table 3. Age-associated distribution of the *cagE* genotype of serotype b. The prevalence of *cagE*-positive and *cagE*-negative strains among the *A. actinomycetemcomitans* serotype b strains (n = 116) sampled from young (≤35 yr; n = 62) and from old patients (>35 yr; n = 54). The numbers and percentages (%) of young, old, and all patients are indicated. The prevalence of *cagE*-positive strains was significantly higher ($p < 0.001$; odds ratio (OR) = 10.5, 95% CI: 4.2–26.1) in the young compared to old patients.

	Young Patients	Old Patients	All Patients
$cagE^+$	40 (64.5)	9 (16.7)	49 (42.2)
$cagE^-$	22 (35.5)	45 (83.3)	67 (57.8)

3. Discussion

In the present work, we used conventional PCR and qPCR to genotypically analyze our collection of 116 *A. actinomycetemcomitans* serotype b strains, collected during 15 years from periodontitis patients living in Sweden, and our present results underline the potential use of *cagE* genotyping in the risk assessment of the development of periodontal attachment loss in adolescents living in Sweden.

Each of the 116 serotype b strains were matched both with its load (% of total viable count) in the respective subgingival plaque sample and with its age-associated prevalence category [27]. As *cagE*-positive, in contrast to *cagE*-negative serotype b *A. actinomycetemcomitans* strains, were found at larger proportions in the plaque samples and exhibited a much higher prevalence in the young compared to in the old patients of this population, our present results are consistent with our findings assessing the longitudinal Ghanaian adolescent cohort [19]. Whereas the proportions of *A. actinomycetemcomitans* genotypes in the total viable counts of subgingival plaque samples had not earlier been assessed in patient cohorts, the ratio of *cagE*-positive among serotype b strains carried by young patients in the Swedish population (64.5%) was similar to that of the adolescents in the Ghanaian cohort, exhibiting an association between the progression of attachment loss and exposure to this particular *cagE*-positive genotype [14,19]. As the *cagE*-positive serotype b strains sampled in both Ghana and Sweden were found at larger proportions in the plaque samples and exhibited a much higher prevalence in the young group of patients [19,27], the results from our present study are consistent with the notion that *cagE*-positive strains (including both the JP2 and non-JP2 genotypes) represent a subgroup of highly virulent *A. actinomycetemcomitans* serotype b.

The genetic similarity of *cagE*$^+$ serotype b strains is supported by the observation that they share the same AP-PCR genotype, as well as the fact that they have all a complete *cdtABC* gene operon [30]. We speculated earlier that they may belong to a clonal lineage that is closely related to the JP2 genotype ancestor [19]. As *cagE*-positive strains include both the JP2 and non-JP2 genotypes but no identified JP2-genotype strain has thus far been found to be *cagE*-negative, it is hypothesized that the JP2 genotype-associated deletion in the *ltxCABD* promoter once originated in a *cagE*-positive serotype b strain (Figure 4). It is tempting to speculate that high leukotoxicity may have been a characteristic of this ancestral *A. actinomycetemcomitans* strain, as that is a property common among *cagE*-positive strains, regardless of whether they are of the JP2 genotype or not.

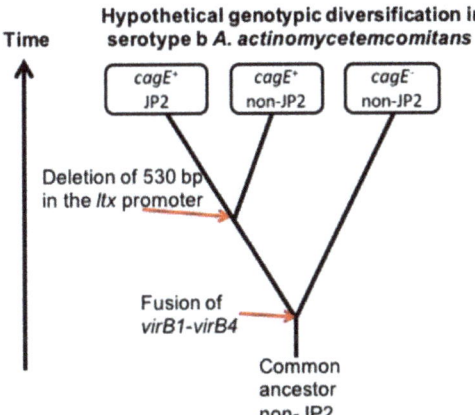

Figure 4. Hypothetical origin of the *cagE* and JP2 genotypes in serotype b *A. actinomycetemcomitans*. The genetic similarity between *cagE*-positive strains and the apparent absence of the JP2 genotype among *cagE*-negative strains suggests the possibility that the JP2-associated 530-bp deletion in the *ltx* promoter might have originated in a *cagE*$^+$ strain. The JP2 genotype of *A. actinomycetemcomitans* initially appeared as a distinct genotype in the Mediterranean part of Africa approximately 2400 years ago [29]. As *cagE*$^+$ strains consistently lack chromosomal copies of *virB1* and *virB4*, an earlier recombination event causing fusion of a *virB1*- and a *virB4*-like gene sequence resulting in the *cagE* determinant might have taken place in a common serotype b *A. actinomycetemcomitans* ancestral strain.

Consistent with our earlier in silico analysis of the genome-sequenced serotype b strains in the NCBI database [19], another property shared between the *cagE*-positive strains assessed in the present work was a lack of chromosomal genes encoding the T4SS-associated proteins VirB1 and VirB4. Based on the homology between VirB1 and VirB4 with the CagE N-, and C-terminus, respectively, we suggested earlier that CagE may represent a fusion product of a VirB1- and a VirB4-like amino acid sequence [19]. A scenario where the origin of the $cagE^+$ serotype b *A. actinomycetemcomitans* strains is a recombination event on the chromosome, generating a fusion of parts of the genes encoding *virB1* and *virB4* (as illustrated in Figure 4), is plausible considering that chimeric proteins do exist in a number of bacterial T4SS gene clusters. For example, it was reported that *H. pylori* VirB3 and VirB4 is a fusion product, i.e., the first 150 amino acids of VirB4 have weak similarity with VirB3 although the motifs are conserved [31]. Similarly, a Western blot assay indicated a CagE-like protein pattern when prototypical *virB3* and *virB4* genes of *A. tumefaciens* were fused together and expressed [32]. Chimeric proteins are also encoded in a number of T4SS gene clusters of other species, including VirB3–VirB4 in *Campylobacter jejuni* [33,34], VirB1–VirB8 in *Bordetella pertussis* [35], and VirB11–VirD4 (MagB11–MagB12) in at least one strain of *A. actinomycetemcomitans* [25]. Moreover, observations with *H. pylori* are consistent with the notion that T4SS gene clusters can include regions that are prone to genetic rearrangements, resulting in the disruption or activation of the secretion system [36]. Results from our present work show that CagE and VirB1/VirB4 can be encoded in the same *A. actinomycetemcomitans* strain, albeit, as supported by PCR, with the T4SS genes most likely encoded on plasmids. The carriage of plasmids encoding T4SS genes, such as *virB1* and *virB4*, has been demonstrated in some *A. actinomycetemcomitans* strains [25,26]. In contrast, *cagE* appears not to be encoded on plasmids. According to the sequences available in the NCBI database, no hitherto sequenced *A. actinomycetemcomitans* plasmid carries a *cagE* gene locus. We were unable to detect by PCR the presence of a T4SS-encoding plasmid in the *cagE*-positive serotype b strain HK1651, which was earlier reported [25]. The reason for this discrepancy is not known but may reflect the possibility that this plasmid was lost in the strain preserved in our stocks upon repeated in vitro cultivation. The loss of plasmids of *A. actinomycetemcomitans* strains during in vitro cultivation is a phenomenon that has been reported earlier, albeit then related to growth in an antibiotic free medium [37].

Taken together, our present results further support the usefulness of the *cagE* gene as a potential diagnostic marker in the risk assessment of the development of attachment loss among young individuals. We conclude that *cagE* positive *A. actinomycetemcomitans* strains of serotype b among periodontitis patients living in Sweden consist of the JP2 and non-JP2 genotypes with phenotypic characteristics similar to the ones seen for the JP2 genotype strains but with a leukotoxin promoter region lacking the 530-bp deletion. Their origin, evolution, and extent of genetic similarity will be further explored by whole genome sequencing.

4. Materials and Methods

4.1. Collection of A. actinomycetemcomitans Strains and Clinical Data Used in the Present Study

For the present work, we used data from our microbiological analyses of 3459 subgingival plaque samples, collected from 1445 patients during 15 years (2000–2014) that included 337 'younger' patients (≤35 years of age) and 1108 'older' patients (>35 years of age) [27]. At the specialist clinics, it is recommended that microbial analysis is performed to study the microbial biofilm profiles of individuals ≤35 years affected by periodontal attachment loss, and of patients >35 years with rapidly progressive periodontitis, not responding to conventional periodontal therapy. The samples were sent from the Specialist Clinic of Periodontology at the Dental School in Umeå, Sweden, and from external specialist dental clinics throughout Sweden to be analyzed at the laboratory for microbiological diagnostics, Dental School, Umeå. The samples were collected from individuals between 9 and 92 years of age that were all diagnosed with periodontitis and referred to specialist clinics for periodontal treatment. However, due to the many clinics involved and the retrospective nature of the present study, clinical and other parameters were not systematically reported in the patient information attached to the referral to the laboratory for microbiological diagnostics. Therefore, the classification of the patients was dichotomized only and was based on the old definition of early onset periodontitis, which distinguished patients ≤35 years versus those >35 years of age [38]. An *A. actinomycetemcomitans* strain was collected and isolated from 347 patients [27]. PCR characterization revealed that 118 (34.0%) of the *A. actinomycetemcomitans* strains were serotype b, and 17 (14.4% of the serotype b strains) were characterized by 530-bp deletion in the promoter region of the leukotoxin gene operon (JP2 genotype). Among these 118 serotype b strains, we were able to cultivate and characterize 116 for use in the present study: 100 non-JP2 genotype and 16 JP2 genotype. For the present work, each of these 116 unique *A. actinomycetemcomitans* strains was combined with recorded clinical data, i.e., the age group of the patient (>35 or ≤35 years), and proportion of *A. actinomycetemcomitans* of the total cultivable microflora (TVC) in the sample.

4.2. Bacterial Strains and Growth Conditions

In the present work, we used a collection of 116 unique *A. actinomycetemcomitans* serotype b strains that were collected from periodontitis patients living in Sweden [27]. A list of these strains is presented in Table S1. The sampling of this collection and the subsequent characterization of the serotype, the AP-PCR genotype, and the leukotoxin promoter type (JP2/non-JP2 genotype) has been described earlier [27]. In the present study, 25 serotype b *A. actinomycetemcomitans* strains were used as reference, as they were subject to prior whole genome sequencing [15,19,39–41] (Table 1). Among these, five belong to a collection of oral *A. actinomycetemcomitans* strains previously reported on by Prof. Sirkka Asikainen: ANH9381, I23C, S23A, SCC1398 and SCC4092. Nine strains belong to the collection of serotype b *A. actinomycetemcomitans* strains, sampled from periodontitis patients living in Sweden: 133A1-08U, 196A1-10U, 115A-11U, 245-12U, 338A1-13U, 304A1-14U, 299A1-15U, 456A1-13U, and 520A-01U [28]. *A. actinomycetemcomitans* strains 443G, 486G, 575G, 605G, and 638G were sampled from a Ghanaian cohort of adolescents [6,42]. Finally, six type strains were included in the study: HK908 [29], HK909 [43], HK912 [29], HK921 [43], HK1651 [39], and Y4 [44,45]. All strains were cultured on blood agar plates (5% defibrinated horse blood, 5 mg of hemin/l, 10 mg of vitamin K/l, Columbia agar base) and incubated in air supplemented with 5% CO_2 at 37 °C.

4.3. DNA Isolation and Polymerase Chain Reaction Analysis

DNA templates for PCR and qPCR analysis were obtained by boiling a loopful of fresh *A. actinomycetemcomitans* colonies in 100 µl of water. *A. actinomycetemcomitans* genomic DNA to be used in AP-PCR was isolated using the GenElute™ Bacterial Genomic DNA kit (Sigma-Aldrich, St. Louis, MO, USA), following the manufacturer's instructions. For the isolation of plasmids from *A. actinomycetemcomitans* strains, a QIAprep®Spin miniprep kit was used (QiaGen, Venlo, The Netherlands). Reaction mixtures for PCR were prepared using illustra™ PuReTaq™ Ready-To-Go™ PCR beads (GF Healthcare, Buckinghamshire, UK), whereas we used a KAPA SYBR®FAST qPCR Kit (KAPA Biosystems, Wilmington, MA, USA) for qPCR. The AP-PCR type was analyzed as earlier described [19,27], using the random sequence oligonucleotide OPB-3 (5′-AGTCAGCCAC-3′) (Invitrogen, Carlsbad, CA, USA) at 0.4 µmol/l and cycling conditions according to Dogan and coworkers [46]. The *cagE* gene was amplified by PCR as a 1020-bp DNA fragment, using a *cagE* forward primer (5′-GGATCCGTCCCTGAAATTTTATTAGCTTG-3′) and a *cagE* reverse primer (5-CTGCAGTTAAACGACCTTTAAACATTTTTTA-3′) [20]. In qPCR analysis, *cagE* was detected as earlier described [19] using the *cagE*_F2 (5′-TGGATTGGGACAAGTGAACA-3′) and *cagE*_R2 (5′-CAATAATGGCTCGTGCAATATC-3′) primers to amplify a 623-bp internal fragment of the *cagE* gene. A ≈630-bp fragment of the lytic transglycosylase, *virB1* gene was amplified using a *cagE* forward primer and a *virB1* reverse primer (5′-GTTTTTAATCAATCTTCCTGATTG-3′). The amplification of the ATP:ase-encoding *virb4* gene, as a ≈900-bp DNA fragment, was carried out by PCR or qPCR using the *virB4* forward primer (5′-GTGCAGAAGCCTGTATTCGTGC-3′), and the *virB4* reverse primer

(5′-CCAGTCATTAGTGGCTTCGCC-3′). The *magB01*-F (5′-GCCATCTACTACGCCTATCGC-3′) and *ssb*-R (5′-TTATCGCCGTCAAGCGGAAG-3′) primers [25] were used in PCR to assess the presence of plasmids encoding T4SS genes. PCR cycling conditions were 94 °C for 1 min, followed by 35 cycles of 94 °C for 30 sec, 54 °C for 30 sec, and 72 °C for 1 min, and then finally 72 °C for 7 min. The cycling conditions for qPCR were 95 °C for 10 min, followed by 45 cycles of 95 °C for 10 sec, 54 °C for 5 sec, and 72 °C for 22 sec. The complete genome sequences of serotype b strains SCC1398 (VirB1; GenBank accession KND83482), and I23C (VirB4; KOE53154) [40] were used as reference in oligonucleotide synthesis.

4.4. Statistical Analysis and Image Processing

The rank test was used to calculate the strength of the association between the *A. actinomycetemcomitans cagE* and JP2 genotypes and proportion of TVC in subgingival plaque samples (IBM SPSS Statistics for Windows, Version 25.0, Armonk, New York). An odds ratio (OR) was used to quantify the strength of the association between the *A. actinomycetemcomitans cagE* genotype and age group (MedCalc for Windows, MedCalc Software, Ostend, Belgium). No normalization of the data or test unit was used in the present work.

4.5. Ethical Considerations

All procedures were conducted according to the guidelines of the local ethics committee at the Medical Faculty of Umeå University, which are in compliance with the Declaration of Helsinki (64th WMA General Assembly, Fortaleza, October 2013). The characterization of the *A. actinomycetemcomitans* strains was made utilizing clinical samples from patients visiting the Specialist Clinic of Periodontology at the Dental School in Umeå. Data from specific strains were grouped in relation to age (>35 or ≤ 35 years) and could not be traced to a specific individual.

Supplementary Materials: The following are available online at http://www.mdpi.com/2076-0817/8/3/153/s1. Table S1. The 116 *A. actinomycetemcomitans* serotype b strains, collected from periodontitis patients living in Sweden, and which were used in the present work.

Author Contributions: Conceptualization, A.J., R.C., and J.O.; methodology, R.C., and J.O.; validation, R.C., M.L., S.J, and J.O; formal Analysis, A.J., R.C., S.J, and J.O.; investigation, R.C., M.L., S.J., and J.O.; resources A.J., R.C., C.H.Å., D.H., and J.O; data curation, A.J., R.C., and J.O.; writing—original draft preparation, A.J., R.C., and J.O.; writing—review and editing, A.J., R.C., C.H.Å., D.H., M.L., S.J., and J.O.; visualization, A.J., R.C., and J.O.; supervision, A.J., R.C., C.H.Å., and J.O.; project administration, A.J. and J.O; funding acquisition, A.J., M.L. and J.O.

Acknowledgments: We are grateful to Elisabeth Granström for valuable technical assistance. This work was supported by TUA grants from the County Council of Västerbotten, Sweden (to J.O. and A.J.), by funds from Insamlingsstiftelsen, Medical Faculty, Umeå University (to J.O. and A.J.), and from Svenska Tandläkare-sällskapet, Kempe Foundation, and Thuréus Foundation (to M.L.).

Conflicts of Interest: The authors declare no competing interests.

References

1. Fine, D.H.; Patil, A.G.; Velusamy, S.K. *Aggregatibacter actinomycetemcomitans* (*Aa*) under the radar: Myths and misunderstandings of *Aa* and its role in aggressive periodontitis. *Front. Immunol.* **2019**, *10*, 728. [CrossRef]
2. Ramich, T.; Asendorf, A.; Nickles, K.; Oremek, G.M.; Schubert, R.; Nibali, L.; Wohlfeil, M.; Eickholz, P. Inflammatory serum markers up to 5 years after comprehensive periodontal therapy of aggressive and chronic periodontitis. *Clin. Oral Investig.* **2018**, *22*, 3079–3089. [CrossRef] [PubMed]
3. van Winkelhoff, A.J.; Slots, J. *Actinobacillus actinomycetemcomitans* and *Porphyromonas gingivalis* in nonoral infections. *Periodontol. 2000* **1999**, *20*, 122–135. [CrossRef] [PubMed]
4. Fine, D.H.; Markowitz, K.; Furgang, D.; Fairlie, K.; Ferrandiz, J.; Nasri, C.; McKiernan, M.; Gunsolley, J. *Aggregatibacter actinomycetemcomitans* and its relationship to initiation of localized aggressive periodontitis: Longitudinal cohort study of initially healthy adolescents. *J. Clin. Microbiol.* **2007**, *45*, 3859–3869. [CrossRef] [PubMed]

5. Haubek, D.; Ennibi, O.K.; Poulsen, K.; Vaeth, M.; Poulsen, S.; Kilian, M. Risk of aggressive periodontitis in adolescent carriers of the JP2 clone of *Aggregatibacter* (*Actinobacillus*) *actinomycetemcomitans* in Morocco: A prospective longitudinal cohort study. *Lancet* **2008**, *371*, 237–242. [CrossRef]
6. Höglund Åberg, C.; Kwamin, F.; Claesson, R.; Dahlen, G.; Johansson, A.; Haubek, D. Progression of attachment loss is strongly associated with presence of the JP2 genotype of *Aggregatibacter actinomycetemcomitans*: A prospective cohort study of a young adolescent population. *J. Clin. Periodontol.* **2014**, *41*, 232–241. [CrossRef] [PubMed]
7. Van der Velden, U.; Abbas, F.; Armand, S.; Loos, B.G.; Timmerman, M.F.; Van der Weijden, G.A.; Van Winkelhoff, A.J.; Winkel, E.G. Java project on periodontal diseases. The natural development of periodontitis: Risk factors, risk predictors and risk determinants. *J. Clin. Periodontol.* **2006**, *33*, 540–548. [CrossRef]
8. DiRienzo, J.M. Breaking the gingival epithelial barrier: Role of the *Aggregatibacter actinomycetemcomitans* cytolethal distending toxin in oral infectious disease. *Cells* **2014**, *3*, 476–499. [CrossRef]
9. Johansson, A. *Aggregatibacter actinomycetemcomitans* leukotoxin: A powerful tool with capacity to cause imbalance in the host inflammatory response. *Toxins* **2011**, *3*, 242–259. [CrossRef]
10. Oscarsson, J.; Claesson, R.; Lindholm, M.; Höglund Åberg, C.; Johansson, A. Tools of *Aggregatibacter actinomycetemcomitans* to evade the host response. *J. Clin. Med.* **2019**, *8*, 1079. [CrossRef]
11. Henderson, B.; Ward, J.M.; Ready, D. *Aggregatibacter* (*Actinobacillus*) *actinomycetemcomitans*: A triple A* periodontopathogen? *Periodontol. 2000* **2010**, *54*, 78–105. [CrossRef]
12. Poulsen, K.; Theilade, E.; Lally, E.T.; Demuth, D.R.; Kilian, M. Population structure of *Actinobacillus actinomycetemcomitans*: A framework for studies of disease-associated properties. *Microbiology* **1994**, *140 Pt 8*, 2049–2060. [CrossRef]
13. Tsuzukibashi, O.; Saito, M.; Kobayashi, T.; Umezawa, K.; Nagahama, F.; Hiroi, T.; Hirasawa, M.; Takada, K. A gene cluster for the synthesis of serotype g-specific polysaccharide antigen in Aggregatibacter actinomycetemcomitans. *Arch. Microbiol.* **2014**, *196*, 261–265. [CrossRef] [PubMed]
14. Höglund Åberg, C.; Haubek, D.; Kwamin, F.; Johansson, A.; Claesson, R. Leukotoxic activity of *Aggregatibacter actinomycetemcomitans* and periodontal attachment loss. *PLoS ONE* **2014**, *9*, e104095. [CrossRef] [PubMed]
15. Kittichotirat, W.; Bumgarner, R.E.; Chen, C. Evolutionary divergence of *Aggregatibacter actinomycetemcomitans*. *J. Dent. Res.* **2016**, *95*, 94–101. [CrossRef]
16. Brogan, J.M.; Lally, E.T.; Poulsen, K.; Kilian, M.; Demuth, D.R. Regulation of *Actinobacillus actinomycetemcomitans* leukotoxin expression: Analysis of the promoter regions of leukotoxic and minimally leukotoxic strains. *Infect. Immun.* **1994**, *62*, 501–508. [PubMed]
17. Haubek, D.; Johansson, A. Pathogenicity of the highly leukotoxic JP2 clone of *Aggregatibacter actinomycetemcomitans* and its geographic dissemination and role in aggressive periodontitis. *J. Oral Microbiol.* **2014**, *6*, 23980. [CrossRef]
18. Poulsen, K.; Ennibi, O.K.; Haubek, D. Improved PCR for detection of the highly leukotoxic JP2 clone of *Actinobacillus actinomycetemcomitans* in subgingival plaque samples. *J. Clin. Microbiol.* **2003**, *41*, 4829–4832. [CrossRef]
19. Johansson, A.; Claesson, R.; Höglund Åberg, C.; Haubek, D.; Oscarsson, J. The *cagE* gene sequence as a diagnostic marker to identify JP2 and non-JP2 highly leukotoxic *Aggregatibacter actinomycetemcomitans* serotype b strains. *J. Periodontal Res.* **2017**, *52*, 903–912. [CrossRef]
20. Teng, Y.T.; Hu, W. Expression cloning of a periodontitis-associated apoptotic effector, *cagE* homologue, in *Actinobacillus actinomycetemcomitans*. *Biochem. Biophys. Res. Commun.* **2003**, *303*, 1086–1094. [CrossRef]
21. Kelk, P.; Claesson, R.; Chen, C.; Sjöstedt, A.; Johansson, A. IL-1β secretion induced by *Aggregatibacter* (*Actinobacillus*) *actinomycetemcomitans* is mainly caused by the leukotoxin. *Int. J. Med. Microbiol.* **2008**, *298*, 529–541. [CrossRef] [PubMed]
22. Christie, P.J.; Whitaker, N.; Gonzalez-Rivera, C. Mechanism and structure of the bacterial type IV secretion systems. *Biochim. Biophys. Acta* **2014**, *1843*, 1578–1591. [CrossRef] [PubMed]
23. Waksman, G.; Orlova, E.V. Structural organisation of the type IV secretion systems. *Curr. Opin. Microbiol.* **2014**, *17*, 24–31. [CrossRef] [PubMed]
24. Galli, D.M.; Chen, J.; Novak, K.F.; Leblanc, D.J. Nucleotide sequence and analysis of conjugative plasmid pVT745. *J. Bacteriol.* **2001**, *183*, 1585–1594. [CrossRef] [PubMed]

25. Liu, C.C.; Chen, C.H.; Tang, C.Y.; Chen, K.H.; Chen, Z.F.; Chang, S.H.; Tsai, C.Y.; Liou, M.L. Prevalence and comparative analysis of the type IV secretion system in *Aggregatibacter actinomycetemcomitan*. *J. Microbiol. Immunol. Infect.* **2018**, *51*, 278–285. [CrossRef] [PubMed]
26. Novak, K.F.; Dougherty, B.; Pelaez, M. *Actinobacillus actinomycetemcomitans* harbours type IV secretion system genes on a plasmid and in the chromosome. *Microbiology* **2001**, *147*, 3027–3035. [CrossRef]
27. Claesson, R.; Höglund-Åberg, C.; Haubek, D.; Johansson, A. Age-related prevalence and characteristics of *Aggregatibacter actinomycetemcomitans* in periodontitis patients living in Sweden. *J. Oral Microbiol.* **2017**, *9*, 1334504. [CrossRef]
28. Claesson, R.; Gudmundson, J.; Höglund Åberg, C.; Haubek, D.; Johansson, A. Detection of a 640-bp deletion in the *Aggregatibacter actinomycetemcomitans* leukotoxin promoter region in isolates from an adolescent of Ethiopian origin. *J. Oral Microbiol.* **2015**, *7*, 26974. [CrossRef]
29. Haubek, D.; Poulsen, K.; Kilian, M. Microevolution and patterns of dissemination of the JP2 clone of *Aggregatibacter (Actinobacillus) actinomycetemcomitans*. *Infect. Immun.* **2007**, *75*, 3080–3088. [CrossRef] [PubMed]
30. Höglund Åberg, C.; Antonoglou, G.; Haubek, D.; Kwamin, F.; Claesson, R.; Johansson, A. Cytolethal distending toxin in isolates of Aggregatibacter actinomycetemcomitans from Ghanaian adolescents and association with serotype and disease progression. *PLoS ONE* **2013**, *8*, e65781.
31. Kutter, S.; Buhrdorf, R.; Haas, J.; Schneider-Brachert, W.; Haas, R.; Fischer, W. Protein subassemblies of the *Helicobacter pylori* Cag type IV secretion system revealed by localization and interaction studies. *J. Bacteriol.* **2008**, *190*, 2161–2171. [CrossRef]
32. Mossey, P.; Hudacek, A.; Das, A. *Agrobacterium tumefaciens* type IV secretion protein VirB3 is an inner membrane protein and requires VirB4, VirB7, and VirB8 for stabilization. *J. Bacteriol.* **2010**, *192*, 2830–2838. [CrossRef] [PubMed]
33. Batchelor, R.A.; Pearson, B.M.; Friis, L.M.; Guerry, P.; Wells, J.M. Nucleotide sequences and comparison of two large conjugative plasmids from different *Campylobacter* species. *Microbiology* **2004**, *150*, 3507–3517. [CrossRef]
34. Fronzes, R.; Christie, P.J.; Waksman, G. The structural biology of type IV secretion systems. *Nat. Rev. Microbiol.* **2009**, *7*, 703–714. [CrossRef] [PubMed]
35. Rambow-Larsen, A.A.; Weiss, A.A. The PtlE protein of *Bordetella pertussis* has peptidoglycanase activity required for Ptl-mediated pertussis toxin secretion. *J. Bacteriol.* **2002**, *184*, 2863–2869. [CrossRef] [PubMed]
36. Christie, P.J. The Mosaic Type IV Secretion Systems. *EcoSal Plus* **2016**, *7*. [CrossRef]
37. Sreenivasan, P.K.; Fives-Taylor, P. Isolation and characterization of deletion derivatives of pDL282, an *Actinobacillus actinomycetemcomitans*/*Escherichia* coli shuttle plasmid. *Plasmid* **1994**, *31*, 207–214. [CrossRef] [PubMed]
38. Loesche, W.J.; Grossman, N.S. Periodontal disease as a specific, albeit chronic, infection: Diagnosis and treatment. *Clin. Microbiol. Rev.* **2001**, *14*, 727–752. [CrossRef]
39. Haubek, D.; Havemose-Poulsen, A.; Westergaard, J. Aggressive periodontitis in a 16-year-old Ghanaian adolescent, the original source of *Actinobacillus actinomycetemcomitans* strain HK1651—A 10-year follow up. *Int. J. Paediatr. Dent.* **2006**, *16*, 370–375. [CrossRef]
40. Kittichotirat, W.; Bumgarner, R.E.; Asikainen, S.; Chen, C. Identification of the pangenome and its components in 14 distinct *Aggregatibacter actinomycetemcomitans* strains by comparative genomic analysis. *PLoS ONE* **2011**, *6*, e22420. [CrossRef]
41. Sun, R.; Kittichotirat, W.; Wang, J.; Jan, M.; Chen, W.; Asikainen, S.; Bumgarner, R.; Chen, C. Genomic stability of *Aggregatibacter actinomycetemcomitans* during persistent oral infection in human. *PLoS ONE* **2013**, *8*, e66472. [CrossRef] [PubMed]
42. Höglund Åberg, C.; Kwamin, F.; Claesson, R.; Johansson, A.; Haubek, D. Presence of JP2 and non-JP2 genotypes of *Aggregatibacter actinomycetemcomitans* and attachment loss in adolescents in Ghana. *J. Periodontol.* **2012**, *83*, 1520–1528. [CrossRef]
43. Haubek, D.; Dirienzo, J.M.; Tinoco, E.M.; Westergaard, J.; Lopez, N.J.; Chung, C.P.; Poulsen, K.; Kilian, M. Racial tropism of a highly toxic clone of *Actinobacillus actinomycetemcomitans* associated with juvenile periodontitis. *J. Clin. Microbiol.* **1997**, *35*, 3037–3042. [PubMed]
44. Kiley, P.; Holt, S.C. Characterization of the lipopolysaccharide from *Actinobacillus actinomycetemcomitans* Y4 and N27. *Infect. Immun.* **1980**, *30*, 862–873. [PubMed]

45. Newman, M.G.; Socransky, S.S. Predominant cultivable microbiota in periodontosis. *J. Periodontal Res.* **1977**, *12*, 120–128. [CrossRef] [PubMed]
46. Dogan, B.; Saarela, M.H.; Jousimies-Somer, H.; Alaluusua, S.; Asikainen, S. *Actinobacillus actinomycetemcomitans* serotype e-biotypes, genetic diversity and distribution in relation to periodontal status. *Oral Microbiol. Immunol.* **1999**, *14*, 98–103. [CrossRef] [PubMed]

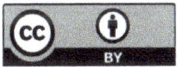

© 2019 by the authors. Licensee MDPI, Basel, Switzerland. This article is an open access article distributed under the terms and conditions of the Creative Commons Attribution (CC BY) license (http://creativecommons.org/licenses/by/4.0/).

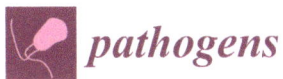

Obituary

In Memoriam: Edward "Ned" Lally

Nataliya Balashova

Department of Basic and Translational Sciences, School of Dental Medicine, University of Pennsylvania, Philadelphia, PA 19104, USA; natbal@upenn.edu

Received: 23 February 2020; Accepted: 27 February 2020; Published: 1 March 2020

On February 11, 2019, we lost a colleague and friend Dr. Edward "Ned" Lally. He was an internationally recognized leader in research on the periodontal pathogen *Aggregatibacter actinomycetemcomitans*.

Ned succeeded in his professional career as a clinical pathologist, scientist and educator. He received his B.S. degree in 1966 and his D.M.D. degree in 1968 from the University of Pittsburgh. He was a resident in both the United States Naval Hospital and the Department of Pathology at the Hospital of the University of Pennsylvania. Ned received his Certificate in Oral Pathology in 1973 and earned a Ph.D. in Immunology in 1978 from the University of Pennsylvania. He then joined the Department of Pathology at the University of Pennsylvania, School of Dental Medicine, where he had grown to the rank of Professor with tenure. In addition to his academic career, Ned distinguished himself in service to the United States Navy and Naval Reserve.

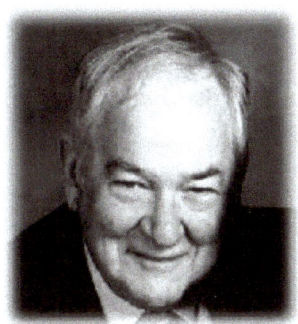

In early years, Ned's research was focused on understanding mucosal immunity. In his practice he met young patients with an aggressive form of periodontal disease and investigated familial aggregation of the disease. Ned had a longstanding interest in the field of microbial pathogenesis and the role of *A. actinomycetemcomitans* in the development of aggressive periodontitis. He was especially intrigued to unravel the mechanism of action of an RTX toxin, LtxA, an immune cell killer. In the 1980s, Ned made his seminal observation that LtxA interacted with β2 integrin receptor LFA-1 on the surface of immune cells. He believed this was the most significant of his contributions related to the field. Following his study, β2 integrin receptors were reported for RTX toxins from other bacteria. In later years, Ned successfully employed various immunological, biophysical, biochemical and molecular techniques for the characterization of the toxin interaction with the host cell membrane. Ned found that the interaction of LtxA with immune cells is both complex and multifaceted, involving both β2 integrin LFA-1 and cell membrane cholesterol. His results provide new insight into the mechanism by which the RTX group of bacterial toxins kill cells. Ned published over 90 peer-reviewed manuscripts and successfully maintained continuous NIH funding.

Ned will be remembered not just for his scientific contributions, but also as a great charismatic teacher for young researchers. Outside his professional career, Ned was a devoted husband, father and grandfather. Personally, I will always remember him as one of the best friends I have ever met in my professional life.

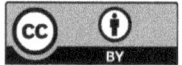 © 2020 by the author. Licensee MDPI, Basel, Switzerland. This article is an open access article distributed under the terms and conditions of the Creative Commons Attribution (CC BY) license (http://creativecommons.org/licenses/by/4.0/).

MDPI
St. Alban-Anlage 66
4052 Basel
Switzerland
Tel. +41 61 683 77 34
Fax +41 61 302 89 18
www.mdpi.com

Pathogens Editorial Office
E-mail: pathogens@mdpi.com
www.mdpi.com/journal/pathogens

www.ingramcontent.com/pod-product-compliance
Lightning Source LLC
LaVergne TN
LVHW070417100526
838202LV00014B/1473